Language in Autism

Language in Autism

Edited by

Jeannette Schaeffer
University of Amsterdam

Rama Novogrodsky
University of Haifa

Alexandra Perovic
University College London

Philippe Prévost
University of Tours

Laurice Tuller
University of Tours

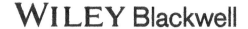

Copyright © 2025 by John Wiley & Sons, Inc. All rights reserved, including rights for text and data mining and training of artificial intelligence technologies or similar technologies.

Published by John Wiley & Sons, Inc., Hoboken, New Jersey.
Published simultaneously in Canada.

No part of this publication may be reproduced, stored in a retrieval system, or transmitted in any form or by any means, electronic, mechanical, photocopying, recording, scanning, or otherwise, except as permitted under Section 107 or 108 of the 1976 United States Copyright Act, without either the prior written permission of the Publisher, or authorization through payment of the appropriate per-copy fee to the Copyright Clearance Center, Inc., 222 Rosewood Drive, Danvers, MA 01923, (978) 750-8400, fax (978) 750-4470, or on the web at www.copyright.com. Requests to the Publisher for permission should be addressed to the Permissions Department, John Wiley & Sons, Inc., 111 River Street, Hoboken, NJ 07030, (201) 748-6011, fax (201) 748-6008, or online at http://www.wiley.com/go/permission.

Trademarks: Wiley and the Wiley logo are trademarks or registered trademarks of John Wiley & Sons, Inc. and/or its affiliates in the United States and other countries and may not be used without written permission. All other trademarks are the property of their respective owners. John Wiley & Sons, Inc. is not associated with any product or vendor mentioned in this book.

Limit of Liability/Disclaimer of Warranty: While the publisher and author have used their best efforts in preparing this book, they make no representations or warranties with respect to the accuracy or completeness of the contents of this book and specifically disclaim any implied warranties of merchantability or fitness for a particular purpose. No warranty may be created or extended by sales representatives or written sales materials. The advice and strategies contained herein may not be suitable for your situation. You should consult with a professional where appropriate. Further, readers should be aware that websites listed in this work may have changed or disappeared between when this work was written and when it is read. Neither the publisher nor authors shall be liable for any loss of profit or any other commercial damages, including but not limited to special, incidental, consequential, or other damages.

For general information on our other products and services or for technical support, please contact our Customer Care Department within the United States at (800) 762-2974, outside the United States at (317) 572-3993 or fax (317) 572-4002.

Wiley also publishes its books in a variety of electronic formats. Some content that appears in print may not be available in electronic formats. For more information about Wiley products, visit our web site at www.wiley.com.

Library of Congress Cataloging-in-Publication Data

Names: Schaeffer, Jeannette, editor. | Novogrodsky, Rama, editor. | Perovic, Alexandra, editor. | Prévost, Philippe, editor. | Tuller, Laurice, editor.
Title: Language in autism / edited by Jeannette Schaeffer, Rama Novogrodsky, Alexandra Perovic, Philippe Prévost, Laurice Tuller.
Description: Hoboken, New Jersey: Wiley, [2025] | Includes bibliographical references and index.
Identifiers: LCCN 2024055007 | ISBN 9781394180363 (paperback) | ISBN 9781394180370 (adobe pdf) | ISBN 9781394180387 (ePub)
Subjects: LCSH: Autism-Language | Language acquisition.
Classification: LCC RC553.A88 L365 2025 | DDC 616.85/8820014–dc23/eng/20250118
LC record available at https://lccn.loc.gov/2024055007

Cover Design: Wiley
Cover Image: © 2024 Désirée Charconnet

SKY10122315_071825

Contents

Preface *vii*
Acknowledgments *ix*
Biographical Notes *xi*

Introduction *1*

1 Putting Language on the Autism Map *3*
Jeannette Schaeffer, Rama Novogrodsky, Alexandra Perovic, Philippe Prévost, and Laurice Tuller

Part 1 Language in Autism: The View Within Language Domains *27*

2 Lexicon *29*
Letitia Naigles and Nufar Sukenik

3 Morphosyntax *49*
Stephanie Durrleman and Theodoros Marinis

4 Phonology *75*
Sandrine Ferré and Christophe dos Santos

5 Semantics *97*
Francesca Foppolo and Francesca Panzeri

6 Implicit Meaning *119*
Napoleon Katsos and Agustín Vicente

7 **Narration** *141*
   Elena Peristeri, Philippine Geelhand, and Ianthi Maria Tsimpli

8 **Discourse** *159*
   Flavia Adani, Petra Hendriks, and Arhonto Terzi

9 **Prosody** *181*
   Sandrine Ferré and Rhea Paul

   Part 2 Language in Autism: The View Across Language Domains *203*

10 **Language Development Across the Autism Spectrum** *205*
   Silvia Silleresi and Laurice Tuller

11 **Language in Autism Compared to Language in Other NDDs** *227*
   Alexandra Perovic and Kenneth Wexler

12 **Language in Autistic Adults** *249*
   Marta Manenti and Philippe Prévost

13 **Multilingualism in Autism** *271*
   Natalia Meir and Rama Novogrodsky

14 **Reading in Autism** *291*
   Racha Zebib and Carole El Akiki

15 **Brain, Language, and Autism** *313*
   Caroline Larson and Inge-Marie Eigsti

   Conclusion *333*

16 **Building a Baseline Battery to Measure Language in Autism** *335*
   Jeannette Schaeffer, Rama Novogrodsky, Alexandra Perovic, Philippe Prévost, and Laurice Tuller

   Author Index *353*
   Subject Index *367*

Preface

We, the editorial team behind this textbook, are linguists. Each of us devotes most of our academic work to the study of language acquisition and development in children, adolescents, and adults, in "extraordinary" contexts, especially autism. Why this book? In a nutshell, we believe that insights from linguistics, the scientific study of human language, are fundamental in advancing knowledge on how autistic individuals develop, produce, and understand language, and, ultimately, navigate in their daily lives.

We belong to a European network of researchers on language development in autistic children (LACA – Language Abilities in Children with Autism) that fosters linguistically informed, in-depth, transnational study of language in autism and its potential relationships with other cognitive abilities and in comparison with other contexts involving language impairment (without autism). A fundamental ingredient in this quest entails methodological streamlining so that studies in different countries (on different languages) give rise to results that can be integrated toward more reliable descriptions and explanations of the nature and development of language abilities in autism.

One of the LACA missions is to "put language on the autism map." As part of this commitment, LACA conducted a survey in 2017 among autism practitioners (including psychiatrists, pediatricians, speech and language therapists) from eight different European countries regarding the role of language in autism (in diagnosis and support). One important gap that was identified was the marginality of the role of language in diagnosis and intervention for autistic individuals. Unfortunately, today, this gap is still far from being closed. A general conclusion was that establishing a detailed linguistic profile of an autistic individual largely depends on which professionals are included in the diagnosis team. For example, in the UK, a speech and language therapist is usually included, but not all private clinics will have one. In Greece, a speech and language therapist is never a part of the team though they often make referrals for autism evaluation. In the

Netherlands, where diagnosis teams often include both speech and language therapists and clinical linguists, language assessments seem to be more sophisticated in the sense that they assess different language domains, including vocabulary, grammar, and linguistic pragmatics. Yet, within and across countries, there is often a lack of agreement between clinicians on the role of language in the diagnosis of autistic children, which is likely to be due to the fact that language abilities are not treated as a core domain of autism in diagnostic manuals. However, language abilities have been put forward as the best predictor of long-term outcomes for autistic individuals (Barthélémy et al. 2019). Consonant with this, the clinicians responding to our survey agreed that it is imperative that language skills be part of autism diagnosis and intervention.

This imperative led the LACA group to the conception of a textbook on Language in Autism, written in accessible language, for all parties interested in autism, including students and professionals from a variety of fields: psychiatry, pediatrics, (neuro)psychology, speech and language pathology, education, and linguistics, and also autistic people themselves, their relatives, and friends. The goal of the book lying in front of you is to contribute to the growing awareness of the crucial role language (development) plays in the lives of autistic people. As such, it is meant to contribute to the understanding of the strengths and weaknesses in the various domains of language in autistic individuals across the spectrum, across the lifespan, across languages, and in relation to the brain and to other conditions. It also provides suggestions for necessary ingredients of language assessment in autism diagnosis.

August 2024

The editorial team:
Jeannette Schaeffer, Rama Novogrodsky,
Alexandra Perovic, Philippe Prévost,
and Laurice Tuller

Acknowledgments

Writing this textbook has been a very pleasant journey, thanks to a number of colleagues and friends, many of whom are part of the LACA Network: Language Abilities in Children with Autism. The LACA Network has laid the basis for a long-term collaboration between linguists from over 12 countries who are all passionate about language, linguistics, and autism. This book and also the proposal for the LACA Baseline Battery as described in Chapter 16 are some of the fruits borne by the LACA Network. We are grateful to NWO (the Dutch Research Council) for funding this pioneering network from 2016 to 2019 with an Internationalization Grant.

We offer our wholehearted thanks to all authors, who include both junior and senior scientists, many of whom have reviewed other chapters as well. Their dedication to this enterprise has been inspiring.

In an effort to ensure maximum accuracy and readability, the reviewing process has included researchers as well as professionals, from a wide range of specialties, working in over a dozen different countries: linguists, neuroscientists, pediatricians, psychiatrists, psycholinguists, psychologists (clinical and research), special education teachers, and speech-language pathologists. We can't thank you enough for joining us in this way: Charlotte Brasset, Frédérique Bonnet-Brilhault, Erik van der Burg, Riley Buijsman, Elena Castroviejo, Maja Cepanec, Tony Charman, Elisabeth Delais-Roussarie, Allison Dodd, Rachel Fiani, Mai Fleetwood-Bird, Rutger-Jan van der Gaag, David Gagnon, Anna Gavarró, Ileana Grama, Jessica Goldberg Florian, Hilde Geurts, Marie Gomot, Marijke Hartemink, Marissa Hartston, Chantal van den Helder, Jasmina Ivšac Pavliša, Stacy John-Legere, Mikhail Kissine, Shasha Kohlmeyer, Edith Kouba Hreich, Varda Kreiser, Vincent van Loenen, Colin Phillips, Sanne Minnee, Rachel Plak, Milena Popović Samardžić, Franck Ramus, Nick Riches, Ana Lúcia Santos, Jo Saul, Anke Scheeren, Sanja Šimleša, Laura Soeters de Kiewit,

Helen Tager-Flusberg, Melanie de Wit, Ariela Yokel, Tim Ziermans, and Hugo Zoppé.

Finally, the five members of the book's editorial team (Jeannette Schaeffer, Rama Novogrodsky, Alexandra Perovic, Philippe Prévost, and Laurice Tuller) would like to thank each other for the fantastic collaboration forged over the past two years: what a team!

Biographical Notes

Editors

Jeannette Schaeffer is Professor of Language Acquisition at the University of Amsterdam. She investigates language acquisition and development across languages and populations, including children with hemispherectomy, Developmental Language Disorder (DLD), autism, and, more recently, in minors in conflict with the law. She founded LACA (Language Abilities in Children with Autism) in 2017, an international, collaborative network focusing on the cross-linguistic investigation of language (development) in autism. She has published in leading journals such as *Language Acquisition, Applied Psycholinguistics, Natural Language & Linguistic Theory*, and *Glossa*.

Rama Novogrodsky is Associate Professor at the University of Haifa, Israel. She studies typical and atypical language development in various populations, including children with autism, hearing impairment (also those who use sign language), and Developmental Language Disorder. Her work has appeared in journals such as *Journal of Speech, Language, and Hearing Research, First Language*, and *Applied Psycholinguistics*.

Alexandra Perovic is Associate Professor at University College London. Her research explores monolingual and multilingual language development in autism, Down syndrome and Williams syndrome, and language difficulties in children within the youth justice system. She has published in *Developmental Science* and *Journal of Speech, Language, and Hearing Research*, among others. She teaches clinical linguistics and language acquisition to postgraduate speech and language therapy students.

Philippe Prévost is Professor of Linguistics at the University of Tours, France. His research, featuring in journals such as *Linguistic Approaches to Bilingualism* and *Autism Research*, spans across several domains of language development, such as second language acquisition and language development in the context of a neurodevelopmental disorder, including Developmental Language Disorder and autism, in both children and adults.

Laurice Tuller is Professor Emerita of Linguistics at the University of Tours, France, with expertise in psycholinguistics, language pathology, and bilingual language acquisition. She has investigated language profiles in contexts including hearing loss, epilepsy, Developmental Language Disorder, and autism. Her work has been published in *Autism Research, Brain and Language*, and *Journal of Speech, Language, and Hearing Research*, among others.

Other Authors

Flavia Adani is Associate Professor of Language Development at the Free University of Berlin, Germany. Her cross-linguistic research focuses on monolingual and bilingual populations of children with typical and atypical language development (Developmental Language Disorder, Autism Spectrum Disorder). Her work has been published in *Journal of Speech, Language, and Hearing Research, Journal of Child Language*, and *Language Learning and Development*.

Stephanie Durrleman leads a group investigating bilingualism in children with and without autism at the Department of Science and Medicine, University of Fribourg, Switzerland. Her work spans diverse languages, age groups, and populations and integrates linguistic theory and empirical methods, to shed light on communication and cognition and to yield concrete applications for language assessment, therapy and policy.

Inge-Marie Eigsti is Professor of Clinical Psychology in the Department of Psychological Sciences at the University of Connecticut, and Director of Research for the Institute for Brain and Cognitive Sciences. Her research on language and communication in autism is funded by multiple grants from the National Institutes of Health and she has authored over 100 peer-reviewed publications.

Carole El Akiki is Associate Professor at the University of Tours, France. Her research focuses on written language acquisition (reading and spelling) in typically developing children and in children with neurodevelopmental disorders

(Autism, Specific Learning Disorder). Her work has been published in journals such as *Frontiers in Psychology* and *Applied Psycholinguistics*.

Sandrine Ferré is Professor of Linguistics at the University of Tours, France. As a phonologist, her research focuses on phonological abilities in typical and atypical contexts such as autism, Developmental Language Disorder and hearing impairment in children and adults. Her work has been published in *Journal of Speech, Language, and Hearing Research, Language Acquisition,* and *Linguistic Approaches to Bilingualism* among others.

Francesca Foppolo is Associate Professor of Psycholinguistics at the University of Milan-Bicocca. Her research focuses on language processing in typically and atypically developing children, bilinguals, and adults by means of off-line and on-line techniques, particularly eye-tracking. She has published in *Journal of Memory and Language, Journal of Child language* and *Journal of Communication Disorders*, among others.

Philippine Geelhand is a scientific collaborator at the Université Libre de Bruxelles. Her research explores how linguistic differences shape social interactions between people of different neurotypes. Her work is published in journals such as *Autism, Autism in Adulthood, Molecular Autism, Clinical Linguistics and Phonetics,* and *Journal of Pragmatics*.

Petra Hendriks is Professor of Semantics and Cognition at the University of Groningen, the Netherlands. Her research focuses on sentence interpretation and processing in typical and atypical populations, including autistic children. She has published in journals such as *Language, Cognition and Neuroscience, Journal of the Acoustical Society of America, Journal of Abnormal Psychology,* and *Cognitive Science*.

Napoleon Katsos is Professor of Experimental Pragmatics at the University of Cambridge. He studies the acquisition and processing of meaning by monolingual, bilingual, neurotypical and neurodivergent individuals. A co-founder of the *Cambridge Bilingualism Network*, Napoleon has co-edited the *Oxford Handbook of Experimental Semantics and Pragmatics* and his research has appeared in journals such as *PNAS, Cognition,* and *Journal of Semantics*.

Caroline Larson is Assistant Professor at the University of Missouri in the Department of Speech, Language, and Hearing Sciences and Interdisciplinary Neuroscience Program. Her research examines relationships between language and other cognitive factors in individuals with language disorders, including developmental language disorder and autism spectrum disorder, using behavioral and functional neuroimaging methodologies.

Marta Manenti is Assistant Professor at the University of Tours, France. Her research explores language development in neurodevelopmental disorders, including Developmental Language Disorder and autism, with a particular focus on the structural language abilities of autistic adults. Her work has been published in autism journals such as *Autism & Developmental Language Impairments* and *Research in Autism Spectrum Disorders*.

Theodoros Marinis is Professor of Multilingualism and Director of the Centre for Multilingualism at the University of Konstanz. His research aims to uncover the nature of language processing in monolingual and multilingual children with typical and atypical language development across languages. He has published in journals such as *Applied Psycholinguistics*, the *Journal of Child Language*, and *Linguistic Approaches to Bilingualism*.

Natalia Meir is Associate Professor at Bar-Ilan University, Israel, coordinating the Linguistics in Clinical Research Program. Her research focuses on language development in monolingual and bilingual populations, including those with ASD and DLD. She studies heritage language maintenance across the lifespan. She co-edited *Methods for Assessing Multilingual Children* and is a member of Bilingualism Matters and IALP.

Letitia Naigles is Professor of Psychological Sciences at University of Connecticut, USA. Her research focuses on child language acquisition across multiple languages, as well as the language development of children with autism, innovating the use of eyetracking methods to assess their language. She has published in the *Journal of Child Language, Cognition, Journal of Autism and Developmental Disorders*, and *Developmental Science*, among others.

Francesca Panzeri is Associate Professor of Philosophy of Language at the University of Milan-Bicocca. Her research focuses on the acquisition of pragmatic phenomena in typical and atypical children, such as the derivation of implicitly conveyed content, presuppositions, and figurative meanings (metaphors and irony). She has published in *Journal of Pragmatics, Journal of Semantics, PLoS ONE*, among others.

Rhea Paul is Founding Chair and Retired Professor of Speech-Language Pathology at Sacred Heart University, Fairfield, Connecticut. She authored over 100 refereed journal articles, over 50 book chapters, and 9 books. She is currently Director of ABCs4ASD, a Personnel Preparation Program, funded by the U.S. Office of Education. She received Honors of the Association in 2014 from ASHA.

Elena Peristeri is Associate Professor at the Aristotle University of Thessaloniki. Her research investigates language and cognitive processing in monolingual and bilingual children with Autism Spectrum Disorder and Developmental Language Disorder. She has published in *Autism* and *Autism Research*, among others. She teaches psycholinguistics, neurolinguistics, and first language acquisition to undergraduate and postgraduate students.

Christophe dos Santos is Assistant Professor at the Linguistics Department of the University of Lyon 2, France. He is a member of the DeNDy axis (Développement, Neurocognition, Dysfonctionnements) of the UMR CNRS 5596 Dynamique Du Langage (DDL). His research focuses on phonological and lexical development in monolingual and bilingual children with and without language disorders.

Silvia Silleresi is Postdoctoral Researcher at the University of Milano-Bicocca, Italy. Her research interests include first and second language acquisition, structural language and cognitive profiles in Developmental Language Disorder and Autism. More recently, her work has focused on the cross-linguistic acquisition of morphosyntax and semantics. Her work has been published in *Autism Research, Autism, Applied Psycholinguistics, Translational Psychiatry*.

Nufar Sukenik is a Lecturer at Bar-Ilan University, at the Graduate Program for Autism Studies. Her research focuses on typical and atypical language development, specializing in semantics and syntax and their relations to language proficiency across ages. She also examines academic profiles in autistic children. Her work has appeared in journals such as *Language Acquisition, Journal of Autism and Developmental Disorders* and *Frontiers in Psychology*.

Arhonto Terzi is Professor of Linguistics at the University of Patras, Greece. She has investigated the morphosyntax and its interfaces in neurotypical populations across the life span along with populations with autism, developmental language disorder and aphasia. Her work has appeared in journals such as *Autism Research* and *Journal of Autism and Developmental Disorders*.

Ianthi Maria Tsimpli is Professor of English and Applied Linguistics at the University of Cambridge, Fellow of Fitzwilliam College and Fellow of the British Academy. Her research focuses on neurotypical and neurodivergent language development, language in education and the interaction between linguistic and cognitive skills in children and adults.

Agustín Vicente is Ikerbasque Research Professor at the University of the Basque Country (UPV/EHU). A philosopher by training, his research in autism is both theoretical and empirical, focusing especially on pragmatics. He has published in venues such as *Journal of Autism and Developmental Disorders*, *Psychonomic Bulletin and Review*, and *Journal of Child Language*.

Kenneth Wexler is Emeritus Professor of Psychology and Linguistics at MIT. After publishing the first mathematical theory of language learnability, he has investigated morphosyntactic development, binding theory, passives, raising, control, etc. in typical language development, Specific Language Impairment, Autism, Williams syndrome and Down syndrome, with many papers in journals like *Journal of Speech, Hearing and Language Development* and *Linguistic Inquiry*.

Racha Zebib is Associate Professor at the University of Tours, France. Her research focuses on language assessment, oral and written language acquisition, and the language-cognition interface in both typically developing children and children with neurodevelopmental disorders (Developmental Language Disorder, Autism Spectrum Disorder, Specific Learning Disorder). Her work has been published in journals such as *Autism Research* and *First Language*.

Introduction

1

Putting Language on the Autism Map

Jeannette Schaeffer, Rama Novogrodsky, Alexandra Perovic, Philippe Prévost, and Laurice Tuller

With approximately 75 million individuals affected worldwide (Schiller 2023), **autism** is the fastest-growing Neurodevelopmental Disorder, with an average prevalence estimated to be at least 1/100 (Zeidan et al. 2022; WHO 2023). Autism Spectrum Disorder entails social communication impairments and restricted, repetitive patterns of behavior, with or without accompanying intellectual disability (APA 2022; WHO 2022) and with or without accompanying **language impairment** (APA 2022; WHO 2022). Around 30% of autistic children remain minimally speaking, meaning that they produce only a few words or phrases or no spoken language at all (Tager-Flusberg and Kasari 2013; Howlin et al. 2014). As for speaking autistic individuals – even if they are perfectly fluent – a sizeable proportion has difficulties in one or more language domains.

To date, it is not clear what factors determine linguistic skills in autism. **Language** in people on the autism spectrum is not systematically assessed for a number of reasons (including time limitations), despite the fact that (i) language difficulties are often the reason for initial parental concerns; (ii) language is one of the strongest predictors of quality of life, including education, employment, autonomy, relationships, etc., in autistic individuals (Barthélémy et al. 2019); (iii) certain language skills in younger children predict social skills later in life (Levinson et al. 2020); (iv) language difficulties pose significant academic and economic challenges for autistic people (Johnson, Beitchman, and Brownlie 2010); and (v) autistic individuals' subtle language difficulties hinder them in expressing emotions (Sturrock et al. 2022). Insufficient focus on language during the diagnostic process can result in a lack of comprehensive language support, which might have been beneficial. Language and language impairment in autism figure repeatedly in the report from the "Lancet Commission on the future of care and clinical research in autism" (Lord et al. 2022): parental initial concerns about language, effects of language level on daily living skills, positive effects of early language intervention, language as a key factor determining the needs and strengths of autistic individuals and predicting the likelihood of change over time, as well as independence and well-being as adults, the role of language in diagnostic assessment and treatment planning, difficulty in selecting (age-appropriate) language tests for individuals across the spectrum, and absence of information about language level in studies on treatment efficacy.

The goal of this book is a better understanding of language in autism and should naturally lead to the development of improved language support for autistic individuals. Quite rightly, students, interns, and professionals, in a variety of fields, are eager to see knowledge translated into actions and attitudes that can be implemented with autistic people and their families. The intention of this book is limited to the first, fundamental step: consolidating current knowledge on language in autism so that these further steps will be truly evidence-based. We hope that the knowledge and understanding accrued through this book can be used as input for the development of improved support methods for language in autism. We encourage students of linguistics to initiate and pursue collaborations with autism actors in this implementation, as well as with health practitioners more generally, as the role of linguistics in health sciences is invaluable whenever language is concerned.

Opinions are divided regarding the classification, or nosography, of language impairment in autism in relation to other types of neurodivergent conditions. We recently raised this question in Schaeffer et al. (2023, p. 433): "Is language impairment in autism the co-occurrence of two distinct conditions (comorbidity), a consequence of autism itself (no comorbidity), or one possible combination from a series of neurodevelopmental properties (dimensional approach)?" So far, the answer to this question is far from clear, partly due to the enormous linguistic heterogeneity we find among autistic individuals, as will be seen in the following chapters. We return more directly to this issue in the conclusion (Chapter 16).

How Is Autism Diagnosed and What Role Does Language Play in the Diagnosis?

There are two internationally adopted nosographic manuals used to **diagnose autism**: the World Health Organization's *International Classification of Diseases*, **ICD-11** (World Health Organization [WHO] 2022), and the American Psychiatric Association's *Diagnostic and Statistical Manual of Mental Disorders Fifth Edition, Text Revised*, **DSM-5-TR** (American Psychiatric Association [APA] 2022). These manuals include how autism is classified within other "mental, behavioral, or neurodevelopmental disorders" (WHO 2022), along with symptom descriptions, diagnostic criteria, specifiers for common co-occurring conditions, and discussions of other clinical features, of boundaries with "normality," of developmental trajectories, of culture-related and sex- and/or gender-related features, and of boundaries with other disorders or conditions.[1] These properties are largely similar between the two manuals, which both utilize the label Autism Spectrum Disorder (ASD) as the diagnostic entity and classify this condition as a Neurodevelopmental Disorder (NDD). NDD is a category that groups behavioral and cognitive conditions whose fundamental features are neurodevelopmental, i.e. having an onset in the developmental period, involving a difference in brain development and with etiologies that are complex or unknown. They involve major difficulties (difficulties that impact daily functioning) in the "acquisition and execution of specific intellectual, motor, language, or social functions" (WHO 2022). These include using ICD-11 terminology, Disorder of Intellectual Development (DID), Developmental Speech or Language Disorders, Developmental Learning Disorder (such as impairment in reading), Attention Deficit Hyperactivity Disorder (ADHD), Stereotyped Movement Disorder, as well as Autism Spectrum Disorder (ASD).

ASD is diagnosed based on two criteria, which must both be present for a diagnosis to be given: (i) persistent deficits in social communication and social interaction, sometimes referred to as SI (for Social Interaction), as Social Communication, or as the First Dimension, and (ii) persistent restricted and repetitive patterns of behavior, interests, or activities, referred to as RRB (for Restricted and Repetitive Behaviors), or the Second Dimension. These criteria include a list of the manifestations of each dimension, with examples (see APA 2022; WHO 2022).

> **Autism Diagnostic Criteria** (APA 2022; WHO 2022)
>
> **First Dimension (SI, Social Interaction):** Persistent deficits in social communication and social interaction across multiple contexts
>
> **Second Dimension (RRB, Restricted and Repetitive Behaviors):** Persistent restricted, repetitive patterns of behavior, interests, or activities

The impact of autism on an individual's daily functioning is indicated separately for each of the two diagnostic criteria. The DSM-5-TR provides three "severity levels" according to whether an individual requires "support" (Level 1), "substantial support" (Level 2), or "very substantial support" (Level 3), with descriptions of what these correspond to for Social Communication and for RRB (APA 2022). It is noteworthy that **language** and **verbal communication skills** figure

---

1 We note that double quotation marks, in keeping with US style, are used throughout this book to signify direct quotations, to refer to terminology, and sometimes to express distance or peculiarity. We point out that in this chapter, the double quotation marks are not used to express irony or to question the validity of the content in quotation marks.

prominently in the severity level descriptions for Social Communication: the description "with few words or intelligible speech" is associated with Level 3, people who "speak in simple sentences" with Level 2, and people who are "able to speak in full sentences" and "engage in communication" with Level 1.

More generally, although language abilities do not constitute a separate criterion for the diagnosis of ASD, mention of language occurs throughout the entry for ASD in the two diagnostic manuals. Notably, specification of whether there is accompanying functional language impairment (see Table 1.1) is an obligatory component of the diagnostic system and, together with whether there is accompanying DID (Disorder of Intellectual Development), gives rise to different diagnostic codes (see Chapter 10). Table 1.1 illustrates the presence of language in the diagnostic process by presenting any mention of language or verbal skills in the ICD-11 entry for ASD, rubric by rubric, either quoted directly (emphasis added) or summarized.

Table 1.1 Reference to language in the ICD-11 entry for ASD.

Rubrics	Mention of language, verbal skills
Description	"Individuals along the spectrum exhibit a **full range of language abilities**."
Essential (required) features	Specific 1st Dimension **manifestations vary according to verbal ability**. "Manifestation may include limitations in [...] understanding of, interest in, or inappropriate responses to the verbal or nonverbal social communication of others, in integration of spoken language with typical complementary nonverbal cues, in understanding and use of language in social contexts and abilities to initiate and sustain reciprocal social conversations."
Specifiers for characterizing features within the autism spectrum	• Degree of **Functional Language Impairment**: "Functional language refers to capacity to use language for instrumental purposes (e.g. to express personal needs and desires). This qualifier is intended to reflect primarily the verbal and nonverbal expressive language deficits present in some individuals with ASD and not the pragmatic language deficits that are a core feature of ASD. The following qualifiers should be applied to indicate the extent of functional language impairment (spoken or signed) relative to the individual's age: with mild or no impairment of functional language, with impaired functional language (i.e. inability to use more than single words or simple phrases), with (almost) complete absence of functional language." • **Loss of previously acquired skills**: language use (second year of life) and regression of language (after age 3)

Rubrics	Mention of language, verbal skills
Additional clinical features	- Common **parental concerns about "problems in language"** - **Pragmatic language difficulties** ("overly literal understanding, speech lacking normal prosody and emotional tone, lack of awareness of appropriateness of choice of language in particular social contexts, pedantic precision in use of language")
Boundary with normality (threshold)	"**Early language delay** alone is not strongly indicative of ASD unless there is also evidence of limited motivation for social communication and limited interaction skills. An essential feature of ASD is **persistent impairment** in ability to understand and use language appropriate for social communication."
Course features	Lifelong disorder whose manifestations and impact are likely to vary, among others, **according to language abilities**
Developmental presentations	"**Plateauing** of social communication and **language skills** and failure to progress in their development is not uncommon."
Culture- and sex-/gender-related features	No mention of language
Boundaries with other disorders and conditions (differential diagnosis)	- **Developmental Language Disorder** with impairment of mainly pragmatic language: individuals with DLD who have mainly impaired pragmatics "are usually able to initiate and respond appropriately to social and emotional cues and to share interests with others, and do not typically exhibit restricted, repetitive, and stereotyped behaviors. An additional diagnosis of DLD should not be assigned to individuals with ASD based solely on pragmatic language impairment. The other forms of DLD (i.e. with impairment of receptive and expressive language) may be assigned in conjunction with a diagnosis of ASD if language abilities are markedly below what would be expected on the basis of age and level of intellectual functioning" - **Selective Mutism** is characterized by normal use of language and patterns of social communication in specific environments but not in others. In ASD, difficulties are evident across all situations and contexts

Source: World Health Organization (WHO), 2022 / CC BY-ND 3.0 IGO.

According to both the ICD-11 and the DSM-5-TR, language should in fact play a pervasive role in the autism diagnostic process. Illustrating this time with the DSM-5-TR, it is explicitly emphasized that "the current level of verbal functioning should be assessed and described," and it is noted that receptive and expressive language skills should be considered separately. In its section on "comorbidity," the DSM-5-TR states that ASD is frequently associated with structural language disorder ("an inability to comprehend and construct sentences with proper grammar") and requires that this be noted under the "accompanying language impairment" specifier (we return to this question in the section "Language and Its Components").

How are these nosographies implemented in the **diagnostic process**? How is it determined that an individual meets SI and RRB criteria? How is it ascertained that an individual has accompanying language impairment? Beginning with the core autism symptoms, SI and RRB, there are a number of standardized, norm-referenced tools, including instruments based on observation of behavior in semi-structured conversation, play, etc., interviews with family, and/or self-administered parent or teacher questionnaires. The most widely used are the Autism Diagnostic Observation Schedule, Second Edition (ADOS-2; Lord et al. 2012), a semi-structured, interaction-based, observational evaluation, and the Autism Diagnostic Interview-Revised (ADI-R; Rutter, Le Couteur, and Lord 2003), a semi-structured caregiver interview. A combination of the ADOS and the ADI-R currently counts as the gold standard for diagnosis. Yet, we cannot simply take scores on these measures and turn them into diagnoses. Expert clinical judgment is needed to complete the diagnostic process (see also below). Another tool often used in the process of diagnosing autism is the Childhood Autism Rating Scale, Second Edition (CARS-2; Schopler et al. 2010), a clinician rating scale. Examples of frequently used questionnaires (in clinical or research settings) include the Autism Quotient Questionnaire (AQ; Baron-Cohen et al. 2001) and the Social Responsiveness Scale, Second Edition (SRS-2; Constantino and Gruber 2012). Another commonly used instrument is the Vineland Behavior Adaptive Scales, Third Edition (VABS-3), an interview caregiver instrument assessing adaptive functioning (including communication skills) that is not specific to autism (Sparrow et al. 2016).

While all of the above-mentioned instruments that are used to detect autism include elements referring to communication or verbal behavior, none of them serve as a dedicated language assessment tool. For instance, the ADOS includes different modules whose use depends on the individuals' age and verbal behavior (e.g. Module 1 – language consisting of a few words, Module 2 – language consisting of a few phrases, and Module 3 – fluent language). In practice, it is not clear how the language specifier required in the ICD-11/DSM-5-TR systems ("extent of functional language impairment" or "impairment of receptive and expressive language") are to be detected in an ASD diagnosis. Besides the fact that proper language screening implies that the diagnostic process includes qualified personnel specialized in language assessment (speech-language pathologists/ therapists), such screening must be carried out with assessment instruments proven to be effective for assessing language in autism. Fulfilling these basic requirements constitutes a significant challenge. The diagnostic process often does not systematically include speech-language pathology consultation, due to a lack of personnel or to time constraints on the diagnostic process. Moreover, as will be highlighted throughout this book, research increasingly indicates that it is unjustified to assume that language assessment tools commonly employed to detect language impairment in nonautistic people are adequate for use in autism (see section "How Is Language Studied in Research on Autism?").

We have presented ASD diagnosis as it is laid out in the ICD-11 and the DSM-5-TR since this is how diagnosis is currently carried out in most contexts or countries, and we have given a succinct presentation of some widely used diagnostic instruments. While these were intended to represent a consensus among clinicians and are based on current research, we believe that it is important to raise two points here. The first one is with regard to commonly used diagnostic instruments. We emphasize again that these are just one part of the diagnostic process, and furthermore that not all of them are appropriate for all autistic individuals. As explicitly and forcefully argued by Bishop and Lord (2023, p. 836), diagnostic instruments are designed to support, inform, and refine the diagnostic process, not replace it: "CLINICIANS make diagnoses, not instruments" [emphasis in original]. In other words, a relevant score on a particular instrument does not entail that an individual is or is not on the autism spectrum. Moreover, they underline that prognosis and intervention rely on an individual's particular profile of symptoms and skills, including language skills. Fombonne (2023, p. 713) likewise warns against overinclusive diagnosis resulting from "reliance on single informants, on isolated administration of instruments [particularly by those having no or little clinical experience], on current only symptomatology, and a failure to adjust for the effect of co-occurring nonautistic conditions."

The second point we would like to raise concerns the notion of a categorical diagnostic entity for autism envisaged as a unitary spectrum in the ICD-11 and DSM-5-TR, and therefore a category that groups together individuals with extremely different profiles. This view has received harsh criticism from some clinicians and researchers, and alternative views have been proposed and given rise to ongoing debate. Mottron and Gagnon (2023), for example, argue that this practice may hinder progress in our understanding of the nature of autism and its underlying mechanisms. They propose that only by studying well-defined subgroups, separately, can progress be made. They argue in particular for a research strategy focusing on "prototypical autism," the readily-identifiable-to-experienced-clinicians subset of children who meet DSM-5-TR criteria, who test positive on commonly used instruments, and who phenotypically are highly similar to each other in showing a unique pattern during the developmental period between ages 2 and 5, notably because they display late language emergence and "apparent verbal intellectual disability."

Both of the points just raised, namely, the proper use of diagnostic instruments and the continuing debate on the construct of ASD, have implications for how we study and understand autism, including language in autism. Scientific papers on autism, including those on language, typically provide information on the diagnosis of autistic participants in the study: what types of professionals gave the diagnoses, in what setting (what type(s) of structure), what the specifier profiles are (whether or not there is Language Impairment, LI, and/or Disorder of Intellectual Development, DID), and, where relevant, what instruments were used. Absence of this information generally raises a red flag for researchers in the field. Knowing who autistic participants are when reading and evaluating a research study is fundamental, as a conclusion about autism could be based on a restricted subset of profiles or just one particular profile.

A final point regarding the autism diagnostic process is the significant variation in practices between countries. These include differences in the availability of culturally adapted norm-referenced tools. Another source of variation is the age at which diagnosis typically takes place. While the global mean age of diagnosis is estimated to be around age 3;6 (ranging from age 2;6 to 6), screening for ASD at age 18 months is recommended in many countries. Nonetheless, initial diagnosis in adulthood is ubiquitous (see Chapter 12).

Language and Its Components

The question of proper assessment of language discussed in the preceding section raises, in turn, the question of what exactly is meant by LANGUAGE, the focus of this book. Language is often regarded as a communication system, be it oral, signed, or written. However, language is much more than a communication system (a system allowing for exchange of information between individuals). It is also the framework for people's thoughts, i.e. it can serve as the expression of thought. We underline, furthermore, that language is not a monolithic entity, but rather a complex construct encompassing a variety of domains. Three main components of language can be distinguished, which will be discussed in more detail in Part 1 of this book: (i) **the Lexicon**, which could be compared to a mental dictionary containing an inventory of words and their properties, e.g. how they are pronounced and what they mean; (ii) **Structural aspects of language**, which correspond to the grammar of a language. This refers not only to the structure of words and sentences (morphosyntax), but also to the structure of sounds (phonology), and the way the meaning of a sentence is organized (semantics). Structural aspects of language are also referred to as the computational system of language since they involve specific linguistic operations necessary for combining elements (for example, combining words in a certain order or attaching the appropriate grammatical markers to make phrases and sentences); (iii) **Pragmatic aspects of language**, which correspond to the way language is used in context and in conversations.

Let us illustrate how these different language domains play out in the sentence given in (1) (the examples we give here are in English, but comparable examples can be given in all human languages).

(1) This dancer worked hard and managed to get a full-time contract at the ballet.

This sentence is made of 14 words drawn from the **lexicon**. Some of these words (*this, work, hard, and, to, get, a, at,* and *the*) contain different speech sounds forming, in each case, one syllable, while all of the other words in (1) contain two syllables. The way speech sounds are organized into syllables is part of **phonology**. Moreover, although both *worked* and *managed* have the same ending – *ed* (called a suffix), whose function is to indicate past tense, this suffix is not pronounced in the same way. It is pronounced as a "t" in *worked* but as a "d" in *managed*. This difference is due to the application of a phonological rule taking into account some specific aspects of the speech sound that appear right before the suffix -*ed* in each of the two words. The fact that the verbs *work* and *manage* end with the suffix -*ed* is part of another language domain, which is **morphosyntax**. Because it is a tense marker, the -*ed* suffix attaches to verbs in order to provide information about the moment the action expressed by the sentence takes place with respect to the moment the sentence is produced (past, present, or future). The sentence itself can be divided into groups of words, or phrases, such as *this dancer* and *a full-time contract*, which each have a particular syntactic function and a specific position in the sentence (typical of the English language). The phrase *this dancer* is the subject of the sentence and appears before the verb *worked*. The phrase *a full-time contract* is the object of the verb *get* and it appears after this verb. Word order in a language is determined via syntactic rules. Finally, each word has a meaning, which contributes to the meaning of the sentence. Yet, in order to understand the full meaning of the sentence, it is not enough to know the meaning of individual words. The ways in which words combine (syntax) determine meaning at the sentence level.

In addition to the mechanics of how linguistic structure is built and how sentence meaning is derived from this, speakers need to pay attention to the context in which language is used: **pragmatics**. While semantics refers to context-independent aspects of meaning, pragmatics refers to how context (including conversations) contributes to meaning. People often use language to share information, tell stories, have an argument, etc. Furthermore, speakers come to a conversation with opinions, desires, and intentions, which they may convey in one way or another. One aspect of pragmatics is **implicit meaning**, which refers to the fact that participants in a conversation do not always express their intentions explicitly. In sentence (1), by talking about a specific dancer, the speaker may implicitly formulate a criticism to the listener, such as *You haven't been working hard enough and this is not getting you anywhere*. Another pragmatic aspect concerns the way people tell stories: **narration**. The sentence in (1) may be the beginning of a story relating the different events that led the dancer to being offered a contract at the ballet. When telling stories, speakers must combine sentences with each other and order the different events with respect to each other, so that conversational partners can keep track of what is happening and why it is happening.

Although language domains are quite independent from each other (for instance, the rules underlying the combination of speech sounds to form syllables (phonology) and words to form phrases and sentences (morphosyntax) are different), they also interact. For example, the way speakers choose to express the information they wish to convey is part of the **interface between morphosyntax and semantics or pragmatics**, playing an important role in **discourse** (how sentences and their content are linked to create larger chunks of language). In the sentence in (1), for example, the fact that *this* is used to talk about a dancer suggests that both the speaker and the listener know who this person is. It could be that the dancer in question was introduced earlier in the conversation or that the speaker is pointing to a dancer who is standing in the vicinity. The speaker may also want to place some parts of the sentence in the foreground, for example, by putting some stress on the word *hard* to insist on what needs to be done in order to be hired at the ballet.

The Language Domains Covered in This Book

Domain	Definition
Lexicon	Knowledge about words: their pronunciation, meaning, grammatical properties, and how they are connected to each other.
Morphosyntax	The structure of words and sentences, i.e. the way words and phrases combine.
Phonology	The structure of sounds, i.e. the way speech sounds combine.
Semantics	The structure of sentence-level meaning, i.e. the way the meaning of a sentence is derived from the meaning of its parts and the way these parts are combined.
Pragmatics	Language use in context (including conversations).
Prosody	Melodic structure, including stress, intonation, and rhythm organization.

Another language domain that this book documents is **prosody**, which has both grammatical and pragmatic aspects. Prosody refers to the melodic structure of a word, phrase, or sentence and is based on stress, intonation, and rhythm. For example, a specific intonation may be used over the whole sentence in (1), ending with a rising tone, to convey the implicit criticism mentioned above. In the noun *contract*, which is made of two syllables, the first syllable is stressed compared to the first syllable (contract). Placing stress on the second syllable (contract) instead would turn the word *contract* into a verb, as in *The dancer contracted a virus, making it impossible to perform for a while*.

The various language domains covered in this book (see text box) are involved in the production, but also in the comprehension of language. Understanding what somebody says requires knowledge about speech sounds, words and their meanings, rules of syllable, word and sentence formation, and how the meaning of sentences is derived, as well as being able to interpret the speaker's intended meaning.

In nosological classifications, such as ICD and DSM (see section "How Is Autism Diagnosed and What Role Does Language Play in the Diagnosis?" above), language or "verbal functioning" is referred to in terms of with or without accompanying "language impairment," "verbal functioning," or "language dysfunctioning." But what does this mean, exactly? Does this refer to all aspects of language, just a few, or even just one? If only a few domains are concerned, which ones are they? Is it the lexicon or are we talking about language domains that are more structural in nature (as they involve rules combining items with each other), such as phonology and morphosyntax? Research has shown that autistic individuals vary in terms of which language components present challenges to them. It is often claimed that autistic people may find pragmatics particularly challenging, due to deficits in social interaction and communication, telling a coherent story, or managing a conversation (e.g. knowing when it is their turn to speak, or providing less or more information than what is expected). Some individuals may also have difficulties with structural aspects of language leading to the production of errors in structures that are particularly complex, such as immediately adjacent consonants forming clusters, as in the first three sounds in the word *strict* (phonology), or sentences containing other sentences (or subordinate clauses), as in *I saw the man who Mary met* (morphosyntax). Yet, other individuals may struggle with the meaning of combinations of words (semantics), displaying ways of categorizing items that differ from those observed in neurotypical individuals. In contrast, in some autistic individuals, language difficulties are almost imperceptible.

This book provides a description of language abilities in autistic individuals by showing, for each of the different language domains, what research says about language development in autism as compared to neurotypical populations. The first part of the book "Within Language Domains" starts with chapters that revolve around the core domains of spoken language that have been identified in more than 70 years of linguistic research: the lexicon, the computational system (structural aspects of language), and pragmatics. In addition, we chose to dedicate a separate chapter to prosody, as it is often claimed to be different in autistic speech.

Extralinguistic Cognition and Other Issues Related to Language in Autism

Similar to the potential interaction between different language domains (as described in the section "Language and its Components"), language can also interact with extralinguistic cognitive domains, some of which are reported to be often different in autism. Examples are **Theory of Mind** (ToM – the ability to infer and understand mental states (e.g. beliefs, true, and false) in oneself and others) and other **social cognition** (perception, processing, interpretation, and response to social stimulus), **Executive Function** (EF – e.g. inhibition, switching, planning, sustained attention, working memory), **central coherence** ("seeing the big picture"), and **intellectual ability**. As these extralinguistic cognitive functions in autistic people may differ from those in neurotypical individuals, their influence on language (development) in autism is explored throughout the book.

Impairment in extralinguistic cognitive domains may result from additional diagnoses, such as ADHD, epilepsy, or Disorder of Intellectual Development (DID; e.g. May et al. 2018). This raises the question as to how these additional conditions affect language outcome in autism. One way to explore these co-occurring conditions is to study language development **across the autism spectrum**, including individuals with and without DID (Silleresi et al. 2020). This can distinguish between the effects of autistic characteristics and the effects of co-occurring conditions. Another direction is to compare language (development) in autism to language (development) in **other neurodevelopmental disorders**. Such comparisons may uncover the language characteristics that are unique to autism. Age is another factor that may influence language in autism (Pickles, Anderson, and Lord 2014). As extralinguistic cognitive functions may be particularly vulnerable in **elderly people** with autism, this may affect their language abilities as well. The study of language-developmental trajectories across the lifespan of autistic people is relatively recent (and still scarce) but provides important additional information to how we understand autism.

The book covers three other important topics related to language in autism, namely, **multilingualism, reading**, and the **brain**. How multilingualism affects language acquisition in developmental disorders is a broad question in the field of multilingualism and education (cf. Franck, Faloppa, and Marinis 2024). Here, focusing on autism, we unfold in detail the mistaken belief that multilingualism exacerbates language and/or cognitive difficulties (Prévost and Tuller 2022). We present studies showing positive relations between exposure and language outcome, and the unexpected path of becoming multilingual through noninteractive sources, such as television and computer games, in autism (Kissine et al. 2019). Reading is directly related to spoken language, although learning how to read generally requires explicit instruction. In the case of autism, individual variability in reading skills is the reality (Brown, Oram-Cardy, and Johnson 2013). We discuss questions relating to reading comprehension, word recognition, Theory of Mind, and other skills that affect reading achievement. Finally, with regard to language and the brain, exploring potentially atypical brain structures in autistic people may help understand how they produce and comprehend language differently from neurotypical individuals (Herbert et al. 2005). Current language and brain studies in autism suggest that the neural network for language in autism is not left-hemisphere dominant as it is in neurotypical people (Peterson et al. 2024). We discuss the implications of this pattern for the diagnosis and language outcomes in autism.

The issues related to language in autism just described make up the core of Part 2 of the book. The chapters in Part 2 integrate topics that are discussed in the first part of the book "Within Language Domains" into a broader view, "Across Language Domains."

How Is Language Studied in Research on Autism?

Regardless of the linguistic domain under investigation, studies on autism commonly report results from standardized language tools in order to provide a background picture of language skills in their samples of autistic children and adults. We use the term "standardized tools" to refer to language assessment instruments that not only follow a strict administration procedure (there is a "standard" for their use), but that are also norm-referenced, and as such are the kind of tool typically used in clinical settings. A norm-referenced assessment is a tool developed through administration to a representative population sample. The established norms, based on average scores and standard deviations, can then be used to generate standard scores (e.g. T-scores or percentile ranks) for a comparison when assessing an individual person. These scores enable comparison of the participant's performance on the test with that of the norming sample. Below, we discuss several standardized language tools, chosen because they are referred to in this book. These include both indirect and direct measures of language comprehension (receptive language) and production (expressive language). Many of these tests were developed for English, and some are adapted for other languages.

Standardized instruments rely on various techniques, similar to those used in the various experimental tasks also reported on in this book. Children's language abilities, both expressive and receptive, can be tested indirectly through the use of questionnaires (usually parental), such as the MacArthur–Bates Communicative Developmental Inventory (MB-CDI-2; Fenson et al. 2006), which is available for over 100 languages (or varieties of same). These can be used with children as young as 12 months, as well as those with little expressive language.

Language abilities can also be assessed directly. Measures of receptive language abilities (comprehension) often include picture selection, where participants are asked to point to one of several pictures presented on a screen or in a picture book, which goes best with the stimulus the experimenter utters (see Chapter 2 for some details concerning vocabulary acquisition). The stimulus can be a word in a vocabulary comprehension test, e.g. Peabody Picture Vocabulary Test-Fifth Edition (PPVT-5; Dunn and Dunn 2018), or a sentence, in tests assessing comprehension of sentence structures, such as Test of Receptive Grammar-Version 2 (TROG-2; Bishop 2003), or the Sentence Comprehension subtest of the Clinical Evaluation of Language Fundamentals–Fifth Edition (CELF-5; Wiig, Semel, and Secord 2013).

To assess expressive language (production), the simplest technique of word naming is used in vocabulary assessments, e.g. Renfrew Expressive Vocabulary Test-Fifth Edition (EVT-5; Renfrew 2023), where the child is asked to produce a word that fits the picture shown. Participants may also be asked to simply repeat a stimulus verbatim: a sentence (for morphosyntax), in the Recalling Sentences subtest in different versions of the CELF-5, or a nonword (for phonology), as in NEPSY Pseudoword Repetition task (Korkman 2004). Other tools use the technique of constrained elicitation (sentence completion), where the experimenter starts the sentence and instructs the participant to finish the sentence off, e.g. Word Structure subtest of CELF-5 (Wiig, Semel, and Secord 2013), Test of Early Grammatical Impairment (TEGI; Rice and Wexler 2000), which assesses verb inflections relevant to tense marking, relies on the same method. To assess narrative production, the child may be asked to tell or retell a story relying on wordless picture books, such as the Bus Story Test (BST, Renfrew 2010), *Frog, where are you?* (Mayer 2003), or the Edmonton Narrative Norms Instrument (ENNI; Schneider, Dubé, and Hayward 2005). These tools involve a sequence of pictures that are organized into episodes forming a story, thus offering a rich context for assessing various aspects of children's language abilities, including their narrative skills, vocabulary knowledge, grammatical proficiency, discourse organization, and pragmatic competence. Some instruments consist of separate subscales assessing receptive and expressive language, relying on methods reviewed above (pointing to or describing pictures, repeating sounds, words or sentences, or answering questions related to pictures, sentences or paragraphs), suitable for both younger, (e.g. Mullen Scales of Early Learning (MSEL; Mullen 1995; Preschool Language Scale, Fourth Edition PLS-4; Zimmerman, Steiner, and Pond 2002) and older children (e.g. CELF-5).

Many language assessment tools are adapted and normed for use in different languages and in different countries. This practice promotes accessibility and cultural relevance of clinical tools, enhances the reliability of results, and allows for more accurate assessment of language abilities across linguistic and cultural contexts (see Chapter 16).

The tools we have discussed here have norms for different ages, with lower age limits ranging from birth (MSEL; PLS-4), to age 2;6 (PPVT-5), 4 (TROG-2), or 5 (CELF-5). The upper age limit also varies from 14 and over (TROG-2), 16 (BPVS-3), 21 (CELF-5), to 90 (PPVT-5). Each tool provides tables that allow conversion of raw scores both to standard scores and to age equivalents. In tests using a mean standard score of 100 (most tests), the lowest standard score can range from 20 (MSEL) to 40 (older versions of BPVS), 55 (TROG-2), or 70 (BPVS-3). Note that the reliability of an instrument falters when participants' language abilities are at the lower end of the spectrum: the lowest standard score of BPVS-3 is 70, but there may be many individuals with very different raw scores who still achieve the same standard score of 70. The implication is that some of these tools may not be sensitive enough to provide a reliable picture of language skills in populations with a heterogeneous range of skills.

While standardized tests designed and used by clinicians offer valuable insights into the general language skills of speakers from diverse language and cultural backgrounds, various chapters in this book also illustrate their limitations. It will become evident that these tests often lack the precision needed to describe an (autistic) individual's linguistic capacities in relevant detail, even when the instrument attempts to cover a range of language skills, such as CELF-5 or PLS-4. Developmental linguists and clinicians build on the background picture provided by these instruments by developing sophisticated experimental tasks to zoom in on a particular area of the language of interest. Some experimental tools developed collaboratively by clinicians and linguists have been subsequently standardized and are now used in clinics: a good example is TEGI (Rice and Wexler 2000), which assesses verb inflections relevant to tense marking, mentioned in Chapter 13. However, even these instruments are not always autism-friendly, a term we use to refer to assessment tools that can be used across the autism spectrum, including individuals with more challenging autistic symptoms, limited intellectual abilities, and/or expressive language. We note that "autism-friendly" does not mean that these considerations are specific to autism, as many other neurodevelopmental disorders may come with similar challenges that require careful selection of language assessment tools. To mention a few, consider tasks with complicated instructions, tasks that entail deciphering detailed pictures that could easily elicit echolalic answers,[2] and/or, at least for some individuals, that require voluntary actions such as pointing. One concerted effort toward

---

2 Echolalia is the spontaneous repetition of something said by another person; it can be immediate (repetition immediately after the utterance) or delayed (repetition sometime after the utterance).

autism-friendly assessment of language involves the use of LITMUS tools (https://www.bi-sli.org/litmus-tools), as explicitly argued in Chapter 16.

An important issue that has consequences for the generalizability of findings reported in research studies is that of **heterogeneity** of language and extralinguistic cognitive skills in autistic individuals. In view of this wide linguistic and extralinguistic cognitive variability, it may be difficult to interpret the results of studies that employ samples of participants with very different language skills, e.g. autism plus language impairment (ALI) versus autism without language impairment (ALN) (Tager-Flusberg 2006).[3] Similarly, if studies do not distinguish between individuals with or without intellectual disability when reporting findings on autistic people's reading abilities, for instance, results may be difficult to interpret as it appears that intellectual disability may affect an individual's ability to read.

A Terminological Note: The Vocabulary of Autism

What are the most **accurate and respectful terms** to use to talk about autism? How to refer to the condition itself, to individuals who have this condition, and to those who do not? How to name the types, intensity, and frequency of the symptoms or characteristics that define and characterize the condition?

In this first, introductory chapter, the reader will have already noticed that a variety of terms have been used to designate all of the above. This **terminological diversity** will be apparent throughout the book: the reader will notice differences in the terms used both between chapters and within given chapters. The editorial team would like to tackle here the question of autism terminology head-on. We will not propose a solution to any waging battles but, rather, explain why this book has adopted a diverse approach.

During the past decades, the vocabulary of autism has evolved considerably and rapidly. While some terms appear to gain consensus, such as using the simple term "autism" to talk about the condition, other terms continue to be the subject of debate. This can be illustrated by a rapid retrospective of how individuals with a diagnosis of autism are referred to (see Vivanti 2020). There was a reaction in the 1970s to the prevailing use of terms, once fully accepted, that were argued to reduce individuals with disabilities to their disability, including, in some cases, terms now

---

3 Language impairment in autism has been noted since at least the 1970s of the previous century (e.g. Allen and Rapin 1980; Churchill 1972; Rapin and Dunn 1997; Rutter 1968; 1970). The distinction between autism plus language impairment and autism without language impairment was coined ALI (Autism Language Impairment) versus ALN (Autism Normal Language) by Helen Tager-Flusberg in 2006.

considered offensive ("retarded," "autistic," etc.), with advocates (including people with lived experience, sometimes referred to as self-advocates, speaking out or acting to defend their interests) asserting the fact that they are people first and foremost. The ensuing widespread (and scientific journal-encouraged/required) use of "person-first" designations ("person with autism") has been criticized in recent years as abnegating an inseparable part of these people's identities through an idiosyncratic and therefore stigmatizing language construction ("person with X"). This shift is in keeping with a broader movement advocating a neurodiversity and cultural approach to differences defined by the medical profession as pathologies. So-called "identity-first language" ("autistic person") has become increasingly endorsed by autistic adults (Bottema-Beutel et al. 2021). These endorsements have been criticized within both autism and wider communities as not being relevant to all concerned individuals and groups, with many individuals being significantly under-represented in community surveys about language choices, notably those with cognitive impairment and/or more complex communication needs and their families.

Vivanti (2020) points out that both person-first and identity-first approaches stem from a will to signify respect for individuals who feel that they are more than their diagnosis and for individuals who are proud of their diagnosis, and notes that both of these approaches appear to be relevant in autistic communities. To this, we can add that terminological preferences observed within the community also vary from culture to culture or country to country. Appellations that appear to be consensual in some countries may not be so in others (e.g. Autism Spectrum Condition [ASC], may be frequent in the UK, but unknown or unaccepted in other cultures or countries). While Kenny et al. (2016) found that autistic adults in the UK preferred identity-first labels ("autistic" or "autistic person"), Buijsman, Begeer, and Scheeren's (2023) survey of Dutch-speaking autistic adults and parents of autistic children showed that the majority preferred person-first designations ("person with autism"). Terminological variation is likewise apparent within sectors within a given country: medical establishment versus educational institutions versus organizations providing resources, support, and advocacy for families and individuals, etc. (see Kenny et al. 2016). Keating et al.'s (2023, p. 406) international survey of English-speaking autistic adults concluded that "there is no universally accepted way to talk about autism," mirroring Buijsman, Begeer, and Scheeren's conclusion that both language and culture may impact language preferences.

It is noteworthy in this regard that the reviews for this book (from reviewers working on autism, and in close contact with autism communities in 12 different countries, in Europe, North America, and the Middle East) have included remarks asking for person-first language to be changed to identity-first language as well as the reverse. Further indication of autism terminological variability is found in Table 1.2, which presents a compilation of terminology from the 2023

Table 1.2 Catalogue of terminology from the 2023 INSAR Meeting handbook.

Reference to the condition	Autism; Autism Spectrum Disorder (ASD); Autism Spectrum Condition (ASC); Neurodevelopmental Disorders (NDD); Neurodevelopmental Conditions; co-occurring conditions; comorbidity
Reference to individuals	Autistic individuals/adults/children/people; ASD individuals/children; children with ASD; individuals/infants/children with or without autism; non-neurodivergent individuals; nonautistic participants/comparisons; TD sample; ASD/no ASD
Reference to symptoms	Symptoms/traits/difficulties/problems/failures/characteristics; clinical factors/clinical features; ASD symptoms; participant characteristics; ASD-associated/related factors; autistic traits; autism severity
	Functionally impactful behaviors and interests; functionally restricting; having a functional impact; having an improved or attenuated impact; increased/decreased symptoms; higher/lower symptoms
	Psychological problems; cognitive failures; reduced multisensorial processing: atypical sensitivity to sensory stimuli; impairment; non-socially biased information processing
	Language deficits/impairment; verbal inability; nonverbal; minimally verbal
	Ameliorate associated issues; improvement; positive effects

International Society for Autism Research (INSAR) meeting. In Table 1.2, note that the diversity in how individuals with autism are referred to reviewed above extends to how individuals without autism are designated. Traditionally, terms such as "control group" and "typically developing (TD) children/adults" have been used; we now find terms that indicate more clearly how comparison groups have been recruited: "nonautistic individuals/participants," "children without autism/ASD," "non-neurodivergent," "neurotypical," or simply "no ASD." Again, terminological diversity appears to be the rule, as there is considerable variety in terms used both between publications and within a single publication.

In light of the differing ways of talking about autism, this book has followed a diverse approach (also followed by some major scientific journals devoted to autism – see Vivanti 2020). In an attempt to ensure clarity, terminology used in the two major diagnostic manuals has frequently been adopted. We believe that diversity in respectful terminology reflects the current state of dialogue within advocacy, academic, and clinical communities. We also acknowledge the likelihood that any terminological decisions made as this publication goes to press might become obsolete in a short time. Given that respectful language has been the intention of all contributors, we humbly ask the reader for their indulgence.

Formal Organization of the Book

This book consists of 16 chapters. To increase readability and to encourage comparison between chapters, all chapters, except for Chapter 1 and Chapter 16, follow the same structure, schematized below:

"What Do You Think?"
Introduction
Anchoring
Main Section (X in Autism)
Focus on a Specific Study
Conclusion
"What Do You Know Now?"
Suggestions for Further Reading
References

Each chapter is flanked by two text boxes, one at the beginning ("What Do You Think?") and one at the end ("What Do You Know Now?").[4] The "What Do You Think?" box includes some anecdotes and questions aiming to make the reader think about their own preconceived ideas. It may also provide a good starting point for a discussion in class. The goal of the "What Do You Know Now?" box is to make the reader realize that their answers to the questions raised in the "What Do You Think?" section at the beginning may be different from the answers they had in mind initially. The "What Do You Know Now?" box summarizes the key learning points and applies these to the "What Do You Think?" section.

Every chapter presents a short introduction, mentioning and illustrating the particular topic (X) and why it is interesting and important to investigate it in autism. The introduction ends with a few questions to be addressed in the main section of the chapter ("X in Autism").

Before delving into the discussion of the particular chapter topic in autism in the main section, each chapter provides an "Anchoring" section, in which some necessary basic knowledge is provided to facilitate understanding of the main section. This often includes linguistic-theoretical background and concepts, the neurotypical situation, including methods, but also aspects of autism relevant to the main section.

Acronyms and technical (linguistic) terminology are defined and explained in the text of each chapter. To help the reader remember those used throughout the relevant chapter, an Acronym and Terminology Reminder text box appears in the

---

4 Inspired by Edward Finegan's (1999) textbook *Language: Its Structure and Use*.

"Anchoring" section of each chapter, which contains colloquial definitions, sometimes illustrated with examples. At the same time, we encourage the reader to look up specific linguistic terminology in available internet glossaries, such as The Internet Grammar of English developed by researchers at the University College London (https://www.ucl.ac.uk/internet-grammar/), Wikipedia (regular editing through the Linguistic Society of America Partnership with Wiki Education Foundation), and SIL (Summer Institute of Linguistics) Glossary of Linguistic Terms (https://glossary.sil.org/). Bold-facing is used for the introduction of a new term or concept throughout the text. Note that bold-faced terms or concepts do not necessarily appear in the Acronym and Terminology Reminder text box. This text box is only meant to remind the reader of certain acronyms and terms that are used repeatedly in the relevant chapter.

The "Anchoring" section is followed by the main section "X in Autism," which highlights what we know to date about the particular topic in autism, including the methods used to establish the empirical foundation for this knowledge. Each chapter then focuses on a specific study illustrating and highlighting promises and pitfalls of the study of X in autism research, including methods. Please note that the lists of studies reviewed and discussed in the anchoring and main sections are not meant to be exhaustive. Rather, they are selected because they highlight important issues regarding the specific topic of the relevant chapter.

The conclusion briefly summarizes the main points and conclusions of the chapter and may provide ideas for future research. At the end of each chapter, there are some suggestions for further reading and a succinct reference list.

References

Allen, D.A. and Rapin, I. (1980). Language disorders in preschool children: predictors of outcome – a preliminary report. *Brain Development* 2 (1): 73–80.

American Psychiatric Association (APA) (2022). *Diagnostic and Statistical Manual of Mental Disorders, Fifth Edition.*, text rev.

Baron-Cohen, S., Wheelwright, S., Skinner, R. et al. (2001). The autism-spectrum quotient (AQ): evidence from Asperger syndrome/high-functioning autism, males and females, scientists and mathematicians. *Journal of Autism and Developmental Disorders* 31: 5–17.

Barthélémy, C., Fuentes, J., Howlin, P. et al. (2019). People with Autism Spectrum Disorder: Identification, Understanding, Intervention. Available at: https://www.autismeurope.org/wp-content/uploads/2019/09/People-with-Autism-Spectrum-Disorder.-Identification-Understanding-Intervention_compressed.pdf.pdf (accessed 11 April 2024).

Bishop, S.L. and Lord, C. (2023). Commentary: best practices and processes for assessment of Autism Spectrum Disorder – the intended role of standardized diagnostic instruments. *Journal of Child Psychology and Psychiatry* 64 (5): 834–838.

References

Bottema-Beutel, K., Kapp, S.K., Lester, J.N. et al. (2021). Avoiding ableist language: suggestions for autism researchers. *Autism in Adulthood* 3 (1):18–29.

Brown, H.M., Oram-Cardy, J., and Johnson, A. (2013). A Meta-analysis of the reading comprehension skills of individuals on the autism spectrum. *Journal of Autism and Developmental Disorders* 43: 932–955.

Buijsman, R., Begeer, S., and Scheeren, A.M. (2023). 'Autistic person' or 'person with autism'? Person-first language preference in Dutch adults with autism and parents. *Autism* 27 (3): 788–795.

Churchill, D.W. (1972). The relation of infantile autism and early childhood schizophrenia to Developmental Language Disorders of childhood. *Journal of Autism and Childhood Schizophrenia* 2: 182–197.

Constantino, J.N. and Gruber, C.P. (2012). *Social Responsiveness Scale, Second Edition (SRS-2)*. Torrance, CA: Western Psychological Services.

Finegan, E. (1999). *Language: Its Structure and Use*. New York: Harcourt.

Fombonne, E. (2023). Is autism overdiagnosed? *Journal of Child Psychology and Psychiatry* 64 (5): 711–714.

Franck, J., Faloppa, F., and Marinis, T. (eds.) (2024). *Myths and facts about multilingualism*. CALEC.

Herbert, M.R., Ziegler, D.A., Deutsch, C.K. et al. (2005). Brain asymmetries in autism and Developmental Language Disorder: a nested whole-brain analysis. *Brain* 128 (1): 213–226.

Howlin, P., Savage, S., Moss, P. et al. (2014). Cognitive and language skills in adults with autism: a 40-year follow-up. *Journal of Child Psychology and Psychiatry* 55 (1): 49–58.

Johnson, C., Beitchman, J., and Brownlie, E. (2010). Twenty-year follow-up of children with and without speech-language impairments: family, educational, occupational, and quality of life outcomes. *American Journal of Speech-Language Pathology* 19: 51–65.

Keating, C.T., Hickman, L., Leung, J. et al. (2023). Autism-related language preferences of English-speaking individuals across the globe: a mixed methods investigation. *Autism Research* 16 (2): 406–428.

Kenny, L., Hattersley, C., Molins, B. et al. (2016). Which terms should be used to describe autism? Perspectives from the UK autism community. *Autism* 20 (4): 442–462.

Kissine, M., Luffin, X., Aiad, F. et al. (2019). Noncolloquial Arabic in Tunisian children with Autism Spectrum Disorder: a possible instance of language acquisition in a noninteractive context. *Language Learning* 69 (1): 44–70.

Levinson, S., Eisenhower, A., Bush, H.H. et al. (2020). Brief report: predicting social skills from semantic, syntactic, and pragmatic language among young children with Autism Spectrum Disorder. *Journal of Autism and Developmental Disorders* 50: 4165–4175.

Lord, C., Charman, T., Havdahl, A. et al. (2022). The Lancet Commission on the future of care and clinical research in autism. *The Lancet* 399 (10321): 271–334.

Lord, C., Rutter, M., DiLavore, P. et al. (2012). *Autism Diagnostic Observation Schedule (ADOS)* Torrance, CA: Western Psychological Services.

May, T., Brignell, A., Hawi, Z. et al. (2018). Trends in the overlap of Autism Spectrum Disorder and attention deficit hyperactivity disorder: prevalence, clinical management, language, and genetics. *Current Developmental Disorders Reports* 5 (1): 49–57.

Mottron, L. and Gagnon, D. (2023). Prototypical autism: new diagnostic criteria and asymmetrical bifurcation model. *Acta Psychologica* 237: 103938.

Peterson, M., Prigge, M.B.D., Floris, D.L. et al. (2024). Reduced lateralization of multiple functional brain networks in autistic males. *Journal of Neurodevelopmental Disorders* 16: 23.

Pickles, A., Anderson, D.K., and Lord, C. (2014). Heterogeneity and plasticity in the development of language: a 17-year follow-up of children referred early for possible autism. *Journal of Child Psychology and Psychiatry* 55 (12): 1354–1362.

Prévost, P. and Tuller, L. (2022). Bilingual language development in autism. *Linguistic Approaches to Bilingualism* 12 (1): 1–32.

Rapin, I. and Dunn, M. (1997). Language disorders in children with autism. *Seminars in Pediatric Neurology* 4 (2): 86–92.

Rutter, M. (1968). Concepts of autism: a review of research. *Child Psychology and Psychiatry and Allied Disciplines* 9 (1): 1–25.

Rutter, M. (1970). Autistic children: infancy to adulthood. *Seminars in Psychiatry* 2: 435–450.

Rutter, M., Le Couteur, A., and Lord, C. (2003). *ADI-R: Autism Diagnostic Interview-Revised*. Torrance, CA: Western Psychological Services.

Schaeffer, J., Abd El-Raziq, M., Castroviejo, E. et al. (2023). Language in autism: domains, profiles and co-occurring conditions. *Journal of Neural Transmission* 130: 433–457.

Schiller, J. (2023) Autism Statistics and Facts – How Many People Have Autism? Available at: https://www.thetreetop.com/statistics/autism-prevalence (accessed 11 April 2024).

Schopler, E., Van Bourgondien, M.E., Wellman, G.J. et al. (2010). *Childhood Autism Rating Scale–Second Edition (CARS-2)*. Los Angeles, CA: Western Psychological Services.

Silleresi, S., Prévost, P., Zebib, R. et al. (2020). Identifying language and cognitive profiles in children with ASD via a cluster analysis exploration: implications for the new ICD-11. *Autism Research* 13 (7): 1155–1167.

Sparrow, S.S., Saulnier, C.A., Cicchetti, D. et al. (2016). *Vineland-3: Vineland Adaptive Behavior Scales*. Minneapolis, MN: Pearson Assessments.

Sturrock, A., Chilton, H., Foy, K. et al. (2022). In their own words: the impact of subtle language and communication difficulties as described by autistic girls and boys without intellectual disability. *Autism* 26 (2): 332–345.

Tager-Flusberg, H. (2006). Defining language phenotypes in autism. *Clinical Neuroscience Research*, 6 (3–4):219–224.

Tager-Flusberg, H. and Kasari, C. (2013). Minimally verbal school-aged children with Autism Spectrum Disorder: the neglected end of the spectrum. *Autism Research* 6 (6): 468–478.

Vivanti, G. (2020). Ask the editor: what is the most appropriate way to talk about individuals with a diagnosis of autism? *Journal of Autism and Developmental Disorders* 50 (2): 691–693.

World Health Organization (WHO) (2022). *ICD-11: International Classification of Diseases* (11th revision). Available at: https://icd.who.int/. (accessed 11 April 2024).

World Health Organization (WHO) (2023). *Autism – Key Facts*. Available at: https://www.un.org/en/academic-impact/un-calls-recognizing-rights-people-autism-make-their-own-decisions (accessed 11 April 2024).

Zeidan, J., Fombonne, E., Scorah, J. et al. (2022). Global prevalence of autism: a systematic review update. *Autism Research* 15 (5): 778–790.

Standardized Language Tests Referred to in This Book, by Acronym

BPVS-3: Dunn, L.M. (2009). *British Picture Vocabulary Scale, Third Edition (BPVS-3)*. G L Assessment Limited.

BST: Renfrew, C.E. (2010). *Bus Story Test, Revised Edition*. Speechmark.

MB-CDI-2: Fenson, L., Marchman, V.A., Thal, D.J. et al. (2006). *MacArthur-Bates Communicative Development Inventories, Second Edition (MB-CDI-2)*. APA PsycTests.

CELF-5: Wiig, E.H., Semel, E., and Secord, W.A. (2013). *Clinical Evaluation of Language Fundamentals–Fifth Edition (CELF-5)*. Pearson.

ENNI: Schneider, P., Dubé, R.V., and Hayward, D. (2005). *The Edmonton Narrative Norms Instrument*. Available at: http://www.rehabresearch.ualberta.ca/enni/ (accessed 15 June 2024).

Frog Story: Mayer, M. (2003). *Frog, where are you?* New York: Penguin.

MSEL: Mullen, E.M. (1995). *Mullen Scales of Early Learning: AGS Edition*. Circle Pines, MN: American Guidance Service.

NEPSY: Korkman, M. (2004). *NEPSY-A Tool* for Comprehensive Assessment of Neurocognitive Disorders in Children. *Comprehensive Handbook of Psychological Assessment, Volume. 1: Intellectual and Neuropsychological Assessment*. Hoboken, NJ: Wiley.

PLS-4: Zimmerman, I.L., Steiner, V.G., and Pond, R.E. (2002). *Preschool Language Scale, Fourth Edition (PLS-4)*. APA PsycTests.

PPVT-5: Dunn, D.M. (2018). *Peabody Picture Vocabulary Test, Fifth Edition (PPVT-5)*. APA PsycTests.

EVT-5: Renfrew, C.E. (2023). *Expressive Vocabulary Test, Fifth Edition (EVT-5)*. Routledge.

TEGI: Rice, M.L. and Wexler, K. (2001). *Test of Early Grammatical Impairment*. San Antonio, TX: The Psychological Corporation.

TROG-2: Bishop, D.V.M. (2003). *Test for Reception of Grammar, Version 2 (TROG-2)*. Pearson.

Part 1

Language in Autism: The View Within Language Domains

2

Lexicon

Letitia Naigles and Nufar Sukenik

> **What Do You Think?**
> Your family recently acquired a collie, and your 4-year-old twins – one with autism and the other neurotypical – have become comfortable with the dog. You are planning to visit your cousins, who have a new dachshund. Your twins have seen pictures. Your child with autism says, "I'm scared; that's not a dog." Your neurotypical child is fine with calling it a dog and expects it to be like your collie. What explains the difference between the children's reactions?
>
> You met your two nieces who have recently visited the zoo. You asked them which animal they liked best. Your 3-year-old niece said she liked "all the really big animals that live in the safari like the elephant and the giraffe." Your 5-year-old niece, with ASD, said that she liked "the one that had a spot on their ear and the one next to the restaurant." Why are these answers different?

Introduction

Your vocabulary is the set of words that you know. What do you think your **mental lexicon** is? If you think it's like a dictionary, then you are probably thinking of words listed according to alphabetic order, with entries that include each word's pronunciation, definition and referents, grammatical form class(es), and possibly etymology. The mental lexicons of neurotypical people may indeed include all these attributes, but they also include connections each word has to other words in the lexicon, connections that are based on pronunciation, based on grammatical characteristics, and based on meaning. The lexicons[1] of individuals on the autism spectrum manifest (some of) these attributes, but these individuals also seem particularly challenged in building the connections amongst words. The degree to which many attributes of the mental lexicon can be observed in individuals with ASD seems to depend at least partially on the task used to study them; as we will discuss below, different tasks target or illuminate different attributes of the mental lexicon.

This chapter covers three questions about the mental lexicons of individuals with ASD. We will largely concentrate on lexical semantics, the meaning of words, as this is the part of research on the lexicon in autism that is so far the most developed.

- How does basic vocabulary development proceed, and what child-internal factors (other abilities the child may have) and child-external factors (properties of the child's environment/input) affect vocabulary growth and composition?
- Which typical word learning strategies are frequently observed, and which are less frequently observed in autistic children?
- How well are category formation and use manifested in the lexicons of autistic individuals?

Anchoring

In order to build their mental lexicons, children need to acquire the sound patterns of words (e.g. which sounds occur in which position), their morphological patterns (e.g. prefixes or suffixes), their meanings, and their myriad relationships to other words. The first stages of this learning process, accomplished during the first year of life in typically developing (TD) children, involve differentiating linguistic sounds from other sounds in the environment and discovering which linguistic sounds distinguish words in their input language. For example, *pat* and *bat* are different words in English, reflecting that /p/ and /b/ are different phonemes; however, whether *pat* is pronounced with an aspirated [pʰat] or unaspirated [pat] /p/ does not affect

---

1 The words "vocabulary" and "lexicon" are closely related and are often used interchangeably in everyday language. A person's vocabulary can vary in size, and it can expand over time as they learn and encounter new words. Vocabulary encompasses a broad range of words, from common everyday terms to more specialized or rare words. In linguistics, the lexicon is a more formal and comprehensive term that covers not only the words people use but also details about each word, such as its meaning, pronunciation, part of speech (e.g. noun, verb), and any associated grammatical information, as well as all of the connections between these components.

its meaning in English but might in other languages. See Chapter 4 on Phonology for more information.

The next hurdle for word learning is often called the **mapping** problem: children need to map words onto their referents in the world, associate a label with an object, a person, an action, an abstract concept, etc. However, the world (the child's environment) is not transparent in revealing which referents go with which words (Gleitman 1990; Suanda et al. 2019). For example, children might hear "dog" in the presence of dogs, but the dogs themselves are also in the presence of fur and tails, toys and food, running and barking, all of which might interfere with mapping "dog" onto *dog*. That TD children solve this problem is documented in their vocabulary growth: first words appear around 9–14 months of age, and vocabulary increases exponentially through preschoolerhood and beyond. Explanations for this speedy rate of vocabulary acquisition point to the use of various word-learning strategies, which have been proposed to help them focus on specific aspects of the world and on the social interaction of the conversation. These are summarized in Table 2.1. For example, TD children have been shown to use a whole object assumption (a word refers to the whole object and not just a tiny part of it), a shape bias (a word is extended to new objects of the same shape rather than color or texture), mutual exclusivity and/or a

---

Acronym and Terminology Reminder

Imageability: Degree of correspondence to a mental/visual representation (e.g. *dog* vs. *collaboration*).

IPL: Intermodal Preferential Looking. Experimental method in which a visual scene is described by auditory stimulus while eye movements of participants are recorded.

Joint Attention: Shared focus of attention between two or more individuals on an object, person, or action.

Lexicon/Mental Lexicon: Knowledge about words – their pronunciation, meaning, grammatical properties, and how they are connected to each other.

Lexical Retrieval: Access and selection of the appropriate word ('getting the right word').

Lexical Semantics: Word meaning.

Mapping: Connecting words (forms) with their referents in the world.

Mutual Exclusivity: Learning principle saying that new words are assumed to have different meanings from already known words.

Phonological Representation: Form of a word, how it is pronounced.

Receptive Vocabulary: Words that an individual can recognize/understand.

Shape Bias: Extending the labels of objects to new objects, based on their shape similarity with the original object.

Semantic Categories: Categories of words based on meaning.

Semantic Network: How word concepts are related to each other.

Semantic Representation: Mental representation of word meaning.

Semantic/verbal fluency: Ability to generate words from a given semantic category.

Syntactic Bootstrapping: Acquiring new words based on associations between a word's syntactic frame (how it appears in a sentence) and its meaning.

TD: Typically developing.

Vocabulary: The set of words a person knows.

Table 2.1 How children acquire words: strategies and cues.

Strategy/Cue	Example
Caregiver input	Frequency of vocabulary input, diversity of types of sentences in which the word occurs.
Joint attention	The father says, "Look at that big dog." The child looks at the place the father pointed out and sees the big dog.
Mutual exclusivity/ principle of contrast	Children assume that objects have only one label: when hearing a new word, they will match it to an unfamiliar object (one they don't have a term for yet). Children assume that words contrast in meaning, so a new word *cat*, cannot have the same meaning as a term already known such as *dog*.
Noun bias	Children's first words will include many more words like *milk*, *dog*, and *book* (nouns) than other kinds of words such as *eat*, *sleep*, and *jump* (verbs) or *big*, *nice*, and *bad* (adjectives).
Shape bias	The word *dog* is not restricted to specific colors or fur textures of dogs (black dogs or short-haired dogs) but is assumed to apply to all animals with a dog shape.
Syntactic bootstrapping	A child hearing "The dog is gorping the cat" will use their syntactic knowledge to determine that "gorping" is an action where a dog is doing an action that affects a cat. Knowing which word is the subject/agent ("dog") and which the object/patient ("cat") is part of children's syntactic knowledge, which scaffolds word learning.
Whole object assumption	A child hearing the word *dog* in the context of a caregiver playing with a dog will assume the word refers to the object *dog* and not just to the dog's tail.

principle of contrast (each new word has a different referent or meaning from known words), a noun bias (preference for nouns/labels for objects), and syntactic bootstrapping (the sentence frames in which a word, especially a verb, is used reveals components of that verb's meaning). In addition, one of the most influential tools available to young children while acquiring words involves the social cues provided by their communication partners (caregivers and others in the conversation). For example, adult eye gaze and gestures can initiate and maintain caregiver-child shared reference to objects or events (Tomasello 2015). Furthermore, caregiver input also influences vocabulary growth, as parents who produce words more frequently, and in complex sentences, have children with larger vocabularies (Hoff and Naigles 2002), and verbs that appear in more diverse sentence frames in parent speech (i.e. providing more opportunities for syntactic bootstrapping) are later produced more frequently by their children (Naigles and Hoff-Ginsberg 1998).

Connecting words with their referents is only the start of building a lexicon, though. The lexicon is organized along a number of parameters, including word form (phonological representations, how a word is pronounced), word structure (morphology, syntax), and word meaning (semantic representations); words are also organized by personal experience.

For example, words are stratified according to their frequency of occurrence, with more frequent words (*dog*) being more easily/quickly retrieved compared to less frequent words (*emu*); this can vary by an individual's experience, so that, e.g. *collie, dachshund, labrador*, and *poodle* are retrieved more quickly by dog lovers than by people with no interest in dogs. Studies have also shown that the phonological structure (see Chapter 4) of the word may have an effect on how fast a word would be acquired and retrieved.

The lexicon is also organized according to word meanings and its semantic organization. One way of thinking about the semantic organization of the lexicon is that the word meanings comprise a web or network (as in Figure 2.1), with words that are more closely related semantically (e.g. *dog/cat* or *doctor/nurse*) connecting more closely and/or strongly to each other than words that are more distantly related. These semantic networks can comprise a wide array of components or dimensions, including imageability (i.e. concrete vs. abstract), function (e.g. kitchenware, vehicles), and perceptual attributes (e.g. shape, which is considered a global feature, as well as color, stripes, etc., which are

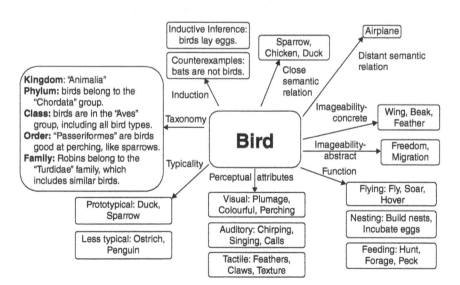

Figure 2.1 Semantic network organization example. *Source:* Letitia Naigles and Nufar Sukenik.

considered local features). Moreover, many word concepts are organized by taxonomy, with superordinate terms (*animal, plant*) connected in a hierarchical relationship to basic-level terms (*dog, tree*), which are further connected in a hierarchical relationship to subordinate terms (*collie, elm*). Such taxonomic category organization reveals a number of additional semantic relationships among words, including typicality, in that some concepts are more typical members of a category than others (e.g. in the US apples are more typical fruits than are kumquats), and induction, in that the properties of one member of a category usually extend to those of another member of that category, especially for natural kind categories, which contain a large number of correlated features (Gelman 2003; e.g. if one rabbit eats grass, then it is likely that other rabbits do so as well). Organizing the words we know systematically into networks allows us to retrieve the right words efficiently (Caramazza 1997) and has been observed in toddlers as young as 2 years of age. For example, toddlers (via their eye gaze, see below) show differential recognition of word-object pairings depending on their frequency and imageability (more frequently used words or words that more easily correspond to a mental/visual representation are recognized faster), whether previously heard words are semantic correlates, and whether the words appear in similar syntactic positions (see Wojcik 2018 for a review).

As we have already seen, researchers use a wide variety of tasks to understand how children learn words and how they organize their mental lexicon. Table 2.2 displays some of the most common tasks that researchers use, organized by their primary area of lexical semantics assessment. We will return to many of these in the rest of this chapter.

Table 2.2 Tasks commonly used to assess lexical semantics.

Area assessed	Task type	Presentation mode (to the child or caregiver)	Child ability assessed
Assessing vocabulary development and composition	Naming	The child is presented with a picture/object and is asked to name it.	Finding the right referent in the mental lexicon and producing the correct word.
	Spontaneous speech samples	The child is engaged in a structured or semi-structured activity with a researcher/parent/another child. The interaction is recorded and later analyzed.	Lexical diversity in terms of a number of different nouns, verbs, adjectives, etc., as well as caregiver speech measures.

Area assessed	Task type	Presentation mode (to the child or caregiver)	Child ability assessed
	Word checklists	The caregiver is presented with lists of words and asked to designate which one(s) their child produces and/or understands.	Vocabulary size and lexical diversity.
	Word–picture matching	The child hears a word and is asked to point to the best corresponding picture out of several choices (usually between 2 and 4 pictures).	Finding the right referent in the mental lexicon.
Assessing word learning strategies	Intermodal Preferential Looking (IPL) or looking-while-listening, with eye-tracking	The child watches one or two videos in which two unfamiliar objects or actions are presented individually, and then side by side, and hears an unfamiliar word. Children's faces are filmed and their eye movements are coded off-line to ascertain which object/action they look at longer. Videos can vary according to the perceptual characteristics of the objects/actions, how the unfamiliar words are presented in sentences, and whether a person is also in the video, looking at one of the two alternatives.	Implicit, time-sensitive strategies about how words are matched with their referents. Both initial gaze speed and duration of looking could be informative about the child's efficiency and certainty of understanding. Unfamiliar objects, events, and words are used so that children will not use prior knowledge in matching words to referents.
	Object or picture selection	The child is presented with an unfamiliar word and asked to point to the best corresponding picture or object out of several choices.	Implicit strategies about how words are matched with their referents.
Assessing lexical organization	Categorical induction	The child is presented with a target object and property and asked whether additional objects also share that property.	Ability to extend properties to objects of similar kinds vs. similar perceptual features.

(Continued)

Table 2.2 (Continued)

Area assessed	Task type	Presentation mode (to the child or caregiver)	Child ability assessed
	Categorization	The child is presented with two categories and asked to sort pictures or objects into those categories, with timing also recorded. Items can vary according to features such as typicality, taxonomy, number, and global vs. local.	Sophistication and efficiency (timing) of sorting preferences.
	Recall	Participants are asked to listen to a list of words and then recall as many words as possible.	Presence of semantic networks. The ability to recall lists of words with shared semantic properties is assumed to be easier than recalling lists of words that are unrelated.
	Verbal fluency	The child is asked to "name all the animals/fruits/vehicles/etc. you can think of" in 60 seconds.	Structure and connections between lexical items in the semantic lexicon as well as the effects of typicality. Responses are coded especially for semantic clustering – the number of subcategories (e.g. different types of animals), the number of words in each subcategory – and for switching – the number of switches between subcategories. Higher numbers for semantic clustering and switching indicate more elaborated and connected lexical-semantic organization.
	Word definition	The child is presented with a picture/object/written word/spoken word and asked to define it.	Selecting the right referent as well as its categorical affiliation, its relations to other words, and its function.

Lexicon in Autism

How Does Basic Vocabulary Development Proceed? What Child-Internal and Child-External Factors Affect Vocabulary Growth and Composition?

Parent reports of toddlers' vocabularies have generally found that toddlers with ASD produce fewer words than their typically developing (TD) age-mates (Charman et al. 2003; but see also Rescorla and Safyer 2013), thus manifesting delayed language onset (Naigles and Tek 2017). Early vocabulary composition, though, seems similar in neurotypical toddlers and those on the autism spectrum, with a preponderance of nouns/object labels in both groups (Rescorla and Safyer 2013). Moreover, overall vocabulary growth after toddler age appears to progress at typical rates in verbal children with ASD, as autistic children without cognitive disabilities score at age-appropriate levels (Naigles and Tek 2017); therefore, receptive vocabulary (word–picture matching tasks, see Table 2.2) is often used in studies as a means of matching between children with ASD and other control groups (commonly children with TD). Children with low scores on receptive vocabulary tasks are often classified as having language impairment; however, the field has not yet resolved whether or how often (i) low vocabulary scores appear in ASD without an accompanying cognitive deficit, and/or (ii) low vocabulary scores appear in ASD without an accompanying grammatical deficit – or the converse, high vocabulary scores in ASD with an accompanying cognitive and/or grammatical deficit (see, for example, Naigles and Tek 2017 and Chapter 10).

Interestingly, vocabulary composition increasingly diverges across childhood from what is observed in nonautistic children, with older children using social words, words for emotions (Jiménez et al. 2021), and mental verbs less frequently and consistently in contexts such as narratives than TD children do (Naigles and Chin 2015). These terms all involve social relationships and are acquired via social interactions, so their paucity is likely traceable to hallmark autistic characteristics.

Further evidence of child-internal contributions to ASD vocabulary development comes from findings that engaging in joint attention, when child and adult are both focused on the same object (see Table 2.1), is often a challenge for children on the autism spectrum (Mundy 2016), and variability in this engagement has been found to be correlated with concurrent and subsequent performance on standardized tests of language and on parent-reported vocabulary (Charman et al. 2003; Mundy 2016); that is, children who have stronger or more consistent joint attention skills also show better language performance on standardized tests and are reported to have larger vocabularies. Moreover, child-external factors, such as caregiver input, also contribute to ASD vocabulary development. As was observed with TD children, parents of children on the autism spectrum who produce more words, and produce longer sentences, have children who subsequently produce a larger and more diverse set of words (Nadig and Bang 2017). However, see Chapter 13 on unusual vocabulary development in a foreign language (variety) based on noninteractive input, which is observed in some autistic children.

Finally, basic vocabulary assessments indicate that verbal children on the autism spectrum, like their TD peers, usually understand more words than they can currently say (Charman et al. 2003; Kwok et al. 2015). Some researchers have claimed that this production/comprehension asymmetry is less pronounced in autistic children than in those who are typically developing; however, their data come primarily from standardized test assessments whose receptive component requires joint attention, which is challenging for children with ASD, as we have seen. Thus, a minimized production/comprehension asymmetry finding is likely due to challenges with testing mode, not core receptive vocabulary challenges (see also Naigles and Chin 2015).

Which Typical Word Learning Strategies Are Frequently vs. Less Frequently Observed in Autistic Children?

Across childhood, children on the autism spectrum have demonstrated generally strong use of word learning strategies. Consistent with the naming patterns described above, preschoolers with ASD who are shown unfamiliar objects engaged in unfamiliar actions, paired with a single novel word, preferentially map that word onto the object over the action, thereby displaying the **noun bias** (Naigles and Tek 2017). **Mutual exclusivity** has been tested across childhood, using IPL methods for toddlers and pointing methods for school-age children and adolescents (de Marchena et al. 2011). Across ages and methods (see Table 2.2), children are presented with an array of two to four objects, some of which are familiar and whose labels the children know (e.g. *truck, dog*), and one of which is unfamiliar and unnamed. Within the experiment, children hear directives containing a novel word such as "look at the dax" or "show me fental," and across studies, they systematically pick up or look longer at the unfamiliar object after controlling for baseline novelty preferences. Compared with a mental or language-age-matched TD group, though, ASD groups sometimes perform less consistently; moreover, those who perform more strongly on the mutual exclusivity task have higher receptive language scores on standardized tests (de Marchena et al. 2011).

Interestingly, experimental studies have revealed that children on the autism spectrum can use eye gaze to focus on specific referents during a labeling task (see Tables 2.1 and 2.2). Again, across ages (preschool, school age) and methods (IPL, pointing), children on the autism spectrum have succeeded in mapping labels onto objects that adults are looking at, even if these objects are less salient or interesting to the children themselves (Bang and Nadig 2020). This pattern of success raises the question, of course, as to the discrepancy with the standardized test findings mentioned in the previous section: if children on the autism spectrum have the capability of using **joint attention** to map unfamiliar words onto unfamiliar objects at levels consistent with their TD mental-age-matched peers, why does their performance on standardized tests and parental checklists suggest that their joint attention abilities are limited? There are a number of possible answers to this question, but perhaps the most straightforward is that just because children with ASD are capable of using joint attention in structured tasks in which 4–8 unfamiliar labels are being presented does not necessarily mean that they consistently do use joint attention in myriad word-learning situations in their daily lives.

An additional strategy observed in verb learning in TD children is **syntactic bootstrapping**, which has also been found to be exploited by children with ASD. The idea is that the sentence frame in which a verb is placed, its syntactic context, varies by the meaning of the verb and so provides clues to that meaning (Gleitman 1990). For example, verbs that appear in transitive frames (i.e. with a direct object, *The girl dropped the ball*, where "the ball" is the direct object) are more likely to refer to causative actions or events (events in which the subject either causes someone or something else to do or be something or causes a change in state – in *The girl dropped the ball*, the girl, the subject, causes the ball to drop), and verbs that appear in intransitive frames (an event which has no object, such as *The ball dropped*) are more likely to refer to noncausative actions or events (in which the participant that caused the event is not mentioned) (Gleitman 1990). Syntactic bootstrapping has been demonstrated in a wide range of studies of TD toddlers and preschoolers (Cao and Lewis 2022), primarily using IPL methods, and these findings have been generally replicated with children with ASD, using both pointing and IPL methods (Naigles and Tek 2017; Horvath et al. 2018).

Thus far, the literature has revealed considerable success on the part of children on the autism spectrum, in using a number of strategies attested in TD children, for learning new words. One strategy, however, has proven to be more challenging: the **shape bias**. Recall that the shape bias involves children extending the labels of objects to new objects based on their shape similarity with the original object (Smith 2000). Thus, this can be considered to reflect an assumption that objects are categorized according to their shapes; moreover, given that object shape is highly indicative of object kind, the shape bias may also reflect the assumption that objects are categorized according to their kinds (Gelman 2003). Potrzeba, Fein, and Naigles (2015) investigated whether children with ASD (average age at the beginning of the study: two and a half) used the shape bias similarly to TD children who were matched on language and cognitive abilities, albeit who were a year younger chronologically. The method was again eye-tracking; these were the same children who participated in the syntactic bootstrapping and noun bias studies reviewed in Naigles and Tek 2017. The children viewed six unfamiliar objects and were asked to match them with new same-shape or same-color objects. Their looking patterns were compared when the target object was unlabeled ("Look at this") vs. labeled ("Look at the dax"). Potrzeba, Fein, and Naigles (2015) found that the children in the TD group demonstrated a shape bias at each of the four visits (spaced four months apart), in which it was tested and increased in their relative looking toward the same-shape object at each subsequent visit. Across all four visits, almost 80% of TD children showed a shape bias consistently (>75% of the visits). In contrast, the children in the ASD group as a whole did not demonstrate a shape bias at any of the six visits in which they viewed the shape bias video, and less than 40% of children with ASD demonstrated a consistent shape bias across visits.

Smith (2000) and her colleagues proposed that the shape bias emerges when (TD) children have acquired 50–100 count nouns. However, analyses of children with ASD demonstrated that this relationship is more complex. Whereas Potrzeba, Fein, and Naigles (2015) found that children with ASD with higher vocabularies overall showed a stronger concurrent and subsequent shape bias, follow-up analyses by Abdelaziz et al. (2018) found that many children with ASD who produced large numbers of nouns that differentiated objects by shape nonetheless did not show a shape bias in the IPL task. In fact, Abdelaziz et al. (2018) reported that the children's duration of joint attention interactions during play sessions with their caregivers, especially those that they themselves initiated, was the strongest predictor of whether or not they subsequently showed a shape bias. Thus, the documented joint attention impairments of children on the autism spectrum seem to diminish their ability to use a shape bias, which may in turn explain their challenges in overall vocabulary development (Bottema-Beutel 2016). These challenges with shape bias might also be reflected in semantic depth, categorization, and organization.

Category Formation and Use as a Window into Lexical Organization: How Are These Manifested in ASD?

Recall that organizing words and concepts into categories allows them to be accessed more quickly and efficiently (Caramazza 1997). See Table 2.2 for an overview of tasks that assess lexical organization. Several studies have found that the sorting accuracy scores of children with ASD are like those of their age-matched TD peers (Ellawadi, Fein, and Naigles 2017); moreover, children on the spectrum consistently distinguish typical members of categories from atypical members at age-appropriate levels (Ellawadi, Fein, and Naigles 2017). In contrast, children with ASD have consistently been found to have slower reaction times while engaged in categorization tasks (Gastgeb, Strauss, and Minshew 2006; Ellawadi, Fein, and Naigles 2017), pointing to a difference between their categorization abilities (their ability to sort pictures or objects into categories) and categorization processing (the processes used to recognize semantic categories).

Additional differences in the categorization performance of children with ASD when compared to neurotypical age-matched children have been observed. For example, some children with ASD are less accurate when sorting stimuli with abstract or complex features compared to perceptual ones (e.g. showing intact sorting of colors or shapes but impaired sorting of trees or beds; Gastgeb, Strauss, and Minshew 2006). Ellawadi, Fein, and Naigles (2017) also reported slowed categorization of somewhat atypical instances in specific contexts by their autistic sample. These findings have not always been replicated, which may be adduced to the hallmark heterogeneity of the ASD population when sample sizes are small and population sampling varies enormously from study to study; however, even in large samples, language characteristics of individuals on the autism spectrum may vary widely (Kjelgaard and Tager-Flusberg 2001).

Developmentally, young neurotypical children usually categorize items based on their shape or function (global features), whereas older children notice subtler differences between items and more specific semantic details (local features). Children with ASD have been observed to show differences in their local and global processing when asked for word definitions; for example, some children with ASD seem to have a very extreme local view, meaning they report small details (e.g. mentioning antennae) but do not put these details together to infer the general shape of the stimulus (e.g. insects). On the other hand, some children with ASD are found to have an extreme global view, meaning they may mention overall shapes (e.g. mentioning pets) but miss out on the details (e.g. not mentioning dogs or tails; Gladfelter and Barron 2020). In both cases, differences in local or global categorization processing may influence which semantic features the child notices and so may have an impact on their word learning abilities as well as the categorization abilities of the child (Ellawadi, Fein, and Naigles 2017; Gladfelter and Barron 2020). Categorical induction tasks (see Table 2.2) have corroborated these challenges, with children with ASD, from school age through adolescence, making category-based inductions less consistent than age- or language-matched neurotypical peers. For example, if they are told that a brown rabbit eats grass, they are unlikely to extend grass-eating to a white rabbit (Tecoulesco, Fein, and Naigles 2021).

Finally, verbal fluency tasks (see Table 2.2) have been very illuminating concerning category structure and use in children with ASD. Studies that tested adults with ASD compared to neurotypicals found no differences in the overall number of words produced, the number of semantic clusters (words that are semantically related to each other), or the number of switches (how often the participant switches between semantic subcategories of words) (see Table 2.2; Foldager et al. 2022). In contrast, results from children with ASD show more challenges. Some studies have found that children with ASD produced overall the same number of words as did TD children, but the groups differed in that the children with ASD produced larger semantic clusters (groups of words or concepts that are closely related to each other within the same category, such as "apple, banana, orange, pear, grape") and made fewer switches (when a person transitions from generating words within one cluster to a new cluster, as in "apple, banana, orange, pear, grape ... strawberry, watermelon, pineapple, kiwi, mango") (Foldager et al. 2022). Other studies found that children with ASD produced fewer words, smaller clusters, and fewer switches (Ehlen et al. 2020). Taken together, these findings suggest that the lexicons of children with ASD may include fewer categories overall, and categories that are smaller (i.e. that include fewer words) and that have fewer subcategories.

Focus on a Specific Study

One of the most common verbal fluency categories that is considered sensitive to differences between children with ASD and neurotypical children is the animal category. Previous studies of children with ASD have reported unusual and atypical productions in this category (e.g. more productions of "emu" and fewer of "dog"; see Dunn, Gomes, and Sebastian 1996). This section focuses on a study by Foldager and colleagues (2022). We chose this study because it highlighted the importance of studying multiple categories and of relating fluency performance to nonlinguistic characteristics. The study reported on the performance of 60 Danish-speaking 7- to 15-year-olds with ASD on semantic fluency with both animals and fruit and on semantic recall of animals, fruits, and unrelated words and examined whether these were related to the children's adaptive behaviors or severity of autism symptoms. The results of the children with ASD were then compared to the performance of 60 TD children matched on IQ scores and age.

On the animal fluency task, the ASD group showed lower levels of fluency, meaning that they produced fewer animal words than the TD group. Unexpectedly, no differences between the groups were found in the typicality of the words produced in the animal category. Within the ASD group, children who produced fewer animal words had higher levels of social communication challenges, more unusual behaviors, and lower adaptive functioning. Different findings emerged in the fruit category of the fluency task, where the participants with ASD produced just as many fruit words as the TD children; however, in this category, children with ASD did produce significantly more atypical words than TD children (e.g. *kumquat, mango,* and *kiwi*). Production of atypical fruits in the ASD group was associated with more unusual behaviors (atypical language, rigidity, stereotypy, and sensory sensitivity).

In the recall task, the children with ASD and children with TD did not differ on the animal words or the unrelated words, but differences were found in recalling fruits. No significant differences between groups were found for the first recall; a trend was found for the second recall, where children with ASD recalled slightly fewer words than TD children, and significantly lower recall rates for the ASD group were found for the third and fourth recalls. Thus, these children with ASD showed a slower learning curve for fruit words.

Foldager et al.'s finding that these children with ASD produced more atypical fruit category members during the fluency task might indicate that their fruit category is not organized with typical items being the most easily retrieved, which might further suggest that their fruit category, at least, is not organized by typicality (Caramazza 1997). At first glance, this seems to be at odds with the results from sorting-type categorization tasks (e.g. Ellawadi, Fein, and Naigles 2017), which have observed graded categorization by typicality in ASD groups. Possibly, the fluency results are further indicators of a distinction in this population between category processing, which appears to be challenged, and category structure, which may be unimpaired. Additionally, Foldager et al.'s findings that the fruit category, but not the animal category, yielded the most atypical instances might have multiple interpretations. For example, it's possible that animal categories are less suitable for demonstrating group differences; however, we think this is unlikely because the animal category has been widely found to differentiate typical and atypical category usage in speakers of languages such as English, French, and Hebrew (see, for example, Riva, Nichelli, and Devoti 2000). Another possibility is that these findings illustrate the cultural context of the lexicon: Foldager and colleagues conducted a study involving Danish speakers, who potentially possess a greater familiarity with animals compared to their knowledge of fruit. This distinction is supported by Wehberg and colleagues (2007), who discovered variations in the early vocabularies of Danish-speaking children, as assessed by the MacArthur-Bates-Communicative Development Inventory questionnaire, in terms of word composition and frequency when compared to age-matched English- and Italian-speaking children. Wehberg et al. attributed these differences to cultural distinctions among the respective countries. Finally, this study signals that the relationships between autistic characteristics and lexical organization are not yet fully understood.

Conclusion

This chapter aimed to address the following questions:
- How does basic vocabulary development proceed, and what child-internal factors (other abilities the child may have) and child-external factors (properties of the child's environment/input) affect vocabulary growth and composition?
- Which typical word learning strategies are frequently observed, and which are less frequently observed in autistic children?
- How well are category formation and use manifested in the lexicons of autistic individuals?

Superficially, many verbal children with ASD may look like they have similar lexicons (mainly regarding the number of words they know) compared to TD peers, but deeper scrutiny reveals differences in lexical acquisition, processing, and structure between ASD and TD. The studies presented here highlight the importance of testing more than just one aspect of lexical functioning. Children with ASD may employ many of the same word-learning strategies but possibly use them less effectively and consistently (Abdelaziz et al. 2018). They may begin to build semantic categories within their lexicons but elaborate or access them less consistently and/or efficiently (Ellawadi, Fein, and Naigles 2017; Foldager et al. 2022). The pervasive heterogeneity across ASD with regard to the different lexical abilities but also with regard to the differences seen in cognitive abilities means that some individuals on the spectrum may indeed manifest lexical semantic knowledge that is indistinguishable from neurotypical peers, whereas many others manifest semantic knowledge and processing that consistently differ from neurotypicals (Naigles and Tek 2017; Sukenik and Tuller 2021). In sum, it is important to consider the totality of task performances to reveal the status of the mental lexicon in ASD.

> **What Do You Know Now?**
> Verbal children with ASD may appear to share similar lexicons with typically developing peers and to use many of the same word-learning strategies, but closer scrutiny reveals diverse lexical acquisition, processing, and structure.
> - TD children's strong category skills allow them to connect different words that are included in a semantic category (e.g. names of different dog breeds grouped under the category "dog"). An autistic child, on the other hand, may have weaker categorical induction abilities and therefore more reluctance to accept that the properties of one word (a particular breed of dog, for example) may transfer to the properties of the inclusive semantic category ("dog").
> - Autistic children and TD children may categorize concepts differently. Returning to the "What Do You Think?" box at the beginning of this chapter, the neurotypical child identified the shared characteristics (global features) of the animals she saw at the zoo (they were big and lived in the safari) and, since her categorization was effective, she was also more efficient in retrieving their names. The child with ASD on the other hand seemed to categorize the animals she saw according to local features (a spot on the animal's ear) or a feature that was not directly related to the animal itself (it was next to the restaurant).

Suggestions for Further Reading

If you want to know more about the shape bias in children with ASD, we recommend reading Abdelaziz et al. 2018. If you are interested in learning more about how children with ASD form categories, see Tecoulesco, Fein, and Naigles 2021. If you would like to learn more about the lexical semantic abilities of children with ASD, we recommend the following review study: Sukenik and Tuller 2021. If you would like to know more about the methods used to study the lexicon in young children, these are good places to start: Pan 2011 and Piotroski and Naigles 2011.

References

Abdelaziz, A., Kover, S.T., Wagner, M. et al. (2018). The shape bias in children with Autism Spectrum Disorder: potential sources of individual differences. *Journal of Speech, Language, and Hearing Research* 61 (11): 2685–2702.

Bang, J.Y. and Nadig, A. (2020). An investigation of word learning in the presence of gaze: evidence from school-age children with typical development or Autism Spectrum Disorder. *Cognitive Development* 54: 100847.

Bottema-Beutel, K. (2016). Associations between joint attention and language in Autism Spectrum Disorder and typical development: a systematic review and meta-regression analysis. *Autism Research* 9 (10): 1021–1035.

Cao, A. and Lewis, M. (2022). Quantifying the syntactic bootstrapping effect in verb learning: a meta-analytic synthesis. *Developmental Science* 25 (2): e13176.

Caramazza, A. (1997). How many levels of processing are there in lexical access? *Cognitive Neuropsychology* 14 (1): 177–208.

Charman, T., Drew, A., Baird, C. et al. (2003). Measuring early language development in preschool children with Autism Spectrum Disorder using the MacArthur Communicative Development Inventory (Infant Form). *Journal of Child Language* 30 (1): 213–236.

de Marchena, A., Eigsti, I.M., Worek, A. et al. (2011). Mutual exclusivity in Autism Spectrum Disorders: testing the pragmatic hypothesis. *Cognition* 119 (1): 96–113.

Dunn, M., Gomes, H., and Sebastian, M.J. (1996). Prototypicality of responses of autistic, language disordered, and normal children in a word fluency task. *Child Neuropsychology* 2: 99–108.

Ehlen, F., Roepke, S., Klostermann, F. et al. (2020). Small semantic networks in individuals with Autism Spectrum Disorder without intellectual impairment: a verbal fluency approach. *Journal of Autism and Developmental Disorders* 50: 3967–3987.

Ellawadi, A., Fein, D., and Naigles, L. (2017). Category structure and processing in 6-year-olds with ASD. *Autism Research* 10: 327–336.

Foldager, M., Vestergaard, M., Lassen, J. et al. (2022). Atypical semantic fluency and recall in children and adolescents with Autism Spectrum Disorders associated with autism symptoms and adaptive functioning. *Journal of Autism and Developmental Disorders* 53 (11): 1–13.

Gastgeb, H.Z., Strauss, M.S., and Minshew, N.J. (2006). Do individuals with autism process categories differently? The effect of typicality and development. *Child Development* 77 (6): 1717–1729.

Gelman, S.A. (2003). *The Essential Child: Origins of Essentialism in Everyday Thought*. New York: Oxford University Press.

Gladfelter, A. and Barron, K.L. (2020). How children with Autism Spectrum Disorder, Developmental Language Disorder, and typical language learn to produce global and local semantic features. *Brain Sciences* 10 (4): 231.

Gleitman, L. (1990). The structural sources of verb meanings. *Language Acquisition* 1 (1): 3–55.

Hoff, E. and Naigles, L. (2002). How children use input to acquire a lexicon. *Child Development* 73 (2): 418–433.

Horvath, S., McDermott, E., Reilly, K. et al. (2018). Acquisition of verb meaning from syntactic distribution in preschoolers with Autism Spectrum Disorder. *Language, Speech, and Hearing Services in School* 49 (3S): 668–680.

Jiménez, E., Haebig, E., and Hills, T.T. (2021). Identifying areas of overlap and distinction in early lexical profiles of children with Autism Spectrum Disorder, late talkers, and typical talkers. *Journal of Autism and Developmental Disorders* 51: 3109–3125.

Kjelgaard, M.M. and Tager-Flusberg, H. (2001). An investigation of language impairment in autism: implications for genetic subgroups. *Language and Cognitive Processes* 16: 287–308.

Kwok, E.Y., Brown, H.M., Smyth, R.E. et al. (2015). Meta-analysis of receptive and expressive language skills in Autism Spectrum Disorder. *Research in Autism Spectrum Disorders* 9: 202–222.

Mundy, P.C. (2016). *Autism and Joint Attention: Development, Neuroscience, and Clinical Fundamentals*. London: Routledge.

Nadig, A. and Bang, J. (2017). Parental input to children with ASD and its influence on later language. In: *Innovative Investigations of Language in Autism* (ed. L. Naigles), 89–114. Washington, DC: APA.

Naigles, L.R. and Chin, I. (2015). Language development in children with autism. In: *Cambridge Handbook of Child Language*, 2e (eds. E. Bavin and L. Naigles), 637–658. Cambridge, UK: Cambridge University Press.

Naigles, L.R. and Hoff-Ginsberg, E. (1998). Why are some verbs learned before other verbs? Effects of input frequency and structure on children's early verb use. *Journal of Child Language* 25 (1): 95–120.

Naigles, L.R. and Tek, S. (2017). 'Form is easy, meaning is hard' revisited: (re) characterizing the strengths and weaknesses of language in children with Autism Spectrum Disorder. *Wiley Interdisciplinary Reviews: Cognitive Science* 8 (4): e1438.

Pan, B.A. (2011). Assessing vocabulary skills. In: *Research Methods in Child Language: A Practical Guide* (ed. E. Hoff), 100–111. New York: Wiley-Blackwell.

Piotroski, J. and Naigles, L.R. (2011). Intermodal preferential looking. In: *Research Methods in Child Language: A Practical Guide* (ed. E. Hoff), 17–28. New York: Wiley-Blackwell.

Potrzeba, E.R., Fein, D., and Naigles, L. (2015). Investigating the shape bias in typically developing children and children with Autism Spectrum Disorders. *Frontiers in Psychology* 6: 446.

Rescorla, L. and Safyer, P. (2013). Lexical composition in children with Autism Spectrum Disorder (ASD). *Journal of Child Language* 40 (1): 47–68.

Riva, D., Nichelli, F., and Devoti, M. (2000). Developmental aspects of verbal fluency and confrontation naming in children. *Brain and Language* 71 (2): 267–284.

Smith, L.B. (2000). Learning how to learn words: an associative crane. In: *Becoming a Word Learner: A Debate on Lexical Acquisition* (eds. R.M. Golinkoff, K. Hirsh-Pasek, N. Akhtar et al.), New York: Oxford Press.

Suanda, S.H., Barnhart, M., Smith, L.B. et al. (2019). The signal in the noise: the visual ecology of parents' object naming. *Infancy* 24 (3): 455–476.

Sukenik, N. and Tuller, L. (2021). Lexical semantic knowledge of children with ASD—a review study. *Review Journal of Autism and Developmental Disorders* 10 (1): 130–143.

Tecoulesco, L., Fein, D., and Naigles, L.R. (2021). What categorical induction variability reveals about typical and atypical development. *Journal of Child Language* 48 (3): 515–540.

Tomasello, M. (2015). The usage-based theory of language acquisition. In: *The Cambridge Handbook of Child Language*, 2e (eds. E.L. Bavin and L.R. Naigles), 89–106. Cambridge, UK: Cambridge University Press.

Wehberg, S., Vach, W., Bleses, D. et al. (2007). Danish children's first words: analysing longitudinal data based on monthly CDI parental reports. *First Language* 27 (4): 361–383.

Wojcik, E.H. (2018). The development of lexical–semantic networks in infants and toddlers. *Child Development Perspectives* 12 (1): 34–38.

3

Morphosyntax

Stephanie Durrleman and Theodoros Marinis

> **What Do You Think?**
> Here is a quote from the 15-year-old main character in the book *The Curious Incident of the Dog in the Night-Time*, who is autistic: "I find people confusing. [...] people often talk using metaphors. These are examples of metaphors: I laughed my socks off. He was the apple of her eye. [...] it is when you describe something by using a word for something that it isn't." Autistic people often have difficulties interpreting figurative language. How about literal language; do you think that they may have difficulties with the grammatical structure of sentences?
>
> Here is a quote from another autistic teenager, describing a picture in which an elephant is pushing a bear: "Bear and elephant playing. Elephant push bear. I don't like elephant, elephant push bear. I like bear that pushed elephant." The last sentence means that the elephant is pushing the bear. What do you think is going on here?

Introduction

The system of sentence structure is called **morphosyntax**, which is part of the structural language domain, as is phonology (see Chapter 4). For example, the verb *push* in *The bear pushes the elephant* consists of a stem (*push*) and an ending, or inflection (*-es*). This ending is determined by the subject *The bear*, which is third-person singular. The order of words in a sentence also matters; some orders are more complex than others, even if they have the same words.

(1) Show me the bear that pushed the elephant.

(2) Show me the bear that the elephant pushed.

What is your intuition? Which sentence is more complex, (1) or (2)?

Language in Autism, First Edition. Edited by Jeannette Schaeffer et al.
© 2025 John Wiley & Sons Ltd. Published 2025 by John Wiley & Sons Ltd.

Autistic individuals who speak were initially hypothesized not to struggle with morphosyntax. However, this may not be entirely correct, especially when it concerns more complex morphosyntax. Complex morphosyntax is attested in various linguistic constructions, including **passives**, **relative clauses** (as in (1) and (2)), ***Wh*-questions**, **complement clauses**, and **clitic constructions**. We will explain below in the Anchoring section what these terms mean.

This chapter discusses how challenging morphosyntax can be for autistic individuals. We focus on studies of morphosyntax in autistic CHILDREN; see Chapter 12 for discussion of morphosyntax in autistic ADULTS. The specific questions we aim to address are:

- Does morphosyntax present challenges for all autistic children?
- How challenging are passives in autism?
- How challenging are relative clauses and *Wh*-questions in autism?
- How challenging are complement clauses in autism?
- How challenging are clitic constructions in autism?

Anchoring

Before delving into the questions formulated above, we first provide some necessary (theoretical) background. Grammatical competence includes knowledge of the system of rules governing different linguistic levels, including sounds (**phonology** – see Chapter 4), words (**morphology**), sentences (**syntax**), and sentence meaning (**semantics** – see Chapter 5). This chapter is concerned with the rules that combine (parts of) words into sentences, a combination of morphology and syntax, called **morphosyntax**. Morphosyntactic competence is implicit/subconscious in most native speakers (except when you're a linguist!) and enables us to determine that (3) is grammatical while (4) is ungrammatical (indicated by the asterisk) because the inflectional ending *-ed* marking past tense is present in (3) and missing in (4).

(3) Show me the bear that pushed the elephant yesterday.

(4) *Show me the bear that push the elephant yesterday.

An example of a complex morphosyntactic structure is the **passive**. Passive sentences are assumed to be derived from active sentences by movement of the original object to sentence-initial position. Often, a by-phrase containing the original subject is also added. This is illustrated in (5) and (6):

(5) The bear pushes the elephant   - active sentence

(6) The elephant is pushed ___ by the bear   - passive sentence

In the active sentence (5), the so-called **agent** of the action (*the bear*) comes first, followed by the so-called **patient** (*the elephant*). This is the most typical or **canonical** order in English. However, this order is switched in the passive sentence (6): the patient (*the elephant*) precedes the agent (*the bear*). As such, a passive has **noncanonical** word order. Noncanonical word order makes sentence structure more complex.

Morphosyntax and (non)canonical word order also allow us to explain why sentence (2) in the Introduction section is more complex than sentence (1). Both (1) and (2) consist of a **main clause** (*Show me the bear*) and an **embedded clause**, which is a **relative clause**, in this case, starting with the **relative pronoun** *that*. In general, sentences with both a main clause and an embedded clause are more complex than sentences consisting of just a main clause. This is because there is a hierarchical relationship between the two clauses that needs to be linguistically computed: the embedded clause depends on the main clause. In other words, the main clause determines the type of embedded clause. Furthermore, there is another factor that contributes to complexity, namely, nonlinguistic cognition. Because sentences with embedded clauses (in this case, complement clauses) are longer, it has been argued that their mastery relates to **Working Memory**, the retention of small amounts of (linguistic) information to be manipulated. If the embedded clause is a relative clause, as in (1) and (2), morphosyntactic complexity can increase even further. The relative pronoun *that* refers to a noun in the main clause, namely, *the bear*. Let us now consider the two different word orders in (1) and (2). The neutral or

> **Acronym and Terminology Reminder**
>
> **ACC1:** 1st person accusative clitic. Dependent direct object pronoun (e.g. *Max me voit* 'Max sees me').
>
> **ACC3:** 3rd person accusative clitic. Dependent direct object pronoun (e.g. *Max le voit* 'Max sees him').
>
> **ALI:** Autism with language impairment.
>
> **ALN:** Autism with normal language.
>
> **Canonical Word Order:** Neutral, default word order.
>
> **Clitic:** Special type of dependent word (always attached to another word) occurring in some languages, e.g. pronouns in languages such as French and Greek.
>
> **Complement Clause:** Embedded clause following a mental state or communication verb (e.g. *Kim believes/says that the marble is in the box*).
>
> **Full Noun (Phrase):** A noun phrase, such as, e.g. *the fork, the girl*.
>
> **Gender:** A morphosyntactic (grammatical) feature, e.g. feminine (*la chaise* 'the-feminine chair') or masculine (*le bureau* 'the-masculine desk').
>
> **Morphosyntax:** Word and sentence structure, i.e. the way words and phrases combine.
>
> **Number:** A morphosyntactic (grammatical) feature, e.g. singular (*plate*) or plural (*plates*).
>
> **Person:** A morphosyntactic (grammatical) feature, e.g. 1st person (*I*), 2nd person (*you*) or 3rd person (*them*).
>
> **Pronoun:** Small words such as *I, me, you, she, they*.
>
> **Relative Clause:** Embedded clause modifying a noun, e.g. *the bear that is white*.
>
> **SVO:** Subject-Verb-Object.
>
> **TD:** Typically developing.
>
> **ToM:** Theory of Mind. Ability to infer and understand mental states (e.g. beliefs, true, and false) in oneself and others.
>
> **Working Memory:** Ability to hold information for a short time while performing a cognitive task.

canonical word order in English is S(ubject)–V(erb)–O(bject) (SVO), and this is what we see in (1): *pushed* (verb) *the elephant* (object). The relative pronoun *that* refers to the SUBJECT of the relative clause, and therefore, this relative clause in (1) is called a **subject relative clause**. In sum, subject relative clauses have canonical word order (Verb–Object (VO)). In contrast, the sentence in (2) includes an **object relative clause**: *that the elephant pushed*. This is because the relative pronoun *that* refers to the OBJECT of the relative clause. In object relative clauses, the canonical order of the verb and the object has changed: Object–Verb (OV), rather than Verb–Object (VO). In linguistic-theoretical terms, we say that in (2), the object *the bear* moves from the underlying, original object position (following the verb) to a position preceding the verb, creating noncanonical word order. This is illustrated in (7).

(7)   Show me the bear that the elephant pushed ___   - object relative clause

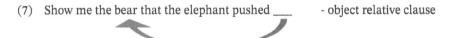

However, the interpretation of the elements in a sentence comes from their original positions. In (7), the phrase *the bear* is the object of the verb *pushed*, and as such, it is interpreted in the original position following the verb (*pushed*), which is designated for objects. This position is indicated by the underscore in (7).

Now, note that the object *the bear* in (7) moves over the subject *the elephant*. Such movement adds to the complexity of a morphosyntactic construction. In turn, the complexity of movement of an object over a subject can vary; some object-over-subject movements are more complex than others. This is captured in a theory called **Featural Intervention** (Rizzi 2018). This theory predicts higher complexity when the moved object shares morphosyntactic features with the subject. In (7), the subject and the object share several morphosyntactic features: they are both full nouns (+Noun), they are both third person (+3rd person), they are both singular (+singular), etc. The schema in (8) illustrates how the subject Z (*the elephant*) **intervenes** when the object Y (*the bear*) moves to a more fronted position (X).

(8)   Featural Intervention

X	Z	Y
+Noun, +3rd person, +singular	+Noun, +3rd person, +singular	
the bear that	**the elephant** pushed	___

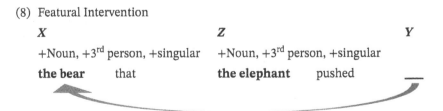

In other words, there is featural intervention by the subject (*the elephant*) in this construction, and the featural intervention is quite strong, because of the high overlap in morphosyntactic features between the subject and the object. The more featural intervention there is, the more complex the structure.

Featural intervention does not occur in subject relative clauses, as in (1) and (9). The subject *the bear* moves from its original position (represented by the underscore) to the main clause, as indicated by the arrow in (9). However, this movement does not affect the English canonical word order in the relative clause; the order remains VO: verb (*pushed*)–object (*the elephant*). Therefore, subject relative clauses are simpler than object relative clauses (in many languages).

(9) Show me the bear that ___ pushed the elephant   - subject relative clause

A morphosyntactic structure similar to relative clauses is the so-called **Wh-question**. Similar to relative clauses, *Wh*-questions can respect canonical word order, namely, in subject questions (10) or the object can move to a noncanonical, preverbal position in object questions (11).

(10) Which bear ___ pushed the elephant   - subject *Wh*-question

(11) Which elephant did the bear push ___   - object *Wh*-question

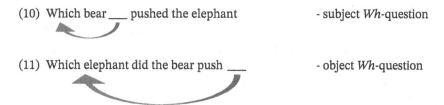

In French, object questions can involve movement of the object as in English (11), but they can also leave the object in its original (*wh*-in situ) position as in (12). This will become relevant in the next section.

(12) L'ours a poussé quel éléphant?
     the bear has pushed which elephant
     'Which elephant did the bear push?'

As already shown with relative clauses, morphosyntactic complexity arises when sentences contain embedded clauses. Other embedded clauses that increase morphosyntactic complexity are **complement clauses**. Complement clauses can be complements of a range of verb types, such as verbs of cognition or mental state verbs (13a) and verbs of communication (13b).

(13) a) Kim believes [that the marble is in the box]
     b) Kim says [that the marble is in the box]

As mentioned above, sentences with embedded clauses are more complex than simple main clauses because they interact with nonlinguistic cognition, such as Working Memory. If the embedded clause is a complement clause (as in (13)), there is another nonlinguistic factor that contributes to complexity, namely, **Theory of Mind** (ToM), the ability to infer and understand mental states (e.g. beliefs) in oneself and others. Indeed, complement clauses are perfect tools to reason about beliefs, which are subjective representations of reality and thus may be false.

A final example of morphosyntactic complexity can be observed in Romance languages whenever an object is a special type of pronoun called a **clitic**, such as the word *le* ('him') in the French example in (14). In these cases, the object moves to a preverbal position as an **object clitic** (14), resulting in noncanonical word order (French is also SVO). Object clitics contrast with objects realized as full nouns (15), which remain in the post-verbal (original) position.

(14) L'ours **le** pousse
the bear **him** pushes
'The bear pushes him.'

(15) L'ours pousse **l'éléphant**
the bear pushes **the elephant**
'The bear pushes the elephant.'

As mentioned above, it has been hypothesized that sentences with embedded clauses and/or syntactic movement yielding noncanonical word order increase complexity because such structures interact with the nonlinguistic domain of Working Memory. This may explain why linguistic structures with complex morphosyntax emerge later than simpler sentences in typically developing (TD) children and are affected in children with so-called **Developmental Language Disorder** (DLD; Jakubowicz 2011; Rizzi 2018; Friedmann and Reznick 2021; see also Chapter 11). The next section discusses how (complex) morphosyntax may also raise challenges in autism.

Morphosyntax in Autism

Does Morphosyntax Present Challenges for All Autistic Children?

Turning to children with ASD, their morphosyntactic abilities are in fact very heterogeneous, ranging from preserved to impaired, and can be potentially dissociated from general cognitive abilities (see Chapter 10) and even other areas of language, such as vocabulary (see Chapter 2). Besides spontaneous speech samples and specific experimental tasks to measure morphosyntactic ability, recent studies on morphosyntax in autism often use standardized omnibus language assessment tools to measure the participants' overall language skills and tasks measuring general cognitive abilities. This has led to the recognition of various (language) profiles within autism, as discussed below.

Kjelgaard and Tager-Flusberg's (2001) seminal study, following work by Rapin and colleagues (e.g. Allen and Rapin 1980; Rapin and Dunn 1997), investigated language subgroups in autistic individuals who speak.[1] Based on data from standardized language assessments, they differentiated between autistic individuals with a language impairment and autistic people who seem to have neurotypical language. Tager-Flusberg (2006) later coined these two phenotypes: **ALI** – Autism with language impairment and **ALN** – Autism with normal language (see Chapter 1). It is important to note that the term "language" here refers to STRUCTURAL LANGUAGE (morphosyntax, (sentence-level) semantics – see Chapter 5, phonology – see Chapter 4) and LEXICON (vocabulary – see Chapter 2), but not pragmatics (see Chapters 6–8) or prosody (see Chapter 9). In a subsequent study, Condouris, Meyer, and Tager-Flusberg (2003) reported a strong correlation between scores on standardized language assessments (CELF and PPVT; see Chapter 1) and measures derived from morphosyntactic analysis of spontaneous speech samples in autistic children age 4–14. This indicates that standardized language measures tap into the same linguistic skills as spontaneous measures do.

Prima facie, individuals with ALI show a language profile similar to what is found in DLD (see Chapter 11). For example, in some languages they often omit tense morphemes (such as *-ed* or *-s*) on the verb or auxiliary verbs (such as a form of *have* or *be*), resulting in so-called Root, or Optional Infinitives. Autistic children produce such infinitive verbs for a much more extended period of time than neurotypical children, who stop doing this around age 3–4 (Roberts, Rice, and Tager-Flusberg 2004). Examples known from child English are *Her go* or *Daddy playing*, and Dutch-acquiring children say, for instance, *Mama toren bouwen* ('Mommy tower build'). For a further discussion of Root/Optional Infinitives in ALI and DLD, see Chapter 11. However, recent research also has pointed to some differences between ALI and DLD (see later in this chapter and Chapter 11). As for the ALN group, it does not seem entirely true that they have neurotypical language in all respects. They have been reported to perform differently on morphosyntactic structures, such as the ones discussed in the Anchoring section, that interact with nonlinguistic cognitive functions (i.e. Working Memory or ToM) or that interface with language domains known to be affected in autism, such as pragmatics (see Chapter 8).

The rest of this section concentrates on the abilities of autistic children regarding the complex morphosyntactic phenomena described and explained in the Anchoring section. It will do so by discussing EXPERIMENTAL studies, which employ experiments that elicit the production or the comprehension of specific morphosyntactic phenomena. While analysis of spontaneous speech yields a

---

[1] Of course, there is also the subgroup of **minimally verbal** or **minimally speaking** autistic individuals. See Chapter 10 for more information on this group.

wealth of information on all domains of language, it also faces the disadvantage that it may not reveal abilities regarding complex morphosyntactic structures, simply because these are often avoided in spontaneous speech. This is particularly the case in children with autism, who may have difficulties sustaining a conversation or telling a story due to general communication impairment, rather than morphosyntactic impairment (Tuller et al. 2017).

How Challenging Are Passives in Autism?

Subsets of autistic children have been reported to struggle with passives, as in example (6) (*The elephant is pushed by the bear*). While two studies on children diagnosed with autism within the normal IQ range report similar performance between autistic children and typically developing (TD) controls (Terzi et al. 2014; Gavarró and Heshmati 2014), other studies show differences (Perovic, Modyanova, and Wexler 2013 and Durrleman et al. 2017).

Interestingly, the study by Durrleman et al. (2017) included 20 French-speaking children with ASD (average age 9;3) of a wide array of IQ levels and compared their performance to 20 TD children of the same age as well as to 65 younger TD children grouped by ages 4–5, 6–7, and 8–9. The study employed a sentence-picture matching task assessing as exemplified in Figure 3.1.

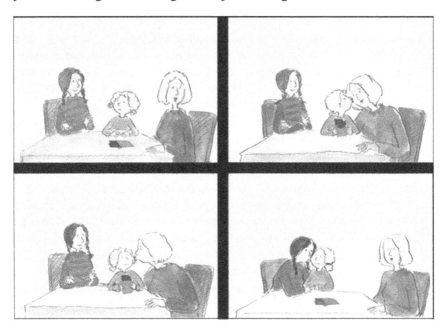

Figure 3.1 Example test item *The little girl is kissed by Mom* from the sentence-picture matching task testing passives. *Source:* Courtesy of Kristine Jensen de López.

Most autistic children struggled with passive constructions compared to their age-matched peers, although their performance followed a similar pattern, which resembled that of younger TD children. A subgroup of autistic children, seemingly proficient in vocabulary and morphosyntax based on omnibus language tests, still showed a subtle delay in passives. Another subgroup, exhibiting broader lexical and morphosyntactic difficulties, displayed a more pronounced delay in passives.

However, the difficulties with passives did not seem linked to nonverbal abilities or Working Memory. The findings suggest that children on the autism spectrum can experience a delay in understanding passive sentence structures rather than a fundamental deviation in the acquisition path of these structures. Even among those apparently proficient in general language skills according to omnibus language tests, subtle difficulties with passives may nevertheless be present and remain unidentified by omnibus language tests that do not place emphasis on structures of syntactic complexity. The fact that performance on passives was not associated with nonverbal abilities aligns with previous studies suggesting that the linguistic characteristics of some children with ASD resemble those with Developmental Language Disorder. This emphasizes the necessity for thorough evaluation of language abilities in autistic children, including those within the normal IQ range.

How Challenging Are Relative Clauses and *Wh*-questions in Autism?

Relative clauses as in (7) (*Show me the bear that the elephant pushed*) and *Wh*-questions as in (11) (*Which elephant did the bear push?*) involving complex movement of the object over the subject remain persistently challenging for groups of autistic children and adolescents.

One study that clearly illustrates this is the study by Durrleman, Marinis, and Franck (2015). To address effects of morphosyntactic complexity in neurotypical and autistic children, this study systematically investigated relative clauses and *Wh*-questions in three groups of French-speaking children: (i) 4-, 6-, and 8-year-old neurotypical children (total = 45, 15 per age), (ii) a group of 6–16-year-old autistic children (total = 20), and (iii) a group of neurotypical children matched on the autistic children in their nonverbal IQ (total = 19).

The study used a sentence-picture matching task, in which participants heard a sentence and were then asked to point to the matching character in a picture (see Figure 3.2). It employed a carefully designed methodology that defines four levels of increasing morphosyntactic complexity in relative clauses and *Wh*-questions, as schematized in Table 3.1.

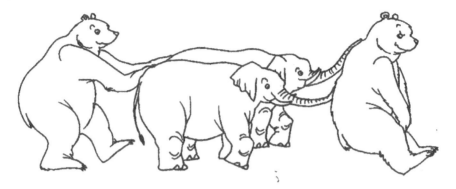

Figure 3.2 Example from the picture sentence-picture matching task testing relative clauses and *Wh*-questions. *Source:* Adapted from Durrleman, Marinis, and Franck (2015). Reproduced with permission of Cambridge University Press.

Table 3.1 Materials and complexity levels sentence-picture matching task testing relative clauses and *Wh*-questions.

Complexity level	Morphosyntactic structure	Example
0	W/o movement (object *Wh*-question)	...*les éléphants poussent qui?* ...the elephants are pushing who?
1	Movement w/o featural intervention (subject *Wh*-question and subject relative clause)	...*qui __ pousse les éléphants?* ...who __ is pushing the elephants? ...*l'ours qui__ pousse les éléphants* ...the bear who __ is pushing the elephants
2	Movement with weak featural intervention (object *Wh*-question)	...*qui les éléphants poussent__?* ...whom the elephants are pushing __?
3	Movement with strong featural intervention (object *Wh*-question and object relative clause)	...*quel ours les éléphants poussent__?* ...which bear the elephants are pushing __? ...*l'ours que les éléphants poussent__* ...the bear that the elephants are pushing __

Source: Adapted from Durrleman et al. (2015).

Questions without movement, such as the Level 0 questions, are the least complex. The next step up (Level 1) includes subject *Wh*-questions and subject relative clauses, in which there is one short movement without intervention: the subject (*qui*) moves to sentence-initial position. This does not change the canonical word order in French, and therefore, Level 1 questions are not that complex. At Level 2, there is featural intervention, which makes the structure more complex: the object (*qui*) moves over the subject (*les éléphants*). This featural intervention is relatively weak because some of the subject's and the object's morphosyntactic features are dissimilar: the subject is a full noun phrase (*les éléphants*), whereas the moved object is a pronoun (*qui*). Finally, questions including movement of an object over a subject with strong featural intervention (Level 3) are the most complex. At Level 3, both the subject (*les éléphants*) and the object (*quel ours* in the *Wh*-questions and *l'ours* in the relative clause) are full noun phrases and third person. As such, they share several morphosyntactic features.

The results of the study suggest that while autistic children obtained lower scores on relative clause comprehension than their TD peers of similar nonverbal abilities, the performance of both autistic and neurotypical children was affected by movement. All groups of children had lower performance in sentences with movement (Levels 1–3) than in those without (Level 0). The effect of intervention (Levels 2 and 3) was stronger in the 4-year-olds than in the 6 and 8-year-olds. The similarity in morphosyntactic features (Level 3) affected 4-year-olds the most and showed that structures with strong featural intervention are the most challenging. The study by Durrleman, Marinis, and Franck (2015) shows that a carefully designed methodology based on linguistic principles can shed light on the morphosyntactic strengths and weaknesses of both neurotypical and autistic children.

In the same vein, Prévost et al. (2017) showed that both children with ASD (aged 6–12, total = 20) and age-matched peers with DLD (total = 20) display similar difficulties in handling the complexity of different question strategies in French; they preferred nonmovement (in situ) strategies, as in example (10), to those involving movement. In the ASD as well as the DLD group, these difficulties were attested across both comprehension and production and were dissociated from nonverbal IQ abilities, which ranged from normal to impaired. While fundamental similarities arose for morphosyntax between these groups, differences could be nevertheless observed regarding the use of language in context, attributable to the well-known pragmatic difference associated with ASD (see Chapters 6–8).

How Challenging Are Complement Clauses in Autism?

Let us now turn to complement clauses as in (13) (*Kim believes/says* [*that the marble is in the box*]). As described in the Anchoring section, complement clauses are a special type of embedded clauses, following verbs of cognition (13a) and verbs of communication (13b). In and of themselves, embedded clauses seem to raise challenges for autistic children. Tuller et al. (2017) show that in spontaneous speech, autistic children with language impairment (ALI) produce much lower rates of clausal embedding than TD children and autistic children without language impairment (ALN). The ALI children in their study either avoid clausal embedding or produce errors in sentences with embedded clauses in their spontaneous language production.

Since complement clauses are embedded clauses, they are already morphosyntactically complex and therefore difficult for autistic children with language impairment (ALI) to produce, as shown by Tuller et al.'s (2017) study described above. Complement clauses have raised considerable additional attention in studies on autistic individuals because it has been proposed that these are important for their success in ToM tasks (de Villiers 2007). The idea here is that autistic individuals have difficulties in ToM that can be overcome if they have good language skills, in particular, complement clauses; they can rely on complement clauses to verbalize ToM and succeed in ToM tasks. In this respect, complementation is a cognitive tool that allows individuals to reason about other people's minds through language.

The results on the success of autistic individuals in the COMPREHENSION of complement clauses are mixed, with some studies showing that they have difficulties with verbs of cognition but not with verbs of communication (e.g. Lind and Bowler 2009), and others showing no differences between autistic and neurotypical individuals (e.g. Durrleman and Franck 2015). Importantly, many studies have demonstrated that complement clauses, especially those with verbs of communication, are strong predictors of autistic individuals' performance in ToM tasks, stronger than in neurotypical individuals (Lind and Bowler 2009), but this does not seem to hold across the board for all types of ToM tasks. Nevertheless, training studies have suggested that enhancing mastery of complement clauses of verbs of communication in autistic children can lead to improved scores in various types of ToM tasks (Durrleman et al. 2023). Future studies need to further investigate the association between ToM and complement clauses in autism, preferably distinguishing between ALI and ALN and between verbs of cognition and verbs of communication. It would be interesting to see if children with ALN – despite the absence of language impairment – systematically have trouble comprehending complement clauses with verbs of cognition (e.g. *believe*) when they have low ToM scores.

How Challenging Are Clitic Constructions in Autism?

Sentences with object clitics, as in (14) (*L'ours **le** pousse* – 'The bear pushes him'), appear to also give rise to difficulties for autistic children. Durrleman and Delage (2016) compared the performance of French-speaking autistic children (total = 21) to French-speaking children diagnosed with DLD (total = 22) on the production of pronominal clitics of the third and first person. The first type of clitic, namely, third-person accusative clitic (ACC3), is a morphosyntactic element renowned for its complexity (see 16b).

(16) a) Jean voit Marie
John sees Mary
'John sees Mary'
b) Jean **la** voit
John her sees
'John sees her'

The sentence in (16a) respects the canonical word order of French, which is exactly like English, namely, SVO. However, when the direct object is a pronoun (as in (22b)), the order becomes noncanonical: SOV. The object clitic pronoun *la* (ACC3) is pronounced before the verb (in contrast to English, where the object pronoun maintains its post-verbal position). The syntactic movement involved in the production of ACC3, namely, from the original post-verbal object position to a preverbal position, moreover, requires holding in Working Memory morphosyntactic features of the direct object (for instance, feminine gender). For all these reasons, the production of ACC3 is difficult, with neurotypical children mastering these only at around 5–8 years old (Varlokosta et al. 2016). Like other areas of morphosyntax that emerge later in neurotypical children, ACC3 clitics remain persistently affected in DLD (Hamann et al. 2003) and are even proposed to be used as clinical markers of this condition in Romance languages (Paradis, Crago, and Genesee 2003; Arosio et al. 2014).

The production of first-person accusative clitics (ACC1), such as French *me* ('me') in (17), is claimed to be simpler than that of ACC3 (such as *la* ('her') in 16b), and indeed they are mastered earlier in both typical development (Coene and Avram 2011; Tuller et al. 2012) and DLD (Tuller et al. 2011).

(17) Jean **me** voit
John me sees
'John sees me'

This may be due to the fact that interpretation of first-person pronouns requires less morphosyntactic computation than interpretation of third-person pronouns: first-person pronouns refer directly to the speaker(s); third-person pronouns require the computation of morphosyntactic features, such as gender, and they require linking to a previously mentioned referent in the discourse. This may solicit Working Memory more extensively.

Production of ACC1 is thus easier than ACC3 in terms of both morphosyntax and Working Memory; however, its correct use interfaces with other cognitive domains as well. Indeed, mastery of ACC1 relies on the ability to understand differences in the perspectives of the discourse participants, in that *me* means one thing when I say it and another when my interlocutor says it. This required shift implied by ACC1 is hypothesized to depend upon the consolidation of a functional ToM. Recall that this is the ability to grasp that people's actions and words relate to their mental states (i.e. perspectives, beliefs, desires, emotions, and intentions), which may differ from our own. As ToM is reportedly a core deficit of individuals on the autism spectrum (Baron-Cohen, Leslie, and Frith 1985), Durrleman and Delage (2016) hypothesize that ACC1 may be affected in autism but relatively spared in DLD.

Durrleman and Delage thus tested ACC3 and ACC1 in 21 autistic children/adolescents (aged 5–16), 22 children/adolescents with DLD (aged 5–16), and also age-matched and younger neurotypical controls (N = 44). They predicted that production of ACC3 would be affected across the board in the DLD group, which is renowned for challenges with (complex) morphosyntax. As for the autistic participants, the prediction was that only autistic children/adolescents with language impairment (ALI) would score relatively low on ACC3. Moreover, as Working Memory is hypothesized to be particularly solicited by ACC3 (which requires computing a movement operation while holding the gender of the referent in mind), performance on this clitic was predicted to relate to Working Memory. Regarding the production of ACC1, because of the simpler morphosyntax of these elements, the authors predicted better performance than on ACC3 by children with DLD. Finally, the dependency of ACC1 clitics on discourse-context/pragmatics and perspective shifting yielded the prediction that they would be problematic for autistic children with compromised ToM (Baron-Cohen, Leslie, and Frith 1985).

A subgroup of seven autistic children (i.e. a third of those tested) was identified as displaying intact grammar (according to standardized scores for global grammar), thus being ALN. The other fourteen autistic children scored relatively low on the global grammar assessment and, as such, were identified as ALI. As expected, the entire DLD group had low standardized scores for global grammar. The ALN group did not demonstrate any difficulty with ACC3 and ACC1. In contrast, their peers with DLD all showed problems with ACC3, although not with ACC1. An interesting difference between the DLD and the ALI group is that the children with DLD managed better with ACC1 than the ALI group. This may be due to the fact that ACC1 is morphosyntactically less complex (easier for children with DLD) but that it does require perspective-shifting skills, which may be weaker in children with ALI. As such, first-person object clitics (ACC1) may be a distinguishing factor between DLD and ALI. Difficulties with Working Memory emerged for both the autistic children (ALI and ALN) and the children with DLD and showed a relation only with performance on ACC3 (as predicted), while better ToM scores went hand-in-hand with better ACC1 scores for 14 out of the 21 autistic children, partially supporting the hypothesis that first-person object clitics (ACC1) require perspective-taking skills.

This study demonstrates the importance of choosing a methodology and experimental design that allows for investigation of the variation in the language profiles of autistic children and, at the same time, the relationship between language and other cognitive abilities, such as Working Memory and ToM (see also Chapter 8). The pattern of performance would not have emerged if this study had not identified subgroups of autistic children, if it had not measured morphosyntactic complexity based on linguistic theory and previous research (ACC1 vs. ACC3), and if it had not included measurements of Working Memory and ToM. This fine-grained design also uncovered an interesting difference between ALI and DLD, which would have otherwise gone unnoticed. As such, the study contributes to providing a foundation on which therapeutic support addressing morphosyntax, Working Memory, and ToM in autism could be elaborated (Durrleman et al. 2023).

Object clitics have also been shown to be challenging in Greek-speaking children with DLD who tend to omit object clitics in their production and are not sensitive to their omission when they process sentences with omitted clitics in real-time (Chondrogianni et al. 2015). This is in contrast to strong pronouns and reflexive pronouns. Terzi et al. (2014) was the first study to investigate how Greek-speaking children with ASD comprehend sentences with object accusative clitics, as in (18) compared to strong pronouns, as in (19), and reflexive pronouns as in (20), as well as how they produce accusative clitics.

(18) I mama **tin** pleni.
    the mum her washes
    'Mum washes her'

(19) I mama pleni **aftin**.
    the mum washes her
    'Mum washes her'

(20) I mama pleni **ton eafto tis**.
    the mother washes the self her
    'Mum washes herself'

The prediction was that children with ASD may also have difficulties with clitics but not with strong pronouns and reflexive pronouns. To test this prediction, 20 children age 5-8 with ASD with nonverbal IQ within the norms and 20 neurotypical children of similar age and individually matched to the children with ASD on their vocabulary abilities participated in a picture-selection task, in which they saw pictures, as the one in Figure 3.3 and listened to sentences, as in (18)–(20) and

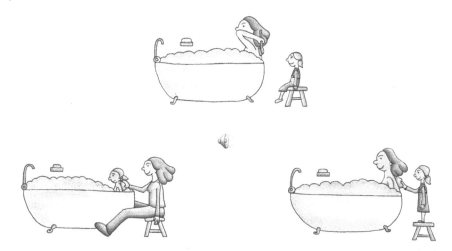

Figure 3.3 Example picture-selection task testing clitics. *Source:* Courtesy of Theodoros Marinis and Arhonto Terzi.

had to select which picture matches the sentence. Although this study did not use the ALN/ALI classification, based on the children's profile, they can be classified as children with ALN.

In the production task, children participated in an elicited production task, in which they saw a picture and had to answer questions about the action in the picture, as exemplified in (21).

(21) Experimenter: Ti kani o likos sti gata?
　　　　　　　　　what does the wolf to-the cat
　　　　　　　　　'What does the wolf do to the cat?'
　　Target:　　　**Ti** filai
　　　　　　　　　her kisses
　　　　　　　　　'He kisses her.'

The results of the comprehension task showed that children with ALN were as accurate as neurotypical children in the comprehension of strong pronouns and reflexive pronouns but were less accurate than neurotypical children in the comprehension of clitics. Although their performance as a group in clitic pronouns was not very low (88.3%), it was lower than the performance of neurotypical children (99.2%) and showed considerable individual variability. The lower accuracy was attributed to 8 out of the 20 children with ALN who scored between 50% and 80%. The remaining 12 children were 100% accurate. The production task showed similar findings. Children with ALN had a lower score (87.39%) compared to the neurotypical children (97.74%), and again, there was also individual variability. The children with ALN performed between 20% and 100%. This suggests that accusative clitics can be a vulnerable structure in Greek but not across all children with ALN.

The study by Terzi et al. (2014) included children with ALN. This suggests that clitics are vulnerable not only in ALI children, but they can be vulnerable also to a subset of ALN children. The study did not use any other measures, such as Working Memory and ToM. Therefore, it is unclear why some children with ALN had a lower score than neurotypical children and what the source of individual variability is. Studies with a more complex methodological design that includes additional measures, such as Working Memory and ToM, are necessary to identify the source of difficulties with clitics in children with ALN that can inform also the necessary therapeutic support to alleviate difficulties with clitics.

Focus on a Specific Study

We focus here on the study reported by Prévost et al. (2018) on object clitics, as this study and Durrleman and Delage (2016), together, illustrate methodological strengths and pitfalls of current studies on morphosyntax in autism. Like Durrleman and Delage, Prévost et al. compared third-person accusative clitics with first-person pronominal clitics in autism and in DLD. As discussed above, third-person clitics require more complex morphosyntactic computation than first-person clitics, as they mark gender in French (and first-person clitics do not) and they require linking to a previously mentioned referent in the discourse (and first-person pronominals do not). First-person pronominals require shifting perspective to take into account the person who is speaking (part of ToM), a skill that is typically weak in autism.

Both of these studies explored pronominal clitics in French-speaking autistic children, through the use of an elicited production task, a task designed to put participants in a context in which the appropriate response entails the production of a pronominal clitic. Moreover, the age range and number of participants with autism were similar in the two studies: 21 participants aged 5–16 in the Durrleman and Delage study and 19 participants aged 6–12 in the Prévost et al. study. Finally, both studies compared participants with autism to age-matched participants with DLD. Like the Durrleman and Delage study, Prévost et al. (2018) also sought to determine whether individuals with autism would have particular difficulty with first-person clitics, which, as outlined above, are morphosyntactically less complex than third-person accusative clitics.

The results of these two studies only partially converged. Both of them found that the ALI subgroup, those autistic children with associated language impairment (14 of the 21 participants in the Durrleman et al. study and 14 of the 19 participants in the Prévost et al. study), resembled the participants with DLD in having difficulties producing third-person accusative clitics. In other words, the ALI children displayed sensitivity to the morphosyntactic complexity of third-person accusative clitics; in this regard, their language impairment resembles known language impairment in French. Both studies also found that the children in the ALN subgroups performed like age controls, reinforcing the fact that they do not have associated language impairment. However, while the Durrleman et al. study found that the ALI subgroup performed worse than the DLD group for production of first-person accusative clitics, the Prévost et al. study found no such difference, with both the DLD and the ALI groups performing in fact better on first-person accusative clitics than on third-person accusative clitics. Durrleman et al. concluded that it was the ALI group's weak perspective-shifting abilities that caused weak performance on first-person accusative clitics, despite their simpler morphosyntax.

Why did two such similar studies arrive at this different result? There are likely a number of reasons that have to do with important methodological issues in studying language in autism. The first issue has to do with population sampling. Linguistically informed study of language in autism entails testing protocols that may be time consuming, limiting the size of population samples. This is a major drawback given the diversity of language skills in children with autism. Both of the studies under question had a modest number of participants (around 20); the subgroups with and without associated language impairment were likely not representative of their proportions in the target population, and, in particular, the ALN subgroups were far too small to yield meaningful ALI/ALN comparisons. Inter-group comparisons, with such small groups, in a condition with such diversity, are perilous at best.

A second issue has to do with the content of the experimental protocols. Very importantly, the Durrleman and Delage study protocol, but not that of Prévost et al., included a task measuring ToM. They were thus able to reinforce their finding that first-person accusative clitics were weak in ALI by showing that the autistic children with weak performance on a verbal false belief ToM task had worse performance on first-person accusative clitics compared to the autistic children who did well on the ToM task. Unfortunately, ToM results were available for only 14 participants, and thus the comparison between ceiling ToM and weak ToM involved comparing five to nine participants. The Prévost et al. study had no such measure and thus no way of examining the eventual influence of this potentially important factor.

The third important issue has to do with the nature of the tasks used to measure morphosyntax. While both studies, guided by linguistic theory, were based on tasks designed to elicit production of pronominal clitics, they differed in many ways, each having advantages and disadvantages. The task used in the Durrleman and Delage was shorter (20 items) than that used by Prévost et al. (32 items), which may have made it more usable with a wider range of children with autism. The Durrleman and Delage task, however, elicited only accusative pronominal clitics ('me', 'him', 'her'), whereas the Prévost et al. task also elicited nominative (subject – 'I', 'he', and 'she') and reflexive ('myself', 'herself/himself') pronouns. In the Prévost et al. task, half of the items (16/32) elicited first-person pronouns, and these included reflexives in which both the subject pronoun and the object reflexive agree in person, reinforcing the perspective shift to first person (e.g. *Je **me** lave* 'I'm washing myself'). In the Durrleman and Delage task, only 8 out of the total 20 items elicited first-person pronominals (e.g. *Il **me** pique* 'It's stinging me'), and there were no items in which both the subject and the object pronouns were first person. It is known that at least some autistic children may be very sensitive to frequency/priming effects, perhaps related to their tendency to perseverate. Having to change perspective for a very small number of items (8/20), with no reinforcing use of first-person subjects or reflexives, may have been especially difficult for some of the children with ASD in the Durrleman and Delage task.

So, why were autistic children's perspective-shifting difficulties not strong enough to prevent them from performing well on the Prévost et al. (2018) elicitation task? The authors argued that their task may have unwittingly provided autistic children with exactly the cues they needed to shift perspective and successfully produce first-person pronouns (which are less complex morphosyntactically). First of all, the pragmatic situation was made particularly salient via the instructions given ("Now you are Marie. What do you answer?") with the temporal clue *now* and an emphatic form of *you*, which was left dislocated and followed by a resumptive pronoun ("Now, YOU, you are Marie.") as well as visual clues in the form of cartoon bubbles (to which the experimenter points), and, in particular, a blank bubble linked to the character with whom the child was supposed to identify (see Figure 3.4). Kissine (2012) noted that autistic children's performance on false belief tasks, which require taking the perspective of the protagonist who is not privy to information the child has witnessed, improves when the perspective of this protagonist is made explicit/focused. Autistic children, in

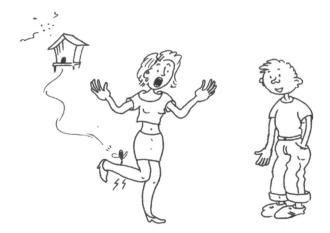

Figure 3.4 Example picture eliciting production of a first-person accusative clitic ('Hey, Marie, what is the bee doing?'). *Source:* Tuller et al. (2011). Reproduced with permission of Elsevier.

this view, would not have problems inhibiting their own perspective and adopting somebody else's, but in doing so spontaneously. If the other perspective is rendered sufficiently salient, they are able to shift perspective. In other words, the task used to determine whether autistic children's perspective-shifting difficulties could affect their production of first-person pronouns may in fact have evacuated this difficulty, making the hypothesis that autistic children have difficulties with perspective-shifting impossible to test with the elicitation task employed in Prévost et al. (2018).

In summary, these two studies both found that French-speaking ALI children are like children with DLD in having particular difficulty with third-person accusative clitics, a syntactic phenomenon known to be a particularly robust marker of language impairment in French. However, they yielded entirely opposite results when seeking to test whether first-person pronouns might be difficult for autistic children due to their reliance on perspective shifting. This focus on the methodology of the two studies has sought to illustrate the methodological limitations of many studies on morphosyntax in autism: population sampling (notably sample size), inclusion of measures of nonlinguistic cognition, and task content. The two studies in question illustrate how such limitations can lead to contradictory results.

Conclusion

This chapter set out to address the following questions:

- Does morphosyntax present challenges for all autistic children?
- How challenging are passives in autism?
- How challenging are relative clauses and *Wh*-questions in autism?
- How challenging are clitic constructions in autism?
- How challenging are complement clauses in autism?

We showed that autistic individuals are a heterogeneous group, who have a range of abilities within the realm of morphosyntax. Autistic individuals with language impairment (ALI subgroup), as measured by standardized omnibus language assessments and morphosyntactic analysis of spontaneous speech, also score lower than neurotypicals in specific morphosyntactic tasks, including passives, object relative clauses, object *Wh*-questions, complement clauses, and clitic constructions. Autistic individuals without language impairment (ALN subgroup) may nevertheless show subtle difficulties with these phenomena as well, because of their morphosyntactic complexity and possibly because of their relationship with Working Memory or ToM.

Given the large heterogeneity and the interface of morphosyntax with other linguistic and nonlinguistic domains, it is important to pay close attention to the methodologies used when assessing morphosyntax. While spontaneous speech provides rich information about abilities in several language domains, it does not always reveal autistic individuals' potential regarding more complex morphosyntactic structures, because such structures are often avoided in spontaneous language production. To assess complex morphosyntactic abilities in autism, complementary experimental tasks are needed.

The chapter also showed that, in addition to testing the specific morphosyntactic phenomenon under investigation, it is crucial to use a general language assessment tool that can distinguish ALI from ALN. It is equally important to measure nonlinguistic domains that have been shown to interact with morphosyntax (e.g. Working Memory and ToM). Such methodology will enable us to profile each autistic individual for their strengths and weaknesses in each domain. Ideally, larger groups of ALI and ALN should be tested and compared on their morphosyntactic and nonlinguistic cognitive skills.

Finally, the chapter demonstrated that it is necessary to screen autistic individuals for aspects of morphosyntax (such as constructions with noncanonical word order or complement clauses) that have been shown to be vulnerable even in individuals who have strong language skills (the ALN group), so as to ensure that adequate support is offered to all individuals that need it, while intact structures can serve as useful structures to build on for these interventions.

> **What Do You Know Now?**
> Portrayals of autism, be they in books and movies, may give rise to the erroneous impression that autistic individuals are mainly characterized by social peculiarities but that once they speak, they have no difficulties with morphosyntax with possibly only challenges with figurative language.
> - Among autistic people who speak, two general morphosyntax subgroups have been identified: ALN (Autism with normal language) and ALI (Autism with language impairment), in which the term "language" mainly refers to structural language (including morphosyntax, (sentence-level) semantics, and phonology).
> - Unsurprisingly, many morphosyntactic phenomena are impaired in the ALI group. The ALI group's language profile superficially resembles that of people with Developmental Language Disorder, but there are subtle differences (see also Chapter 11).
> - Nevertheless, the ALN group may also show difficulty with morphosyntax. This is particularly the case in complex morphosyntactic constructions with noncanonical word order or embedding, for example, passives, object relative clauses, object *Wh*-questions, complement clauses, and clitic constructions.
>
> Adequate screening for areas to be addressed by therapeutic support should include assessments targeting complex morphosyntax. Structures that are intact can be used for scaffolding to assist language interventions.

Suggestions for Further Reading

If you want to know more about morphosyntax in autism, we suggest reading the collection of articles in Durrleman and Gavarró 2018. We recommend a book, Guasti 2017, if you want to know more about how nonautistic children acquire morphosyntax.

References

Allen, D.A. and Rapin, I. (1980). Language disorders in preschool children: predictors of outcome - a preliminary report. *Brain Development* 2 (1): 73–80.

References

Arosio, F., Branchini, C., Barbieri, L. et al. (2014). Failure to produce direct object clitic pronouns as a clinical marker of SLI in school-aged Italian-speaking children. *Clinical Linguistics and Phonetics* 28 (9): 639–663.

Baron-Cohen, S., Leslie, A.M., and Frith, U. (1985). Does the autistic child have a "Theory of Mind"? *Cognition* 21 (1): 37–46.

Chondrogianni, V., Marinis, T., Edwards, S. et al. (2015). Production and on-line comprehension of definite articles and clitic pronouns by Greek sequential bilingual children and monolingual children with Specific Language Impairment. *Applied Psycholinguistics* 36 (5): 1155–1191.

Coene, M. and Avram, L. (2011). An asymmetry in the acquisition of accusative clitics in child Romanian. *Studies on Language Acquisition* 43: 39–68.

Condouris, K., Meyer, E., and Tager-Flusberg, H. (2003). The relationship between standardized measures of language and measures of spontaneous speech in children with autism. *American Journal of Speech-Lang Pathology* 12 (3): 349–58.

de Villiers, J.G. (2007). The interface of language and Theory of Mind. *Lingua* 177 (11): 1858–1878.

Durrleman, S., Bentea, A., Prisecaru, A. et al. (2023). Training syntax to enhance Theory of Mind in children with ASD. *Journal of Autism and Developmental Disorders* 53: 2444–2457.

Durrleman, S. and Delage, H. (2016). Autism Spectrum Disorder and Specific Language Impairment: overlaps in syntactic profiles. *Language Acquisition* 23 (4): 361–386.

Durrleman, S., Delage, H., Prévost, P. et al. (2017). The comprehension of passives in Autism Spectrum Disorder. *Glossa: A Journal of General Linguistics* 2 (1): 88.

Durrleman, S. and Franck, J. (2015). Exploring links between language and cognition in Autism Spectrum Disorders: complement sentences, false belief, and executive functioning. *Journal of Communication Disorders* 54: 15–31.

Durrleman, S. and Gavarró, A. (2018). Investigating grammar in Autism Spectrum Disorders. *Frontiers in Psychology* 9: 1004.

Durrleman, S., Marinis, T., and Franck, J. (2015). Syntactic complexity in the comprehension of Wh-questions and relative clauses in typical language development and autism. *Applied Psycholinguistics* 37 (6): 1501–1527.

Friedmann, N. and Reznick, J. (2021). Stages rather than ages in the acquisition of movement structures: data from sentence repetition and spontaneous clauses. *Glossa: A Journal of General Linguistics* 39 (1): 143.

Gavarró, A. and Heshmati, Y. (2014). An investigation on the comprehension of Persian passives in typical development and autism. *Catalan Journal of Linguistics* 13: 79–98.

Guasti, M.T. (2017). *Language Acquisition, Second Edition: The Growth of Grammar.* Cambridge, MA: MIT Press.

Hamann, C., Ohayon, S., Dubé, S. et al. (2003). Aspects of grammatical development in young French children with SLI. *Developmental Science* 6 (2): 151–158.

Jakubowicz, C. (2011). Measuring derivational complexity: new evidence from typically developing and SLI learners of L1 French. *Lingua* 121 (3): 339–351.

Kissine, M. (2012). Pragmatics, cognitive flexibility and Autism Spectrum Disorders. *Mind & Language* 27 (1): 1–28.

Kjelgaard, M.M. and Tager-Flusberg, H. (2001). An investigation of language impairment in autism: implications for genetic subgroups. *Language and Cognitive Processes* 16 (2–3): 287–308.

Lind, S. and Bowler, D. (2009). Language and Theory of Mind in Autism Spectrum Disorder: the relationship between complement syntax and false belief task performance. *Journal of Autism and Developmental Disorders* 39 (6): 929–937.

Paradis, J., Crago, M., and Genesee, F. (2003). Object clitics as a clinical marker of SLI in French: evidence from French-English bilingual children. In: *Proceedings of the 27th Annual Boston University Conference on Language Development* (eds. B. Beachley, A. Brown, and F. Conlin), 638–649. Somerville, MA: Cascadilla Press.

Perovic, A., Modyanova, N., and Wexler, K. (2013). Comparison of grammar in Neurodevelopmental Disorders: the case of binding in Williams Syndrome and Autism with and without Language Impairment. *Language Acquisition* 20 (2): 133–154.

Prévost, P., Tuller, L., Barthez, M.A. et al. (2017). Production and comprehension of French Wh-questions by children with Autism Spectrum Disorder: a comparative study with Specific Language Impairment. *Applied Psycholinguistics* 38 (5): 1095–1131.

Prévost, P., Tuller, L., Zebib, R. et al. (2018). Pragmatic versus structural difficulties in the production of pronominal clitics in French-speaking children with Autism Spectrum Disorder. *Autism & Developmental Language Impairments* 3: 1–17.

Rapin, I. and Dunn, M. (1997). Language disorders in children with autism. *Seminars in Pediatric Neurology* 4 (2): 86–92.

Rizzi, L. (2018). Intervention effects in grammar and language acquisition. *Probus* 30 (2): 339–367.

Roberts, J.A., Rice, M.L., and Tager-Flusberg, H. (2004). Tense marking in children with autism. *Applied Psycholinguistics* 25 (3): 429–448.

Tager-Flusberg, H. (2006). Defining language phenotypes in autism. *Clinical Neuroscience Research* 6 (3–4): 219–224.

Terzi, A., Marinis, T., Francis, K. et al. (2014). Grammatical abilities of Greek-speaking children with autism. *Language Acquisition* 21 (1): 4–44.

Tuller, L., Delage, H., Monjauze, C. et al. (2011). Clitic pronoun production as a measure of atypical language development in French. *Lingua* 121 (3): 423–441.

Tuller, L., Ferré, S., Prévost, P. et al. (2017). The effect of computational complexity on the acquisition of French by children with ASD. In: *Innovative investigations of language in Autism Spectrum Disorder* (ed. L.R. Naigles), 115–140. Washington, DC: de Gruyter Mouton; American Psychological Association.

Tuller, L., Henry, C., Sizaret, E. et al. (2012). Specific Language Impairment at adolescence: avoiding complexity. *Applied Psycholinguistics* 33 (1): 161–184.

Varlokosta, S., Belletti, A., Costa, J. et al. (2016). A cross-linguistic study of the acquisition of clitic and pronoun production. *Language Acquisition* 23 (1): 1–26.

4

Phonology

Sandrine Ferré and Christophe dos Santos

> **What Do You Think?**
> Your mother is watching a documentary on TV in which a child with autism is explaining his difficulties at school. The child is really hard to understand because he makes a number of pronunciation errors. Your mother is very surprised and says that this child may have some other impairment besides ASD. What would you tell her?
>
> You are chatting with one of your friends, and he tells you that this morning he had a conversation with one of the IT support staff at the university. He learned that this person is autistic. He told you that it was the first time he had ever met an autistic person, and it seemed to him that this condition was not a big deal because all he noticed was a funny way of talking. You remember that one of your distant cousins is also autistic but that he is unable to speak without leaving out some consonants or changing some vowels. You tell your friend that mastering the sounds of language for individuals with autism is more complicated than one may think. How do you explain to your friend why mastering language sounds is not an easy task?

Introduction

Phonology is part of structural language competence, just like morphosyntax is. Phonology is important to study in autism because it concerns small units (sounds) that are part of the foundations of word structure. If these foundations are not mastered, this could lead to major difficulties in other language domains. The traditional assumption is that **sound structure** is not a problem for speakers with autism; that is, they do not have difficulty with the sounds needed to say words and comprehend them. As a result, phonological development in children with autism has not been a major concern for clinicians or researchers.

Moreover, when phonology is assessed, the tools that are used are sometimes not specific to it.

However, some studies suggest that phonology may in fact be impaired in autistic individuals, both children and adults, like other structural aspects of language, such as sentence structure (syntax) or word structure (morphology). Deficits in phonology can lead to communication difficulties due to significant alteration and perception of sound structure, such as **phonemes** and **syllables** (see Anchoring section). To talk about phonology in autism, it is important to understand the difference between a **phonetic** (or **speech**) **disorder** and a **phonological** (or sound structure) **disorder**. This distinction can be confusing and can lead to false conclusions about what kind of difficulties an individual with autism may have.

This chapter provides an overview of current knowledge about phonetic and phonological abilities in individuals with autism by addressing the following questions:

- What are the phonetic abilities of individuals with autism?
- What are the phonological abilities of individuals with autism?
- What are the limitations of phonological assessment in autism?

Anchoring

For those who have never studied or worked in the field of linguistics, it is easy to get confused between phonetics and phonology. **Phonetics** is the study of the sounds of speech,[1] in particular, how they are produced by the speech production system, including articulatory organs (e.g. vocal cords, tongue, lips, teeth, upper gum ridge, palate, etc. – articulatory phonetics), how they propagate in the form of waves (acoustic phonetics), and how they are perceived (auditory phonetics/speech perception). **Phonology**, on the other hand, is not related to speech but to language (see Figure 4.1). As such, phonology concerns how sound is structured, just like morphosyntax is about how words are structured into sentences. Phonology is not concerned with physical sounds but with abstract units, called phonemes, syllables, etc.

A **phoneme** is an abstract sound category (a phonological unit) that can be produced in different ways (at the phonetic level), notably according to the context in

---

[1] Be careful not to confuse sounds with letters! In an alphabetic writing system, letters may not be pronounced (e.g. the so-called silent "e" in English, as in *done*), and if they are, they may represent different categories of sounds, depending on the word being produced. For example, the letter "i" can be produced in American English as [ɪ] in *kit*, or as [ə] in *pencil*, or as [aɪ] in *wine* (which also contains a silent "e").

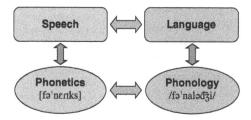

Figure 4.1 The relations between phonetics and phonology. *Source:* Sandrine Ferré and Christophe dos Santos.

which the sound appears, but also according to the performance of the speaker at a specific time. For instance, in English, the phoneme /p/ can be produced with an accompanying puff of air, noted [pʰ], as in *pit* [pʰit], which is not the case in *stop* [stɑp].[2] A phoneme can be described as a set of **phonological features**, which correspond mainly to sound properties such as place of articulation or manner of articulation that make it distinctive from other phonemes (see Figure 4.2 for an overview of how manner and place of articulation interact in the production of consonants). Features are generally based on a description of the articulatory system and are often presented as binary. For instance, /b/ is [+voiced] (meaning that the vocal cords vibrate when it is produced), whereas /p/ is [−voiced] (with no vibration of the vocal cords). Features are extremely useful to describe phonological processes (see below). For example, suppose a child says *tebiatrician* instead of *pediatrician*. How can

Acronym and Terminology Reminder
ALI: Autism with language impairment.
ALN: Autism with normal language.
Articulation (articulatory): Ability to physically move the tongue, lips, teeth, and jaw to produce sequences of speech sounds.
CAS: Childhood Apraxia of Speech. Motor speech neurological condition resulting in difficulties with speech movement, in the absence of neuromuscular deficits.
Coda: Consonant(s) appearing at the end of a syllable.
DLD: Developmental Language Disorder. Language abilities below age expectations are not attributable to any other condition.
Motor Speech Disorder: Difficulties in planning, programming, controlling, coordinating, and executing speech productions.
Phoneme: Abstract sound category.
Phonetics: Production and perception of speech sounds.
Phonological process: An error pattern that affects the way a phoneme is being produced.
Phonology: The structure of sounds, i.e. the way speech sounds combine.
Speech: The expression of language by means of articulating sounds.
Speech Sounds: Vocal sounds used in spoken language.

---

2 It is standard practice to use square brackets to indicate a speech sound and a pair of slashes to indicate that the symbol between the slashes is a phoneme.

we describe what happened? Instead of saying that /p/ has been replaced by /t/ and /d/ by /b/, we can simply say that the features related to the places of articulation (roughly, lips for /p/ and /b/ and upper gum ridge for /t/ and /d/) of these two consonants have been swapped, all other features remaining equal.

> **Stop (obstruent, plosive):** Consonant produced with complete obstruction of the airflow in the mouth.
>
> **Syllable:** Sequence of speech sounds organized into a unit that includes a nucleus (usually a vowel) and may be preceded or followed by one or more consonants.

Another important abstract unit in phonology is the **syllable**. It contains a much higher level of formalization than what speakers think they know when asked what a syllable is. Indeed, everyone can tell how many syllables there are in a word like *sonority*, but it becomes more difficult for words like *strict* or *first*. A syllable can be seen as a constituent that provides a template limiting how phonemes can be combined to form words. For example, in English, the

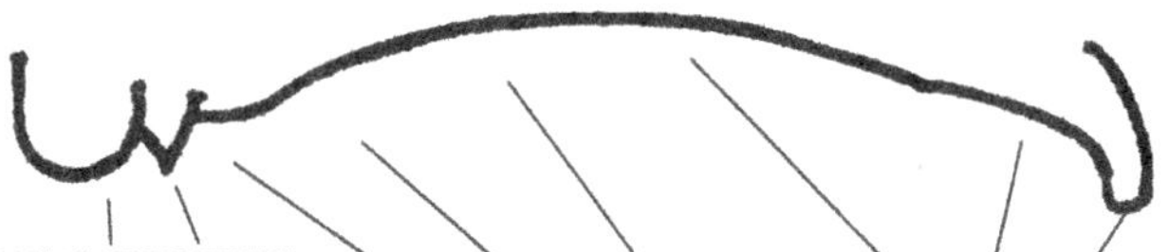

CONSONANTS (PULMONIC)

	Bilabial	Labio-dental	Dental	Alveolar	Postalveolar	Retroflex	Palatal	Velar	Uvular	Pharyngeal	Glottal
Plosive	p b			t d		ʈ ɖ	c ɟ	k ɡ	q ɢ		ʔ
Nasal	m	ɱ		n		ɳ	ɲ	ŋ	ɴ		
Trill	ʙ			r					ʀ		
Tap or Flap		ⱱ		ɾ		ɽ					
Fricative	ɸ β	f v	θ ð	s z	ʃ ʒ	ʂ ʐ	ç ʝ	x ɣ	χ ʁ	ħ ʕ	h ɦ
Lateral fricative				ɬ ɮ							
Approximant		ʋ		ɹ		ɻ	j	ɰ			
Lateral approximant				l		ɭ	ʎ	ʟ			

Symbols to the right in a cell are voiced, to the left are voiceless. Shaded areas denote articulations judged impossible.

(CC-BY-SA) 2020 IPA Typefaces: Doulos SIL (metatext): Doulos SIL, IPA Kiel, IPA LS Uni (symbols)

Figure 4.2 Consonant manner (rows) and place (columns) of articulation. Places of articulation are aligned under a side view of a mouth shape, from front (lips) to back (uvula). *Source:* Adapted from International Phonetic Association (2015) (IPA Chart).

sequence /pl/ can occur at the beginning of a word, as in *plum*, but not in Japanese. On the other hand, the sequence /ps/ never occurs word-initially in English, but it does occur in that position in German. Most of the restrictions on possible phoneme combinations within syllables are due to the properties of the syllable in a given language. A classical view of syllable structure relies in part on the abstract notion of **sonority**. In phonology, sonority is based on acoustic and articulatory criteria, as well as on the behavior of sounds in languages. Sound categories can then be placed along a scale of sonority from least to most sonorous, with the least sonorous being **stops** (consonants in which there is complete blockage of the air during production), such as [p] or [t], and the most sonorous being vowels, such as [a] or [e]. In the classical view, the most sonorous element of a syllable is considered to be the nucleus of that syllable, which is the only obligatory element in a syllable. In general, the syllable nucleus is a vowel. From the nucleus, the sonority can only go down, never up. In the example for the word *plum*, given in Figure 4.3, to the left of the nucleus (the vowel /ʌ/), there is a /l/, which is less sonorous than the vowel /ʌ/ in the nucleus, and a /p/, which is less sonorous than /l/. The same goes for the right side of the nucleus, with /m/ being less sonorous than the vowel in the nucleus. The part to the left of the syllable nucleus is called the **onset**, and the part to the right of the syllable nucleus is called the **coda**. The nucleus and the coda together form what is called a **rhyme**. If the rhyme has a segment in the coda position, it is called a branching rhyme, which is the case in *plum* (see Figure 4.3). The same goes for the onset: if the onset contains two segments, it is called a **branching onset**, which is also the case in our example. When a syllable constituent branches (is associated with two segments), it is considered to be complex, so there can be complex onsets (/pl/ in *plum*), complex rhymes (/ʌm/ in *plum*), and complex codas (/mz/ in *plums*). As will become clear below, complexity plays a major role in phonological impairment.

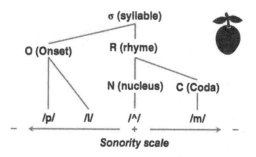

Figure 4.3 The syllable structure of the word *plum*. *Source:* Sandrine Ferré and Christophe dos Santos.

Some languages, for example, Japanese, do not allow for certain sequences to appear in the onset, such as /pl/. In other words, complex onsets do not occur in Japanese and some other languages. The same goes for branching rhymes, which are allowed in some languages but not in others. In addition, there may be other restrictions on the proper formation of a branching onset in languages that do allow branching onsets. For example, the branching onset /pl/ is possible in English, but the branching onset /ps/ is not; in contrast, both of them are possible in German. The difference between the two languages has to do with the **sonority hierarchy**: /p/ is less sonorous than /s/, which is less sonorous than /l/, and the sonority difference between /p/ and /l/ is larger than between /p/ and /s/. In English, two consonants that are too close in terms of sonority cannot appear in the same branching onset; yet, this restriction does not apply to German.

In addition to phonological units, such as phonemes and syllables, phonology includes **phonological processes**, a fundamental aspect of human languages. All human languages have phonological processes. When speaking, humans, including children, use phonological processes all the time that either conform to what is expected in their language or not. In the latter case, it results in productions that are judged as errors, which may correspond, in the case of children, to the early stages of typical language development. In the case of children with language impairment, phonological processes that do not conform to the target language persist beyond the typical age and/or involve unusual patterns. Phonological processes arise because languages are spoken and therefore are subject to constraints linked to spoken communication (articulatory, auditory, temporal, etc.). One way of characterizing phonological processes is that they are the result of speakers using just enough energy so that the contrasts between segments (phonemes) are perceived and thus understood, but no more. One of the most common phonological processes is **assimilation**. Assimilation most commonly takes place between two segments that are adjacent to each other. Let's take the case of the palatal consonant [ç] (see Figure 4.2) in German, as in the word *ich* 'I' [ıç]. When this consonant is preceded by a back vowel like /u/, it assimilates the [back] feature of the vowel and is produced further back in the mouth as a velar consonant [x], as in the word *Buch* 'book' [buːx] or in the word *Bach* 'brook' [bax].

Children also display assimilation processes during language acquisition that do not always conform to the adult phonology. Assimilation in fact frequently takes place before the child's phonology is fully adult-like. For instance, the French word *trop* 'too much' [tχo] is often produced as [kχo] by children in the early stages of development. In this example, [t] is produced as [k], a sound whose place of articulation is further back in the mouth (velar) (see Figure 4.2). In other words, /t/ assimilates (in this case, changes its place of articulation) the backness of the following consonant, the uvular rhotic [χ]. As illustrated in Table 4.1, other common phonological processes include epenthesis (where a segment is inserted between two

Table 4.1 Examples of phonological processes from child production.

Process	Language	Word	Target	Child production
Assimilation	French	*drôle* 'funny'	/dʁol/	[gʁol]
Epenthesis	Portuguese	*livro* 'book'	/ˈlivru/	[ˈlivɨru]
Deletion	English	*Book*	/bʊk/	[bʊ]
Metathesis	English	*Cup*	/kʌp/	[pʌk]

consonants), deletion (where a segment is deleted), and metathesis (where a switch occurs between two features, as in the *pediatrician/tebiatrician* example above).

During the developmental period, a child's language approaches adult phonology gradually. Along the way, several different phonological processes can be observed. Some productions are stable for several months, while others are quite variable, depending, for example, on the child's fatigue. When productions are stable over several months, it is said to reflect the child's current phonological system. The majority of phonological patterns found in child production are observed in most children.

Developmental phonological patterns also follow a determined order. With respect to phonemes, vowels are mastered before consonants. For vowels, there is a general tendency for open vowels (/a/) to be acquired before closed ones (/i, u/). Oral vowels also tend to be produced accurately before nasal vowels are. At a young age, children often tend to denasalize nasal vowels when they are part of the phonological system to be acquired (e.g. in French, *pense* 'think' /pãs/ → [pɔs]). The first consonants acquired are generally voiceless **plosives** (or stops) (e.g. /p/, /t/, /k/), namely sounds that involve complete stopping of the airflow and that are produced with no accompanying vibration of the vocal cords. The most stable consonant is /p/, whereas /k/ and /t/ may undergo substitutions in some young children's production. For example, some children show velar fronting (e.g. *cup* /kʌp/ → [tʌp]), where a consonant normally pronounced in the back of the mouth, such as /k/, is "moved forward" in articulation, and others display coronal backing (e.g. *eat* /it/ → [ik]), which results in coronal consonants such as /t/ being pronounced further back in the mouth. **Fricatives**, i.e. sounds in which the vocal tract is narrow enough to create turbulent airflow (e.g. [s] and [z]), are generally acquired after stops (e.g. [p] and [k]), although some children may be able to produce fricatives at the end of words at an early age. Early on, fricatives are often replaced by stops (a process commonly referred to as stopping) (e.g. *zoo* /zu/ → [du]). In many languages, the most unstable consonants correspond to the natural class of liquids, which include rhotics (/r/-like sounds) and laterals (/l/-like sounds). These consonants are generally deleted in early acquisition and tend to be acquired last.

When children attempt to produce them, the semivowels [j] or [w] are often produced instead. Finally, when coronal fricatives (/θ, ð/, /s, z/, /ʃ, ʒ/) are part of the phonological system of a language, such as English, the contrast between them is acquired later. All these developmental steps can be understood in terms of **segmental complexity**: stops are less complex than fricatives, front stops are less complex than backstops, etc.

Concerning syllables, children generally produce only basic syllable types in early acquisition stages: vowel only (e.g. in French *eau*, 'water' /o/) or a consonant followed by a vowel (e.g. *tea* /tiː/). Branching syllable constituents, such as branching onsets, which are a type of **consonant clusters**, are rarely produced in the initial stages of development. For example, the word *block* [blɑk] would likely be produced as [bɑk]. Children generally acquire all the vowels and consonants that occur in words composed of basic syllable types between the ages of 2.5 and 4.5, even though there is a great deal of individual variation. In more complex syllables, the lack of production of a phoneme could be due to one of two scenarios. It could be due to the application of a phonological process, such as phoneme deletion, to reduce the complexity of the syllable structure, such as complex onsets or complex rhymes. Alternatively, the phoneme in question may not have been acquired yet.

Like other linguistic domains (lexicon, morphology, syntax, semantics, and pragmatics), phonology may be impaired (see Figure 4.4). Phonological disorders are associated with a deficit in phonological representations and structures that result in errors that apply across a class of sounds, such as stopping (where fricatives are replaced by stops) or simplifying a branching constituent. In some cases, however, it may be difficult to distinguish between a phonetic disorder and a phonological disorder.[3] The term **Speech Sound Disorder** includes both types of disorders, as shown in Figure 4.4. How can phonological impairment be identified, then? Individuals with phonological disorder show significantly lower performance at the segmental level (individual phonemes) than those with no phonological disorder, for example, on measures such as percentage of phonemes correctly produced. This is partly because these individuals struggle with syllable structure, with, for example, consonants not being produced in coda (syllable-final) position. Even though individuals with phonological impairment show most of the same phonological patterns seen during typical language acquisition, they tend to delete or add segments or syllables much more often than typically developing (TD) children, and they do so for a longer period. Another way of classifying phonological

---

3 Readers can refer to American Speech-Language-Hearing Association (ASHA) website pages to learn more about classification criteria:
   https://www.asha.org/practice-portal/clinical-topics/articulation-and-phonology
   https://www.asha.org/practice-portal/clinical-topics/spoken-language-disorders

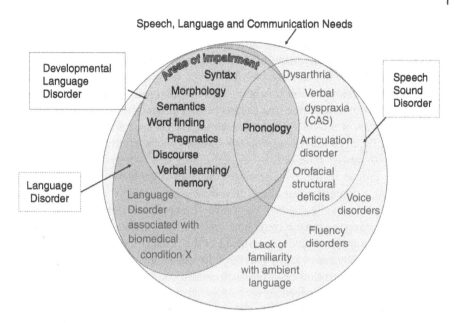

Figure 4.4 Venn diagram illustrating the relationship between different diagnostic terms. *Source:* Bishop et al. (2017).

difficulties as part of a language disorder is to see whether other domains of language are impaired as well. When this is the case, it is an indication that structural aspects of language are particularly impacted in such individuals.

Phonology in Autism

As seen above, speech (phonetics) is distinct from phonology. However, since both of these domains are based on the same material (sounds), it is sometimes hard to distinguish how they affect the way a person speaks and understands. The literature on speech sounds in autism suffers from the confusion between phonetics and phonology. In this chapter, we propose to clarify this issue, separating what we know about the phonetic abilities of individuals with autism from what we know about their phonological abilities.

What Are the Phonetic Abilities of Individuals with Autism?

Most studies focusing on speech sounds in autism have been concerned with articulatory aspects. In general, articulatory skills are said to be relatively spared in children with ASD. Yet, a majority of autistic individuals (50–79% according to Green et al. 2009) have motor difficulties, such as deficits in preparation and planning, timing and organization, muscle tone, balance, and gait. The question thus arises as to whether orofacial difficulties have consequences on **verbal praxis**, which refers to the voluntary movements used to make speech gestures and movements. These movements involve programming articulators and rapid sequences of muscle firings that are required for speech sound production. Orofacial difficulties indeed seem to affect verbal praxis in autism. In particular, children with autism have difficulties performing oral movements, such as elevating the tongue to the alveolar ridge, the gum ridge behind the front teeth (Adams 1998). Moreover, variability in tongue movements is larger in children with autism than in TD children (McKeever, Cleland, and Delafield-Butt 2022). Difficulty moving the tongue could have an important impact on articulation, as the tongue is a major articulator involved in the production of most consonants and all vowels. Tongue mobility and flexibility also allow for more precise **coarticulation** (the transition from one articulatory configuration to another) and more accurate phonemic sequences.

Some studies have concluded that there is a dyspraxia-type disorder (i.e. a motor speech disorder) in ASD or even **Childhood Apraxia of Speech** (CAS) associated with ASD (see Figure 4.4).[4] Some authors have even suggested that this verbal praxis deficit should be included in the diagnosis of autism, as it is observed in a large majority of individuals with autism, including **minimally verbal** children (Chenausky et al. 2019). Errors found in some children with ASD are indeed similar to those identified in children with CAS, as listed in (1) (Prizant 1996).

(1) Errors identified in ASD and CAS:
   a. Primarily vowel-like vocalizations
   b. Limited consonant inventory
   c. Difficulty in sequencing phonemes in multisyllabic words
   d. Reduction of intelligibility as word length increases
   e. Better intelligibility in automatic, rote speech (such as echolalia) than in spontaneous speech.

Phonetic skills of autistic children have been described via the Kaufman Speech Praxis Test (KPST; Kaufman 1995). It has been observed that children with ASD produce simple items as well as TD children but make errors on complex items

---

4 According to ASHA's definition, CAS is a "neurological speech sound disorder in which the precision and consistency of movements underlying speech are impaired in the absence of neuromuscular deficits. The core impairment in planning and/or programming spatiotemporal parameters of movements sequences results in errors in speech sound productions and prosody" (American Speech-Language-Hearing Association 2017).

(Adams 1998). Production of simple items includes production of isolated vowels (/a, ɛ, ɔ, ɪ, ʌ, u, i/), simple consonants /m, b, p, t, d, n, h/), and syllables with no consonant cluster (e.g. Consonant–Vowel – CV /da, me, do/, CVCV /mama, papa/, and VCV /opa, apo, obo/). Complex items include complex consonants (/k, g, f, s, z, l, r, w, v, j, ʃ, tʃ, dʒ, θ, ð/) and complex syllables displaying consonant clusters (e.g. *stop, window*). Adams (1998) draws a parallel between the errors found in ASD with those frequently observed in children with CAS, such as Phoneme distortion (*sun:* [sʌn] > [ɫʌn]), Fronting (*cookie:* [kʊki] > [tʊki]), and Consonant substitution (*so:* [so] > [to]). Results on the KPST have in fact been used to reinforce the hypothesis that CAS affects children with ASD. It has been proposed that CAS is a sufficient cause for lack of speech development in at least some autistic children classified as nonverbal, and it could contribute to inappropriate speech or prosody (see Chapter 9) and to particular voice features in children and adults with ASD (Shriberg 2009). However, acoustic evidence has shown that autistic children with dyspraxia do not seem to display all of the CAS warning signs. In particular, they do not display slow speaking and articulation rates, spatiotemporal vowel errors, vowel lengthening, and distorted consonants (due to the planning and programming of movement gestures for speech) (see Strand 2017).

Some authors have also hypothesized that general **Motor speech disorders** predict later expressive language (especially in minimally verbal children) (Chenausky and Tager-Flusberg 2022; LeBarton and Landa 2019). The development of fine or gross motor skills can indeed impact language development, particularly since children, by exploring their world and manipulating objects, develop their cognitive abilities, their interactional skills with others (e.g. by handing an object to those close to them), and their vocabulary skills (e.g. by naming new objects). However, communication development is complex, and motor dysfunction alone cannot explain atypical language development. First of all, there are (nonautistic) children with severe motor deficits who have intact language skills (Rivière, Lécuyer, and Hickmann 2009). Moreover, even though significant correlations may be found in children with autism between gross and fine motor skills and language communication skills, these correlations do not explain the underlying mechanisms at play between motor and language skills, nor are they indicative of the way their directionality should be interpreted (West 2019). In other words, we do not know whether poor language development is responsible for poor motor performance or whether the reverse is true. Questions can also be raised concerning the language measures used in studies reporting correlations between motor and language skills. For example, some studies have used the Vineland (see Chapter 1), which is a parental questionnaire and therefore does not allow for fine and direct measurement of the different language domains. Others have used general expressive language scores, such as the Expressive Language score from

The Mullen Scales of Early Learning (MSEL; see Chapter 1), as in LeBarton and Landa's (2019) study, which concludes that motor skills at age 6 months predict expressive language at 30 and 36 months. However, the Expressive Language score is partly based on vocabulary skills, which are very different from abilities in structural language such as phonology or syntax, in that they develop throughout the lifespan. In particular, lexical knowledge is dependent on the exploration of the child's environment, as this exploration allows children to discover the world and acquire new words. It is thus unsurprising that the Expressive Language score should increase between the ages of 6 and 30 months. Finally, the KPST, which is often used to investigate the production of speech sounds in ASD, focuses mainly on the segmental level. Notably, this test does not aim to explore, in any meaningful way, the structural reasons (e.g. where the segment appears in the syllable structure) that may be underlying the deletion of a phoneme or the substitution of a phoneme by another. This means that it is impossible to determine whether production errors are phonetic/articulatory (a speech sound disorder) or phonological (a **developmental language disorder**).

In summary, current evidence suggests that we should be cautious in our interpretation of speech errors produced by children with autism. The distinction between phonetic/articulatory disorders (which may be related to motor speech disorders) and language disorders (e.g. phonological disorders) is important to maintain because these two disorders probably do not have the same origin and do not have the same impact on language development.

What Are the Phonological Abilities of Individuals with Autism?

We now consider phonological difficulties from the vantage point of language disorders rather than speech sound disorders (recall Figure 4.4). Phonological disorders, unlike phonetic/articulatory disorders, involve difficulties not only in place and mode of articulation, as we will see, but also in maintaining the syllabic structure of a word. They are therefore language disorders. To make this clearer, regarding the phonemic level, consider a child who always fronts back consonants, meaning that words starting with the sound /k/ are systematically pronounced with a starting /t/ regardless of the following vowel. This is an articulatory difficulty. On the other hand, systematically substituting the place of articulation of a back consonant due to a specific, supportive (i.e. front) phonological context (see Figure 4.2) can be interpreted as a phonemic error – in other words, a phonological and therefore structural error. Regarding the syllabic level, the same could be said for lengthening a vowel instead of producing a liquid (/r, l/) in a specific syllabic position (e.g. the coda position). Imagine a child producing [paːti] instead of [paʁti] for the French word *parti* 'left', and at the same time producing [ʁ] correctly in other contexts, for instance in a simple onset position (*rat* 'rat' [ʁa]). Difficulties producing [ʁ] in the coda position can be seen as a sign of immature syllabic development or of difficulties with syllabic complexity in the case of impaired development, rather than an articulatory problem, as the child is unable to produce a phoneme in a specific syllabic position (the coda, or syllable-final position).

The prevalence of phonological disorders in autistic children has been reported to range between 25% and 50% from study to study. This variation has been claimed to depend on various factors, such as age, autism severity, and the presence of an associated disorder. For instance, Rapin et al. (2009) found severe and persistent phonological disorders in 24% of autistic children aged 7–9 years, while in Tuller et al. (2017) phonological disorders were observed in 50% of autistic children aged 6–12 years. For Boucher (2003), only a subset of children with autism have ("mild to moderate") phonological impairment, those with "Low Functioning Autism." In contrast, according to her, children with "Asperger Syndrome" or "High Functioning Autism" do not have any phonological impairment. The implication is that phonological impairment could be linked to **autism severity** (see below). Other explanations for phonological disorders include immature syllabic development (Paul et al. 2011) and a **chronological shift** in phonemic development, whereby a sound develops earlier or later compared to typical language acquisition (see the explanation for this particularity in the "Focus on a specific study" section) (Wolk and Edwards 1993). Low performance in phonology could also be due to the type of task used for assessment. In particular, tasks may call on extralinguistic skills, such as Short-Term Memory or Executive Function (e.g. inhibition), which is deficient or immature in many autistic children (see below).

Particular phonological characteristics appear very early in children at risk for autism who are later positively diagnosed. For instance, these children tend to have fewer vocalizations than TD children. Canonical **babbling** (i.e. the first adult-like syllable production period) is often delayed in autistic children. Canonical babbling is considered a developmental milestone, independent of environmental factors, which, if not initiated by 10 months of age, is a predictor of language delay or developmental disabilities. Moreover, babbling in autism generally contains a lower rate of canonical syllable production (CV syllables) (from 9 to 48 months), besides a lower rate of syllable types (i.e. diversity of syllable types) (Paul et al. 2011). These differences have been correlated with autism symptoms at age 2. A delay in canonical babbling may also lead to a delay, or even a deficit, in the construction of the most complex phonological structures later on. Another possible consequence of delayed canonical babbling is that as toddlers with autism vocalize less often, they have fewer opportunities to benefit from adult feedback.

Regarding **phonemic inventory**, which is the set of distinctive sound units (phonemes) that a speaker has at a specific age and which is used as a basic measure of phonological knowledge, fewer consonants and fewer consonant types are observed in very young children at high risk for autism, whose general developmental indices are nevertheless within norms (Paul et al. 2011; Pokorny et al. 2017).

When considering structural aspects of language in autism, it is necessary to look at reported results in a nuanced way. We know that language is not uniformly impaired in autistic individuals, be they adults or children. The lack of consensus regarding the existence of phonological impairment in this population is based primarily on group assessments of individuals with autism considered to form homogeneous language groups, whereas heterogeneity is at the very heart of autism. It is therefore very difficult to characterize language in individuals with autism in a uniform way. In recent research, individuals with autism are typically divided into two basic language groups: those with language impairment (ALI) and those for whom structural aspects of language are normal (ALN). In ALI, phonological performance is similar, quantitatively and qualitatively, to that observed in children without autism but with **Developmental Language Disorder** (DLD) (Riches et al. 2011; Tuller et al. 2017). Similarities in performance and errors (in type and proportion: about 45% substitution and 45% omission) have been observed in ALI children (see Chapter 1 for the distinction between ALI and ALN) and children with DLD (Tuller et al. 2017). In the same study, ALN children and TD younger children were found to score significantly higher than the first two groups on measures of expressive phonology. Additionally, errors on liquids /r, l/ were found in ALI children, which cannot be explained by age.

In ALI children, the phonological structures that are most affected are generally identical to those observed in DLD, and they always involve a higher degree of phonological complexity (Tuller et al. 2017). In particular, these children may have difficulties due to consonant clusters, especially in word-final position (e.g. in French, *thermomètre* 'thermometer' [tɛʁmomɛtʁ]) and those involving two stops (*tractor* 'tracteur' [tʁaktœʁ]), as well as internal codas (e.g. *horloge* 'clock' [ɔʁlɔʒ]). Yet, some structures that are extremely difficult for children with DLD may not be so for ALI children, such as consonant clusters containing /s/ (e.g. /sp/ and /sk/). This has been found in the word-final position (e.g. *casque* 'helmet' [kask]) and word-initial position (e.g. *spectacle* 'show' [spɛktakl]). In brief, impairment of complex syllabic structure is systematically found in some autistic children in studies that focus on phonology in fine detail. The findings reported above suggest that phonological complexity plays a major role in performance and could be used as a marker of language disorder in autistic individuals.

Zooming in on phonological processes reported for autistic children, atypical patterns of phonological acquisition have been found, such as segmental coalescence, whereby two sounds in contact combine into a single sound[5] (as in [wi] 'spring') and substitution of an intervocalic consonant (appearing between two vowels) by a glottal stop (as in *butter* [bʌʔə], for American English [ˈbʌɾɚ]). These would not be considered unusual (by therapists, for instance) if the focus was on the phonemes alone. Yet, these atypical patterns are observed at each level of the phonological structure, from the phonemic to the syllabic structure, very early in phonological development and throughout the autism spectrum. Finally, by manipulating the coarticulation effect between words, it has been shown that some children with autism (those with sufficient receptive language) use phonological information very efficiently to process speech as it is being produced. The effect of coarticulation on word recognition efficiency can even be greater in children with autism than in TD children with equal receptive language ability (Pomper et al. 2021). As children grow older, these atypical patterns tend to disappear, and the processes observed are similar to those of children with DLD without autism (see also Chapter 11 for other ASD/DLD comparisons).

Finally, some studies looked at a potential link between autism severity and phonological impairment. Boucher's (2003) claim that such a relationship exists, as seen above, has not been confirmed in recent studies, either for autistic children (Silleresi et al. 2020) or autistic adults (Manenti et al. 2024). These other studies identified language profiles based on the performance of the autistic participants on phonological measures or a combination of phonological and morphosyntactic measures (see also Chapter 10). With respect to autism severity, they reported no differences between the language profiles, and crucially, between the profiles with low and high phonological performance. Importantly, unlike Boucher (2003), these two studies used experimental tasks that specifically targeted structural phonological skills (specifically, syllabic complexity).

What Are the Limitations of Phonological Assessment in Autism?

As with studies of children with DLD, results depend more or less directly on how phonological skills are tested and how test performance is analyzed. Existing standardized, normed tests typically do not allow for fine-toothed assessment of phonological structures that may cause difficulties, or for distinguishing between processing or task management difficulties and underlying language impairment. We illustrate this issue by taking a look at the NEPSY Pseudoword Repetition task (Korkman 2004), a standardized test frequently used in studies on sound production in autism. This test was designed to assess Short-Term Memory, but it is frequently used as a proxy for phonological skills. It is composed of 13 items of

---

5 Coalescence involves both lenition (weakening of a sound that can make it more sonorous or to entirely disappear) and assimilation processes. It is also known as contraction or fusion.

two to five syllables. These pseudowords are close to English words (e.g. *crumsee*). Moreover, within items and across the task, phonological complexity is not balanced, meaning that some items contain one complex syllable and others several (e.g. ***pwaidumay***, ***bwelextiss***, ***pledgyfriskree***). Finally, some items contain sequences of sounds that correspond to affixes or true English words (e.g. *inkewsment*). All these characteristics mean that it is not possible to be sure that impaired phonology is the source of low scores for this task. Poor performance may also be due to difficulties in memory because of the very long items, those consisting of four or five syllables. It could also be due to articulatory difficulties because of motor programming challenges for some items. Another reason could be lexical difficulties because of items resembling English words or containing affixes, and therefore performance may be affected in individuals with poor lexical knowledge. Any combination of these factors could also contribute to low performance.

These observations can apply to other methods of language assessment. For example, Whitehouse, Barry, and Bishop (2008) assessed oromotor skills in children with ASD compared to children with DLD using difficult-to-pronounce sequences (e.g. *squish squash*) and tongue twisters (e.g. *put the pepper beads in the paper bag*), also from the NEPSY oromotor sequences subtest, and a sentence repetition task composed of sentences of increasing length and complexity (NEPSY Sentence repetition subtest). Their results showed that the children with DLD performed much worse on these tasks than the children with ASD. Since, for these authors, impairment in children with DLD is only due to a deficit in **Short-Term Memory**, the results were interpreted as suggesting that language disorders in autistic children have a different origin, i.e. they are not related to a deficit in Short-Term Memory. However, language deficits in children with DLD may also be related to phonological (and syntactic) difficulties, as shown in various studies. It is therefore not clear that impairment in autistic children and children with DLD should be different. While the question of the origin of language disorders is important, it is equally important to identify and characterize a possible phonological impairment in children with ASD in comparison with that of children with DLD, which may exist alongside a deficit in verbal Short-Term Memory. This is suggested by studies reporting that only ALI children show difficulties in verbal Short-Term Memory, which are related to the severity of their language deficits when compared to ALN children (Hill et al. 2015).

Focus on a Specific Study

Wolk and Giesen (2000) present a systematic phonological analysis of spontaneous language in autistic children by observing their phonological system and the phonological processes that they use. This article is important in that it highlights well-identified phonological processes by distinguishing between processes that are linked to articulation (phonetic) and those that are phonological. Another merit of the study is that it brings together previous work that uses the same type of phonological analysis. Moreover, this study is valuable because it observes four siblings with ASD, which allows for comparisons of autistic children with various degrees of language impairment who are growing up within the same linguistic context. The authors raise the difficulty of collecting analyzable language data in autistic children, particularly phonological data, and point out three nonexclusive explanations for this difficulty: production is sometimes unintelligible, jargon may be used, making the target to be transcribed opaque, and the quantity of language data produced may be very small.

The study analyses the language production of a group of siblings, including four with autism (one girl and three boys), aged 2.3–9.0 years, diagnosed at 2 years of age. They belong to a sibship of eight children, with the other four being described as having typical language development. The four children with autism all showed delays in both gross motor and fine motor skills (delay of one to four years depending on the child). For receptive and expressive language, the gap was even greater: between one and five years of delay. Articulatory and phonetic skills were described as being severely to moderately impaired.

Two methods of language elicitation were used: object naming via the Assessment of Phonological Process (APP; Hodson 1980) and spontaneous language based on toys and cards. For each of the children, the total number of words obtained by combining the production collected in the two tasks was computed. These values varied across the four autistic children due to heterogeneous language levels, from 2 to 100 words per child. This discrepancy is important to note as it highlights the difficulty of eliciting language production for some children. Indeed, studies on language in autism have tended not to include participants who have low IQ or who are minimally verbal because they are expected to have difficulties performing the tasks to be administered. The efforts deployed by the authors of this study to elicit and analyze language production by such children are therefore particularly noteworthy.

Two levels of phonological analysis were carried out: phonemic inventory of sounds in different word positions and analysis of phonological processes. In general, the results show that at least for the most severely impaired children, delayed phonological expression and atypical patterns that rarely occur in typical development were observed. Phonemic inventories varied greatly from one child to another, ranging from a complete inventory to a near-empty inventory for the child who produced only two words (*yes* /jɛ/ and *no* /ŋʌŋ/) and was considered primarily nonverbal. The most striking fact about these inventories was the presence of sounds that are normally acquired after sounds that were nonetheless absent (which is referred to as chronological shift). For example,

/θ, ʃ/ were present in the youngest child's inventory, but this child did not produce normally earlier-appearing nasals (/m, n, ɲ/) and voiceless stops (/p, t, k/). Similarly, /m/ was absent in the inventory of the child who was aged 3;9, who nevertheless had all sound classes (it was replaced by the sound /j/, as in *music box* [jujubɔks]). The analysis of phonological processes shows that phonological processes found in typical development often appeared in the production data of these children: vocalization (e.g. *get out* [geə]), liquid and /s/ cluster reduction (e.g. *clown* [kaʊn], *screwdriver* [kudaɪvə]), velar fronting (e.g. *can* [dʌn]), gliding of liquids (e.g. *fly* [fwai]), final consonant deletion (e.g. *dad* [dæ]), and initial voicing (e.g. *play* [bʌ]). However, unusual patterns also appeared, such as frication of stops (e.g. *crayon* [fwejɔn]), segment coalescence (e.g. *truck* [tʃʌk]), and velarization and frication of liquids (e.g. *ball* [bæθ]). In summary, the authors presented five general phonological patterns seen in these children, as listed in (2):

(2) General phonological patterns observed by Wolk and Giesen (2000):
- Evidence of several phonological processes equivalent to those found in typical development
- Persistence of phonological processes beyond typical age, such as labialization, cluster reduction, and final consonant deletion
- Evidence of unusual sound changes, such as extensive segment coalescence, frication of liquids, and velarization
- Evidence of chronological mismatch: absence of earlier sounds co-occurring with characteristics of later development
- Restricted use of contrasts between sounds (i.e. reduced phonemic inventory).

The authors also noted that the more language was affected, the more atypical the phonological processes and inventories were when compared to either typical development or language impairment. The authors therefore advocated for a phonological rather than a sound-by-sound analysis, as this allows unusual patterns to be observed so that conclusions beyond delayed phonology can be drawn.

While the proposed analysis is fundamentally what is expected of a phonological analysis, it has a crucial drawback. Analyzing spontaneous speech is labor-intensive since it is time consuming to transcribe and code speech samples. However, such precise and detailed observations of phonology allow us to go further in understanding what language impairment may look like in autism. An analysis based on a task built on specific phonological variables known to be sensitive to phonological impairment, as shown in Wolk and Giesen's study, would make it possible to draw detailed conclusions about the phonological strengths and weaknesses of autistic individuals. Such a tool could then be easily used by non-phonologists without the need for in-depth analysis of structures (see Chapter 16).

Conclusion

This chapter set out to address the following questions:

- What are the phonetic abilities of individuals with autism?
- What are the phonological abilities of individuals with autism?
- What are the limitations of phonological assessment in autism?

First of all, it is extremely important to bear in mind and to operationalize the distinction between speech (phonetics) and language (phonology) in analyzing and understanding the language production of children, especially those with language impairment. Unfortunately, the tools that are used across published studies do not always adequately distinguish between these two aspects, leading to interpretations that tend to overdiagnose (motor) speech deficits, that is, phonological deficits tend to be interpreted as (motor) speech deficits.

In children with autism, both motor speech (phonetic) disorders and phonological disorders can be observed, although they are not present in every child: some display typical speech-sound development, while others show difficulties in one or both of these domains from a very early age. Carefully distinguishing between these two types of impairment is also important because findings suggest that these disorders do not have the same origins (articulatory vs. structural language) and the same impact on language development.

Focusing on phonology, observations of children with autism are congruent: difficulties occur at every level, from the phoneme to the syllable. Similarities are found with children with DLD, although convergence in the structures affected and in the processes used does not appear to be absolute. It is noteworthy that autism severity seems to have little to do with the presence or absence of phonological impairment, as some children with a high severity do not show any impairment in phonology, and vice versa.

The inclusion of phonology in language assessment would contribute to a better understanding of overall language abilities, as well as the relation between phonology and other structural language domains (e.g. morphosyntax) in autism.

What Do You Know Now?
Phonology and phonetics are two different domains, and phonology can be impaired in ASD, with characteristics that resemble what is found in Developmental Language Disorder.
- Phonology is part of structural language. It deals with the organization and the role of abstract units such as sound classes (phonemes) and syllables.
- Motor speech impairment is distinct from phonological impairment; they may affect children with and without autism independently.
- Speakers with autism may have difficulties with sounds. This may be due to various reasons: they may have a motor speech (phonetic) deficit and/or a phonological deficit.
- Not all children with autism show such deficits. The severity of autism does not appear to determine whether a child has a speech sound disorder.
- Impaired sound structure in children with autism is similar to that observed in children with DLD, but they do not show exactly the same phonological processes and structures.
- There is a need for more studies with dedicated tools for the assessment of phonology.

Suggestions for Further Reading

If you want to know more about the early sound development of children at risk for autism, we recommend that you read Paul et al. 2011. It is one of the rare studies that investigate very early language development in infants at risk for ASD. If you want to read a synthesis of the work by Wolk and colleagues, read Wolk, Edwards, and Brennan 2016. It presents detailed and solid phonological analyses that avoid confusion with other aspects of language assessment. If you want to read more about the link between phonology and other language domains, we recommend that you read Pomper et al. 2021. It is a recent study that will allow you to understand how abilities in other domains contribute to phonological skills in children with autism.

References

Adams, L. (1998). Oral-motor and motor-speech characteristics of children with autism. *Focus on Autism and Other Developmental Disabilities* 13 (2): 108–112.

American Speech-Language-Hearing Association. (2017). *Child Apraxia of Speech*. Available at https://www.asha.org/policy/ps2007-00277/ (accessed 1 July 2024).

Bishop, D.V.M., Snowling, M.J., Thompson, P.A. et al. (2017). Phase 2 of CATALISE: a multinational and multidisciplinary Delphi consensus study of problems with language development: terminology. *The Journal of Child Psychology and Psychiatry* 58 (10): 1068–1080.

Boucher, J. (2003). Language development in autism. *International Congress Series* 1254: 247–253.

Chenausky, K., Brignell, A., Morgan, A. et al. (2019). Motor speech impairment predicts expressive language in minimally verbal, but not low verbal, individuals with autism spectrum disorder. *Autism and Developmental Language Impairments* 4: 10.

Chenausky, K.V. and Tager-Flusberg, H. (2022). The importance of deep speech phenotyping for neurodevelopmental and genetic disorders: a conceptual review. *Journal of Neurodevelopmental Disorders* 14 (1): 36.

Green, D., Charman, T., Pickles, A. et al. (2009). Impairment in movement skills of children with autistic spectrum disorders. *Developmental Medicine and Child Neurology* 51 (4): 311–316.

Hill, A.P., Van Santen, J., Gorman, K. et al. (2015). Memory in language-impaired children with and without autism. *Journal of Neurodevelopmental Disorders* 7 (1): 19.

Hodson, B.W. (1980). *The Assessment of Phonological Processes*. Danville, IL: The Interstate Printers & Publishers.

International Phonetic Association. (2015). *IPA Chart*. Available at: https://www.internationalphoneticassociation.org/content/ipa-chart (accessed 1 July 2024).

Kaufman, N.R. (1995). *Kaufman Speech Praxis Test for Children*. Wayne State: University Press.

Korkman, M. (2004). NEPSY-A tool for comprehensive assessment of neurocognitive disorders in children. In: *Comprehensive Handbook of Psychological Assessment, Vol. 1: Intellectual and Neuropsychological Assessment* (eds. M. Hersen, G. Goldstein, and S. Beers), 1: 157–176. Hoboken, NJ: Wiley.

LeBarton, E.S. and Landa, R.J. (2019). Infant motor skill predicts later expressive language and autism spectrum disorder diagnosis. *Infant Behavior and Development* 54: 37–47.

Manenti, M., Ferré, S., Tuller, L. et al. (2024). Profiles of structural language and nonverbal intellectual abilities in verbal autistic adults. *Research in Autism Spectrum Disorders* 114: 102361.

McKeever, L., Cleland, J., and Delafield-Butt, J. (2022). Using ultrasound tongue imaging to analyse maximum performance tasks in children with Autism: a pilot study. *Clinical Linguistics and Phonetics* 36 (2–3): 127–145.

Paul, R., Fuerst, Y., Ramsay, G. et al. (2011). Out of the mouths of babes: vocal production in infant siblings of children with ASD. *Journal of Child Psychology and Psychiatry* 52 (5): 588–598.

Pokorny, F.B., Schuller, B., Marschik, P.B. et al. (2017). Earlier identification of children with Autism Spectrum Disorder: an automatic vocalisation-based approach. *Proceedings Interspeech* 2017: 309–313.

Pomper, R., Ellis Weismer, S., Saffran, J. et al. (2021). Coarticulation facilitates lexical processing for toddlers with autism. *Cognition* 214: 104799.

Prizant, B.M. (1996). Brief report: communication, language, social, and emotional development. *Journal of Autism and Developmental Disorders* 26 (2): 173–178.

Rapin, I., Dunn, M.A., Allen, D.A. et al. (2009). Subtypes of language disorders in school-age children with autism. *Developmental Neuropsychology* 34 (1): 66–84.

Riches, N.G., Loucas, T., Baird, G. et al. (2011). Non-word repetition in adolescents with specific language impairment and autism plus language impairments: a qualitative analysis. *Journal of Communation Disorders* 44 (1): 23–36.

Rivière, J., Lécuyer, R., and Hickmann, M. (2009). Early locomotion and the development of spatial language: evidence from young children with motor impairments. *European Journal of Developmental Psychology* 6 (5): 548–566.

Shriberg, L.D. (2009). Childhood speech sound disorders: from postbehaviorism to the postgenomic era. In: *Speech Sound Disorders in Children: In Honor of Lawrence D. Shriberg* (eds. R. Paul and P. Flipsen), 1–33. San Diego, CA: Plural Pub.

Silleresi, S., Prévost, P., Zebib, R. et al. (2020). Identifying language and cognitive profiles in children with ASD via a cluster analysis exploration: implications for the new ICD-11. *Autism Research* 13: 155–1167. Strand, E. (2017). Appraising apraxia when a speech-sound disorder is severe. How do you know if it's childhood apraxia of speech? *ASHA Leader* 22 (3): 50–58.

Tuller, L., Ferré, S., Prévost, P. et al. (2017). The effect of computational complexity on the acquisition of French by children with ASD. In: *Innovative Investigations of Language in Autism Spectrum Disorder* (ed. L.R. Naigles), 115–140. Berlin: de Gruyter.

West, K.L. (2019). Infant motor development in Autism Spectrum Disorder: a synthesis and meta-analysis. *Child Development* 90 (6): 2053–2070.

Whitehouse, A.J., Barry, J.G., and Bishop, D.V. (2008). Further defining the language impairment of autism: is there a specific language impairment subtype? *Journal of Communication Disorders* 41 (4): 319–336.

Wolk, L. and Edwards, M.L. (1993). The emerging phonological system of an autistic child. *Journal of Communication Disorders* 26 (3): 161–177.

Wolk, L., Edwards, M.L., and Brennan, C. (2016). Phonological difficulties in children with autism: an overview. *Speech, Language and Hearing* 19 (2): 121–129.

Wolk, L. and Giesen, J. (2000). A phonological investigation of four siblings with childhood autism. *Journal of Communication Disorders* 33 (5): 371–389.

5

Semantics

Francesca Foppolo and Francesca Panzeri

> **What Do You Think?**
> Leo and Ann are talking about their son Ed, who is autistic and will soon start school. Ann is worried that he may have problems attending regular schools because she read that many autistic individuals have language difficulties. Leo is convinced that since Ed knows a lot of words, he won't have any problems. What do you think?
>
> Susan and Max are chatting about Susan's birthday party. Susan says that she is a bit disappointed because every guest did not bring a present. Max is surprised and says that all her friends are impolite given that none of them brought anything. Susan laughs because she meant that not all the guests brought a present (although some did). Which interpretation would you have given? Which interpretation do you think an autistic individual might prefer? Why?

Introduction

While Chapter 2 discusses words, including their meaning (lexical semantics), this chapter focuses on the meaning of sentences, which is called **semantics**: how the meaning of a sentence is derived from the meaning of its parts and the way these parts are combined. For example, in (1), depending on how the word *not* is combined with the word *every*, the sentence means "some but not all the guests brought a present" or "none of the guests brought a present":

(1) Every guest did not bring a present.

Semantics explains how we derive the meaning of a sentence compositionally, taking into account (i) lexical semantics, e.g. the meaning of **content words** (words with intrinsic meaning, lexically defined), such as *chair* (noun), *swim* (verb), *small* (adjective), *carefully* (adverb) (see Chapter 2); (ii) syntax, the way elements are combined in a sentence, including **function words** (words/phrases that express relationships between other words or phrases), such as the quantifier *all* or the connective *and*, and their interactions; (iii) morphology, i.e. word structure, including elements such as the temporal marker *-ed* or the aspectual marker *-ing* on English verbs; and (iv) pragmatics, i.e. language in context, including world knowledge and other discourse factors (see Chapters 6–8).

This chapter presents and discusses existing research on semantics and autism and identifies gaps and limitations that need to be taken into account in future research. Focusing on the influence of syntax and morphology on semantics, we address the following questions:

- Are combinatorial rules of sentential elements challenging for autistic individuals?
- Are function words such as quantifiers and connectives and their interactions challenging for autistic individuals?
- Are temporal and aspectual markers challenging for autistic individuals?

Anchoring

One of the defining characteristics of human language is its productivity. This encompasses the fact that competent speakers are able to produce and understand a potentially infinite number of sentences that they have never heard before in their native language(s). Semantics, the discipline that studies the meaning of linguistic expressions, explains this ability with the **Principle of Compositionality**. This principle states that the meaning of an expression is a function of the meaning of its parts (the words) and of the way they are syntactically and morphologically combined. This section introduces some basic semantic operations involved in the derivation of the meaning of complex expressions, and it indicates when these are acquired by neurotypical children. We restrict our attention to those semantic phenomena that have been investigated in autism and that are not covered by other chapters in this book.

One basic principle underlying semantic composition is the

Acronym and Terminology Reminder
ALI: Autism with language impairment.
ALN: Autism with normal language.
Aspect (Aspectual): Expression of how an action, event, or state extends over time (i.e. if it is ongoing or completed).
Compound: Combination of two words to make another word (e.g. *dishwasher*).
Connective: Word/phrase that links words, phrases, or clauses (e.g. conjunction *and*, disjunction *or*, negation *not*).
Content Word: Word with intrinsic meaning, lexically defined (e.g. *chair*).

combination of words. For instance, adjectives combine with nouns (e.g. *blue square*), and **compounds** are combinations of two words that make another word (e.g. *dishwasher*). To understand the meaning of a compound expression, it is necessary not only to identify the two parts but also the semantic relationship between them. So, for example, the word *bread* in *breadknife* modifies the word *knife* to make it a type of knife (which is used to cut bread), and the word *cinnamon* in the compound *cinnamon bread* modifies the word *bread* to make it a type of bread. McGregor et al. (2010) suggest that the identification of the semantic relationship between the two words that form a compound may be challenging for children with Developmental Language Disorder (DLD – language abilities below age expectations not attributable to any other condition): even if they can correctly identify the nouns in conventional noun–noun compounds such as *bookshelf*, they struggle describing the semantic relation between them (they may say, for example, "books go on shelves"). We will see in the main section that some autistic children experience similar challenges.

Another example of semantic composition concerns verb phrases, which combine a verb and its complement, for example, an object. A transitive verb may restrict the range of possible objects, something

---

DLD: Developmental Language Disorder. Language abilities below age expectations not attributable to any other condition.

Existential Quantifier: Function word such as *some* that places at least one element in the set to which the noun belongs.

Function Word: Word/phrase that expresses a relationship between other words or phrases (e.g. *every, and, not*).

Inverse Scope: When the order in which function words are logically combined is the opposite of the order in which they appear in the sentence.

IPL: Intermodal Preferential Looking – experimental method in which a visual scene is described by auditory stimulus while eye movements of participants are recorded.

Lexical Restriction: Requirement imposed by the lexical meaning of a verb on the type/class of nouns that can follow it (e.g. the verb *eat* requires edible objects).

LI: Language impairment.

Morpheme: The smallest unit of language that has meaning, either a word (e.g. *work*) or a part of a word (*-er* or *-s*, in *work-er-s*).

Quantifier: Word/phrase expressing relations of quantity between sets of objects or individuals, e.g. *all, some, each*.

Scope: Part of sentence to which a function word applies.

Semantics (sentence-level): How the meaning of a sentence is derived from the meaning of its parts and the way these parts are combined.

Surface Scope: When the order in which function words are logically combined follows the order in which they appear in the sentence.

SVO: Subject-verb-object word order.

Temporal Marker/Morpheme: Word or part of the word that expresses collocation in time of the event (its **Tense**, i.e. if it occurs in the past, present, or future).

Thematic Role: Semantic role noun phrase has in an event (e.g. agent, patient, …); who-does-what-to-whom?

Universal Quantifier: Function word such as *every* or *all* that refers to the entire set to which the noun belongs.

that is referred to as **lexical restriction**. This is a requirement imposed by the lexical meaning of a verb on the type/class of nouns that can follow it. For example, the verb *eat* can take edible objects only, which is why example (2b) is perceived as semantically anomalous (marked with a #), despite it being syntactically well-formed.

(2) a. Lia *ate* a cake.
    b. # Lia *ate* a book.

Mani and Huettig (2012) show that, already by age 2, neurotypical toddlers interpret sentences incrementally, based on the lexical restrictions of the verb. They used the **Intermodal Preferential Looking (IPL) paradigm,** an experimental method in which a visual scene is described by auditory stimulus while eye movements of participants are recorded. Mani and Huettig (2012) presented sentences auditorily, such as *The boy eats/sees the big cake*, along with a visual scenario depicting a cake on one side and a nonedible object on the other (Figure 5.1). After hearing *eats*, but not after hearing *sees*, the 2-year-olds looked at the image of the cake (before hearing the word *cake*). In other words, at hearing *eats*, they predicted the type of object that could follow, namely, an edible object. Importantly, the children's prediction skills were significantly correlated with their productive vocabulary size assessed by parental communicative inventory reports but not with their receptive vocabulary size assessed in a similar manner.

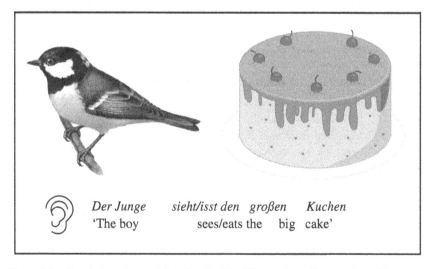

Figure 5.1 Simulation of one of the stimuli of the IPL paradigm. *Source:* Adapted from Mani and Huettig (2012) by Francesca Panzeri.

At sentence level, word order provides fundamental information to interpret a sentence (see also Chapter 3):

(3) a. The dog is biting the girl.
  b. The girl is biting the dog.

To interpret the sentences in (3), we need to understand who is doing what to whom. This requires the identification of **thematic roles**: semantic roles that noun phrases have in an event. For example, we must associate the thematic roles of **Agent** (the doer of the action, the dog in (3a)) and **Patient** (the undergoer/target of the action, the girl in (3a)) with the noun phrases of the sentence. The manner in which thematic roles are associated with noun phrases differs per language. Languages such as English, which have a strict subject–verb–object (SVO) order, identify thematic roles based on the order in which the elements appear in the sentence (see (3)). Other languages may depend on other cues for the identification of thematic roles. For instance, Turkish allows for various word orders, but the direct object can be identified by **accusative** case (inflection attached to the object). In Mandarin Chinese, where word order is flexible and subject and/or object are frequently omitted, thematic roles are often recovered from the context.

Candan et al. (2012) tested the ability to identify thematic roles (Agent, Patient, ...) based on word order in neurotypical children aged 1–3 years, in English, Turkish, and Mandarin Chinese. To assess comprehension in children of this age, they used the IPL paradigm, presenting sentences describing an event and two videos showing the event with correct and inverted thematic roles. Increased looks at the video matching the sentence are interpreted as evidence that participants understand the sentence. The results show that infants acquiring English, a language that has strict SVO order, can identify the agent and patient of action on the basis of word order already at age 1;6, whereas more time is required for children who are learning a language with more flexible word order, such as Turkish (2 years) or Mandarin Chinese (almost 3 years).

Another case in which words serve as instructions on how to combine linguistic units is that of function words such as quantifiers and connectives. **Quantifiers** are words or phrases that express relations of quantity between sets of objects or individuals. Consider (4):

(4) (Two/Some/All/None) of the girls ate the cake.

Simplifying, *girls* denotes the set of individuals who are girls, and *ate the cake* is also a set of individuals, the cake-eaters. The semantic contribution of the quantifiers follows from set-theoretic operations on these two sets: the **numerical** quantifier *two* requires the two sets to have (at least) two elements in common; the **existential quantifier** *some* requires that the set of *girls* is not disjoint from the set of *cake-eaters* (i.e. they have at least one element in common); the **universal quantifier** *all* requires that the set of *girls* is included in the set of *cake-eaters*; the **negative quantifier** *none* requires that the two sets are disjoint (i.e. they have no element in common). Other types of function words are **connectives**. A connective is a word or phrase that links words, phrases, or sentences (e.g. conjunction *and*, disjunction *or*, negation *not*).

In general, neurotypical children as young as 2 already use negation to deny statements. They also master conjunctions and numerical and universal quantifiers by the age of 3, while they struggle with the various interpretations of disjunction (*or*) and of the existential quantifier (*some*) up to at least age 5 (Chierchia et al. 2001; Hurewitz et al. 2006) (see also Chapter 6).

Quantifiers can also contribute to sentence meaning by interacting with other function words. When two (or more) function words (such as *every* and *not*) appear in the same sentence, as in (5), **semantic ambiguity** arises, as in (6), making sentence (5) true and false in different situations:

(5) *Every* horse did *not* jump over the fence.

(6) a. Not every horse jumped over the fence.
b. Every horse is such that it did not jump over the fence.

If two of four horses (Figure 5.2) did not jump over the fence but the others did, (5) is true under the reading in (6a) – since horses 3 and 4 did not jump – while it is false under (6b) – since horses 1 and 2 did jump. Considering the linear order in which the two function words appear in the sentence (*every...not*), (6a) represents what is called the **inverse scope** reading: when the order in which the function words are logically combined is the opposite of the order in which they appear in the sentence. **Scope** is the part of the sentence to which a function word applies. In (6a), negation (*not*) **takes scope** over the universal quantifier (*every*), thus inverting the linear order of the elements (NOT>EVERY), as they appear in (5). Conversely, the meaning in (6b) represents what is called the **surface scope** reading, when the order in which function words are logically combined follows the order in which they appear in the sentence (EVERY>NOT).

Semantic ambiguity ensuing from the interaction of two (or more) function words in the same sentence constitutes a challenge for semantic composition. Several studies in language acquisition report that, while adults accept (5) in a situation in which two out of three horses jump over a fence, compatible with the inverse scope interpretation (6a), children typically reject it, favoring the surface scope interpretation (6b) (Musolino and Lidz 2002; see Gualmini 2008 for a pragmatic explanation).

Some words or parts of words, called **morphemes**, contribute to sentence meaning by operating on other linguistic elements. A morpheme is the smallest

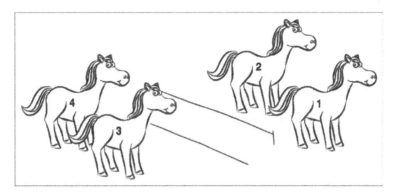

Figure 5.2 Example of a scenario accompanying the sentence in (5). *Source:* Scontras and Pearl (2021).

unit of language that has meaning. Consider (7), in which the lexical verb *to bake* appears in the **progressive**, with morpheme -*ing* (a), or the **perfective**, with morpheme -*ed* (b):

(7) a. Yesterday, Lia *was baking* a cake.
    b. Yesterday, Lia *baked* a cake.

When verbs appear in a sentence, morphosemantic information is added. For example, **temporal** markers or morphemes express the collocation of an event in time (its **Tense**, i.e. if it occurs in the past, present, or future). **Aspectual** markers or morphemes express how an action, event, or state extends over time, i.e. if it is ongoing or completed. In (7a), the aspectual progressive morpheme -*ing* contributes the meaning that the cake-baking event was in progress at the time at which the sentence was uttered and, possibly, is still incomplete (e.g. the oven broke down before the cake was fully baked). The morpheme -*ed* (representing both past tense and perfective aspect) on the verb *bake* in (7b) presents the event as completed in the past.

Neurotypical children use tense/aspect morphemes (such as -*ed*, -*ing*) from an early age. However, full mastery of aspectual properties develops around age 3, or even later. Wagner, Swensen, and Naigles (2009) tested American English-speaking neurotypical children aged 2 and 3 by monitoring children's eye movements in an IPL paradigm. The children heard sentences such as *She is picking the flowers* (progressive) or *She picked the flowers* (perfective) while two videos were shown simultaneously: one in which a woman was still in the process of picking flowers and one in which she picked them all. Both groups reliably looked more at the ongoing event with the progressive (-*ing*) and at the completed event with a perfective morpheme (-*ed*).

Semantics in Autism

Research to date on the sentence-level semantic abilities of autistic individuals is relatively scarce. Existing studies have often been based on small participant groups and have almost exclusively focused on autistic individuals with typical language (ALN), as opposed to autistic people with language impairment (ALI) and minimally verbal people. One notable exception to the latter is Vicente, Barbarroja, and Castroviejo (2023).

Are Combinatorial Rules of Sentential Elements Challenging for Autistic Individuals?

Vicente, Barbarroja, and Castroviejo (2023) tested a small sample of seven Spanish-speaking autistic adults (age range: 21–60) with intellectual disability and minimal receptive vocabulary (their mean mental age was 1;2–3;10, as assessed by the PPVT-III [see Chapter 1] for Spanish). The authors investigated whether these autistic participants could understand basic semantic adjective+noun combinations such as *red broom* by pointing to the red broom in a scenario with two brooms (one red, one green) and two drums (one red, one green). They tested color and size (*big, small*) adjectives. Only one participant demonstrated full understanding of this basic semantic operation, while another one understood the combination of a noun with size, but not color, adjectives. Even though the small sample of participants limits conclusions, this study suggests that semantic composition may be particularly challenging for autistic individuals with minimal receptive vocabulary, even though it is not yet clear whether the problems are to be imputed to the diagnosis of autism or to linguistic and/or intellectual disability.

Compound words are another way in which basic semantic composition can be represented. Kambanaros, Christou, and Grohmann (2019) investigated implicit and explicit knowledge of compound words in four Greek autistic children aged between 6;3 and 8;9, diagnosed as language impaired and with a nonverbal IQ within the norms. Focusing on noun+noun compounds (e.g. *domatoximós* 'tomato juice'), they tested the children's ability to recognize the two noun constituents and to explain the relation between them (e.g. by saying that *tomato juice* is a juice made of tomatoes, and a *mouse trap* is a trap for mice). Even if autistic children had no difficulty in recognizing the nouns constituting the compound, they struggled to explain the compound's meaning, similar to what was found for children with DLD (as discussed in the Anchoring section). For example, they said that *avlóporta* ('yard gate') is "the gate that has a yard." The authors hypothesize that this difficulty in explaining compounds may be related to weaker lexical-semantic knowledge.

These first two studies, conducted on small samples of participants with minimal receptive vocabulary or general language impairment (LI), found weaknesses in basic semantic composition. What about autistic children whose language development is typical? As seen in the Anchoring section, neurotypical children are able to use a verb's lexical restriction: the verb's meaning restricts the range of its possible objects. For instance, they look for edible objects as soon as they hear the verb *eat*. This anticipation requires the integration of linguistic meaning with perceptually accessible objects. Autistic individuals have often been described as experiencing difficulties in integrating information from different sources, which has been formulated as the **Weak Central Coherence Hypothesis** (Frith 1989). Brock et al. (2008) investigated whether weakness in central coherence may impact the ability of predicting the object of a verb. They tested 24 autistic adolescents aged 15 and a control group matched on age, nonverbal intelligence, and language skills (vocabulary and grammar comprehension). Similar to Mani and Huettig (2012), they monitored participants' eye gazes during sentences with highly constraining verbs ("Sam stroked the…," where *stroke* requires an animate object) or neutral verbs ("Sam chose the…," where *chose* can be followed by either an animate or inanimate object). The authors found that autistic participants looked at the animate object (a hamster) upon hearing *stroke*, showing that they were able to integrate linguistic and visual cues incrementally. Inspecting the correlation of this ability with linguistic scores (by considering a composite score of language) and autistic characteristics, they report that participants with poorer language showed reduced ability to integrate verbal and visual cues, irrespective of their autism diagnosis. This suggests that language competence, and not central coherence, predicts autistic children's performance in online tasks on lexical restriction. With the same paradigm, Zhou, Zhan, and Ma (2019) tested Mandarin-speaking autistic children (mean age 5;7) and two neurotypical control groups: one matched on age and one on both Mean-Length-of-Utterance (MLU) and verbal IQ. They report that autistic 5-year-olds, like neurotypicals, showed anticipatory eye movements during real-time sentence comprehension, thus using lexical-semantic information of verbs to predict upcoming linguistic input. Nonetheless, the 5-year-old autistic children exhibited fewer looks to the target area than their neurotypical peers and patterned like 4-year-old neurotypical children in this respect. The authors interpret this pattern as a developmental delay rather than as a language processing deficit, which may be due to lower cognitive control of visual attention and not to linguistic knowledge per se.

Bavin et al. (2016) investigated another case of semantic integration, namely the combination of an adjective with a noun. They presented sentences such as *Look at the blue square with dots* in a visual display with four squares: the target, two distractors (squares that were not blue), and a competitor (a blue square but without dots). If participants integrated the meaning of the adjective (*blue*) with that of the noun it refers to (*square*), they should immediately look away from the two distractors, focusing on the two blue squares only, and then wait until the disambiguating prepositional phrase (*with the dots*) to converge on the target. Bavin et al. tested 48 autistic children and 56 neurotypical children (aged 5–9) and found that both groups of children performed well in terms of the order of looks. Nevertheless, the autistic children were slower than the neurotypical group in both phases, namely, in ignoring the distractors and in converging on the target. Also, participants who were older or had higher scores on sustained attention performed better. The authors linked these results to autistic children's difficulties in performing a fast integration of the auditory stimuli, to their style of visual processing, or to problems integrating auditory and visual information. However, the fact that performance improved with age suggests that the incremental processing of words' meanings may be delayed but not impaired in the developmental trajectory of autistic children.

Turning to word order, and to the mapping of noun phrases to thematic roles, autistic children demonstrate an intact, even if delayed, comprehension of SVO order in English. Swensen et al. (2007) used the IPL paradigm to test autistic infants (mean age = 33 months) and a group of younger neurotypical children of 21 months matched on vocabulary with the MacArthur-Bates Communicative Developmental Inventory. They found that both groups looked longer at the video matching the target sentence, without significant group differences. Interestingly, both groups showed evidence of comprehension of the SVO order before being able to produce full sentences.

Su and Naigles (2019) investigated sensitivity to word order in Mandarin Chinese, a language in which, as discussed in the Anchoring section, word order is not fixed, and in which the subject and/or the object are frequently omitted if they are recoverable from the context. Given the difficulties experienced by some autistic individuals in considering contextual and discourse cues (see also Chapter 6), they may have problems understanding bare verb sentences (i.e. sentences with omitted subjects and objects), thus failing to use them to learn the SVO construction. The study tested a large cohort (N = 70) of autistic children, with a mean age of 50 months and variable linguistic profiles, and 52 younger neurotypical children (33 months) who were more proficient than the autistic group in both vocabulary and sentence production. With the IPL paradigm, the experimenters presented sentences such as "The bird is pushing the horse!" and monitored eye movements directed to the matching video or its competitor (a video of a horse pushing a bird). Overall, while both groups of children looked longer at the matching video, autistic children showed reliable-looking preferences for the matching video during the second half of the test trials only. Moreover, autistic children with higher linguistic abilities performed better, even if some of the minimally verbal children (cf. Chapter 10) demonstrated comprehension of SVO order too.

In summary, there is evidence that autistic individuals are able to use semantic operations that require the combination of words or phrases. Autistic children: (i) recognize the elements of a compound expression (Kambanaros, Christou, and Grohmann 2019); (ii) integrate the lexical meaning of a verb to predict its object (Brock et al. 2008; Bavin et al. 2016; Zhou, Zhan, and Ma 2019); (iii) rely on word order to understand who-did-what-to-whom not only in English (Swensen et al. 2007) but also in Mandarin Chinese (Su and Naigles 2019). Importantly, semantic challenges in autistic individuals seem more tied to their language abilities (vocabulary and/or morphosyntax) than to their autism diagnosis. They have difficulty explaining the meaning of compounds, similar to children with DLD. Their performance in predicting the object of a highly restrictive verb correlates with their language scores and not with autism severity (Brock et al. 2008). However, one study suggests that semantic composition may be particularly challenging for autistic participants with both impaired language and intellectual disability (Vicente, Barbarroja, and Castroviejo 2023).

Are Function Words Such as Quantifiers and Connectives and Their Interactions Challenging for Autistic Individuals?

As seen in the Anchoring section, neurotypical children show early mastery of the universal quantifiers *every/all* and of the conjunction *and*, but tend to struggle with the interpretations of the existential quantifier *some* and disjunction *or* until the age of about five. Since the derivation of the enriched meaning of *some* and *or* (*some but not all* and *A or B, but not both*) is linked to pragmatic considerations, many studies have focused on autistic individuals' interpretation of these function words (see Chapter 6). All these studies also included quantifiers and connectives as control items, tested in conditions in which they were blatantly true or false. Given that knowing the basic semantic (logical) meaning of quantifiers and connectives is crucial to understanding the mechanisms involved in semantics (independently of pragmatics), it is important to assess this knowledge in autistic individuals.

Behavioral experimental studies conducted with Dutch-speaking adults (Pijnacker et al. 2009) and children (Schaeken, Van Haeren, and Bambini 2018) have shown that autistic individuals know the semantic meaning of the universal quantifier *all* and of the existential quantifier *some*. They accept *all* in true and informative situations (e.g. *Some birds are sparrows*; Pijnacker et al. 2009) and reject *all* in false situations (e.g. *He picked some of the yellow flowers* in a context in which he picked only red flowers; Schaeken, Van Haeren, and Bambini 2018). Studies by Chevallier et al. (2010), with English-speaking adolescents, and Pijnacker et al. (2009), with Dutch-speaking adults, indicate that semantic knowledge of connectives (*and* and *or*) does not differ between autistic and neurotypical participants.

Different results were obtained by Su and Su (2015) with Mandarin-speaking autistic children and adolescents aged 4–15 (and further divided into two groups based on age: 14 between 4;2 and 8;5; 14 between 9;4 and 15;2). The study also included two comparison groups of neurotypical children, one matching the younger autistic group on age, gender, and receptive vocabulary and nonverbal IQ, and the other one matching the older autistic group on age and gender only. Su and Su used a Truth Value Judgment task in which participants had to evaluate statements containing the quantifier *some* and the connective *or*. In one condition, *or* interacted with the universal quantifier *every*, as in *Every child got a starfish or a shell*. This sentence had to be evaluated at the end of a story that made the sentence true (two of the children found a starfish and the other two a shell), false (one child found a starfish, one child a shell, but two of the children found nothing), or under informative (all children found both a shell and a starfish). While the performance of the neurotypical children in both groups was at ceiling in all the true and false conditions, the autistic children in both age groups performed at ceiling only with *some* but lagged behind their peers in the case of *or* interacting with the universal quantifier (*every*). Specifically, children in the two autistic groups rejected the sentence *Every child got a starfish or a shell* when two of the children found a starfish and the other two a shell: the rejection rate was 59% in the younger group and 34% in the older group, compared to 7% for their neurotypical peers. Additionally, the younger autistic children had a higher acceptance rate (26%) of the same sentence in the scenario that made it false; all the children in the other groups correctly rejected it 100% of the time.

To summarize, autistic individuals with typical language (vocabulary and/or morphosyntax) abilities seem to display relative strengths in the semantic interpretation of quantifiers (*some, all*) and connectives (*and, or*) across languages. Meanwhile, autistic children and adolescents have shown delayed semantic knowledge when two function words interact, for example, *every* and *or* (Su and Su 2015). We return to this latter point below.

Are Temporal and Aspectual Markers Challenging for Autistic Individuals?

The Anchoring section discussed how morphological cues contribute important semantic information. So, for instance, a past can be presented as completed (*baked the cake*) or as ongoing (*was baking the cake*). It has been claimed that autistic children have difficulty producing temporal (e.g. -*ed*) and aspectual morphemes (e.g. -*ing*). Bartolucci, Pierce, and Streiner (1980) found high omission rates in 10-year-old autistic children, though Roberts, Rice, and Tager-Flusberg (2004), Tek et al. (2014), and Modyanova, Perovic, and Wexler (2017) reported that these omissions seem limited to those autistic children with LI. Hypothesizing that such difficulties were due to study task demands in young children (e.g. participants had to talk about nonpresent events or to provide a pragmatically appropriate response), Tovar, Fein, and Naigles (2015) used the IPL paradigm. They tested 22 English-speaking 4-year-old autistic children using the same experimental design as in Wagner, Swensen, and Naigles (2009) (see the Anchoring section). They found that autistic 4-year-olds behaved like the (younger) neurotypical children in that study, looking significantly more quickly at the matching than the mismatching scene for both progressive -*ing* and past perfective -*ed* morphemes. Moreover, children's performance on the progressive marker correlated significantly with their production of aspectual markers and with their vocabulary knowledge (scores in the Receptive language scale of the Mullen Scales of Early Learning), but not with their ADOS score.

Chen et al. (2022) investigated the comprehension and production of aspectual morphemes in Mandarin Chinese: the imperfective markers *zai* and *zhe* (indicating that the event is ongoing and that it has a duration, respectively) and the perfective markers -*le* and -*guo* (signaling that the event is completed and that it has been experienced at least once in the past, respectively). They tested three groups of Mandarin-speaking 5-year-olds: 20 autistic children with LI, 20 children with DLD, and 20 neurotypical children. For comprehension, they employed a sentence-picture matching task: participants were shown three images depicting the initial, middle, and final stages of an event while hearing a sentence in which the verb was accompanied by one of the aspectual morphemes described above. The participants' task was to indicate the image corresponding to the sentence. Only the durative marker *zhe* was understood well in all groups. Regarding the comprehension of *zai* (ongoing), -*le* (completion), and -*guo* (at least once), the autistic children with LI and the children with DLD performed significantly more poorly than the neurotypical children, and there were no significant differences between the two clinical groups. Regarding production, an elicitation task was used, providing participants with specific sentences to describe (ongoing or completed) events in pictures (e.g. *A little girl is drinking a cup of juice*) and prompting them to use similar sentences to describe a picture depicting a similar event (e.g. *The man is building a house*). The two clinical groups performed more poorly than their neurotypical peers, with the autistic children producing more irrelevant or ungrammatical sentences than the other two groups. Interestingly though, a study using the IPL paradigm found different results. Su and Naigles (2021) tested the comprehension of the perfective and the progressive markers in 56 autistic

Mandarin-speaking children aged 2–6, who had dramatically delayed vocabulary production levels (21 of them were minimally verbal). These children rarely produced any aspectual markers, but they looked reliably longer at the videos matching sentences containing the progressive and perfective aspectual markers.

These studies suggest that autistic children may experience difficulties in **explicit** tasks, which require a behavioral response (such as pointing at an image or producing a sentence), at least when the children have LI (Roberts, Rice, and Tager-Flusberg 2004; Tek et al. 2014; Modyanova, Perovic, and Wexler 2017). This could be the case in, for example, the studies by Chen et al. (2022) and Bartolucci, Pierce, and Streiner (1980), which explicitly tap both comprehension and production of some aspectual morphemes. Nevertheless, when **implicit** measures are used (as in the IPL paradigm, which monitors eye gaze), autistic children do demonstrate an understanding of the semantic contribution of aspectual morphemes (Tovar, Fein, and Naigles 2015; Su and Naigles 2021). The use of implicit measures may attenuate social or pragmatic demands that may be independently challenging for individuals on the autism spectrum, yielding results otherwise unobtainable.

Focus on a Specific Study

This section focuses on the study by Noveck et al. (2007) because it tackles a core question in semantic composition, namely the interaction between function words in a sentence. It constitutes a crucial test case to understand how function words interact in a sentence, yielding different interpretations. Despite their derivational complexity, sentences of this kind are frequently used in communication, so it is important to assess the challenges they may present to autistic individuals.

We have seen that neurotypical children seem to prefer to interpret sentences such as *Every horse did not jump over the fence* (cf. (5)) according to the order in which the function words appear (EVERY>NOT), whereas adults prefer the inverse interpretation (NOT>EVERY). Noveck et al. took this semantic puzzle as a starting point to test a group of 15 French-speaking autistic adolescents (mean chronological age: 16;3 and mean mental age of 8;9). These were compared to a group of 19 French-speaking neurotypical 4-year-olds and a group of French-speaking neurotypical adults. The authors employed a Truth Value Judgment task comprising 10 stories about three people or three objects. Each story was accompanied by a drawing depicting one of two possible interpretations in which either two out of three characters performed the action mentioned in

Statement	Presentation condition	
	2-of-3 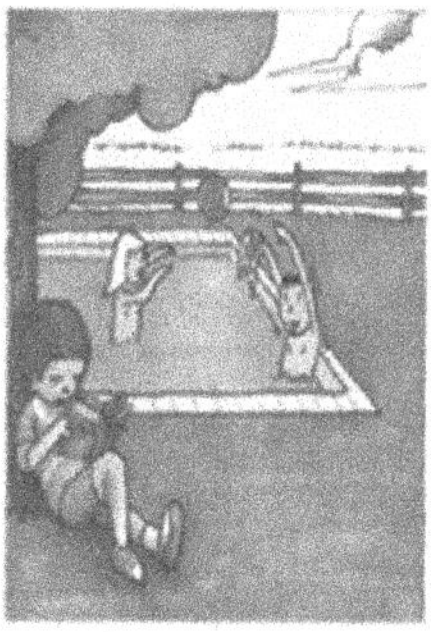	3-of-3 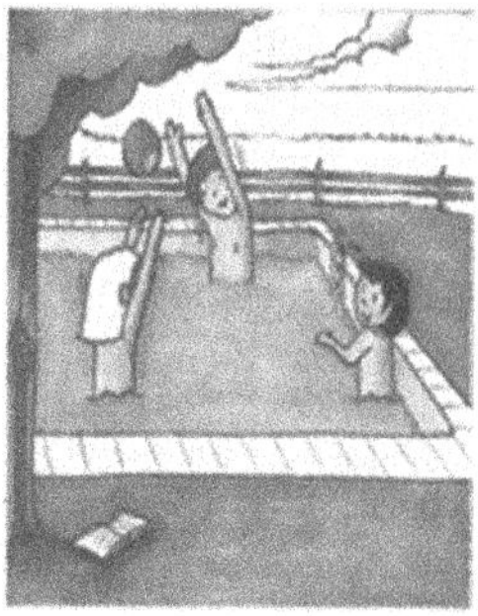
QN: All the children are not in the pool.	?	F
QP: All the children are in the pool.	F	T

Notes. The ? indicates that this is the main test statement and that the truth value depends on the participant's reading. It would be true with a *Not > every* reading (*Not all the children are in the pool*) and false with an *Every > not* reading (*None of the children are in the pool*).

Figure 5.3 Example of an experimental item in a test on the interaction of function words *all* and *not*. Source: Noveck et al. (2007). Reproduced with permission of Oxford University Press.

the sentence or all three did. For example, one story is about children playing in a pool (see Figure 5.3). In one scenario, all three boys are playing in the pool (3-of-3 scenario); and in the other scenario, two boys are playing in the pool, while a third boy remains outside (2-of-3 scenario). At the end of each story, the experimenter presented either a quantified positive sentence (QP) as in (8) or a quantified negative sentence (QN) as in (9), which involves the universal quantifier (*tous* in French)[1] and negation. The participants were asked to judge this statement as true or false in the depicted scenario.

(8) QP: All the children are in the pool.
(9) QN: All the children are not in the pool.

---

1 The study was conducted in French, using the universal quantifier *tous*, which can be translated as *all* or *every* in English. Note that the interaction between a universal quantifier and negation takes place in the same way for both *all* and *every*.

In the 3-of-3 scenario, sentence (8) is blatantly true and sentence (9) is false under any interpretation. The 2-of-3 scenario provides the critical case: while sentence (8) is false this time (since one boy is not in the pool), the truth value of sentence (9) depends on one of its interpretations in (10):

(10) a. Not all the children are in the pool (NOT>EVERY).
b. None of the children are in the pool (EVERY>NOT).

Under the surface scope interpretation (10b), the sentence is false (two boys are in the pool); under the inverse scope interpretation (10a), the sentence is true (one boy is not in the pool).

The accuracy rates for QP statements (as in (8)) were comparably high for neurotypical adults (95%), neurotypical children (92%), and autistic participants (88%). Similarly, the rate of accuracy (i.e. "false" responses) in the QN statements in scenario 3-of-3 was high and comparable among neurotypical adults (93%), neurotypical children (81%), and autistic participants (82%). In other words, the autistic adolescents did not show particular problems in interpreting sentences that contained quantifiers and negation; even in the case in which the sentence was falsified by the context, they were able to reject it, demonstrating that they could perform semantic composition of complex sentences.

A crucial difference emerged in the case of QN statements (as in (9)) in scenario 2-of-3, which are ambiguous between interpretations (10a) and (10b), depending on the scope interaction between negation and the universal quantifier *every/all*. In this case, the rates of "true" responses were higher for the neurotypical adults (88%) than for either the neurotypical children (45%) or the autistic adolescents (40%), who did not significantly differ from each other. So, the French adults consistently preferred the inverse scope reading of this sentence, similar to what has been found for English adult speakers. In the case of the neurotypical children and the autistic adolescents, the responses were more equivocal: 5/19 neurotypical children and 6/15 autistic adolescents consistently preferred the surface scope reading, which makes the sentence false based on the fact that there are two boys playing in the pool. Only two of the neurotypical children and three of the autistic adolescents preferred the inverse scope (adult) reading; the rest of the participants were inconsistent across the three items in the critical condition. The distribution of non-adult-like responses is different from that found in the original experiments by Lidz and Musolino (2002) discussed above: in that study, English-speaking children were consistently selecting the surface scope reading. In the experiment by Noveck et al. (2007), instead, both neurotypical children and autistic adolescents oscillated between the two possible interpretations.

So, in the authors' words, what does autism reveal about *every... not* sentences? These sentences are interesting from a semantic point of view because of the interaction of scope-bearing elements (such as *not, all, every*), which play a crucial role in deriving sentence meaning via semantic composition. The study conducted with autistic adolescents suggests that some of them rely solely on linear order (surface scope) to derive sentence meaning. This is consistent with the strategy adopted by some of the neurotypical children in this and previous studies. However, the majority of neurotypical children and half of the autistic adolescents in this study are not consistent in their responses. What does this mean? It is unlikely that these participants answered at random because their accuracy scores on the nonambiguous conditions were generally high, though, we note, individual patterns were not discussed in the study. The inconsistent response pattern may suggest, instead, that these participants were aware of the ambiguity of the sentence and responded to each item on the basis of some pragmatic factors. One of the two readings may be more pragmatically appropriate in a certain scenario or situation. This may override the tendency toward surface scope interpretation, as also observed by Gualmini (2008) for neurotypical children. Alternatively, the inconsistency found in the autistic (and neurotypical child) participants' responses may indicate a general difficulty with the interaction between function words. This may be due to limited availability of cognitive resources, particularly the **Executive Functions** inhibition and switching. Inhibition and switching are likely to be involved in the process of handling two competing meanings in the mind, selecting the one that matches the situation and/or inhibiting the other. Unfortunately, a Truth Value Judgment task (as used in this study) cannot disentangle the underlying cognitive processes involved in the decision. To investigate these, an online measure of processing is necessary. Finally, we cannot exclude the possibility that morphosyntactic difficulties, not analyzed in this study, may have played a role (ALI).

Conclusion

This chapter aimed to address the following questions:

- Are combinatorial rules of sentential elements challenging for autistic individuals?
- Are function words, such as quantifiers and connectives and their interactions, challenging for autistic individuals?
- Are temporal and aspectual markers challenging for autistic individuals?

Before answering these questions, we showed how the meaning of sentences or phrases is derived by the combination and interaction of the different elements in the sentence. The lexical meaning of content words (see Chapter 2) is the first step in the compositional derivation of meaning, but syntactic and morphological factors contribute to sentence meaning as well. For example, the same words can change their semantic contribution to the sentence by virtue of their word order (syntax); function words (e.g. *every, not, and*) introduce operations on phrases and sentences, and their interaction can create ambiguities, as in the sentence *Every guest did not bring a present* from the "What do you think?" box (syntax). Furthermore, the same verbs can locate events differently on the timeline by virtue of their aspectual/temporal properties (morphology).

Considering research with autistic individuals without language impairment (ALN), studies so far suggest that sentence-level semantics, including combinatorial rules, quantifiers, connectives, temporal and aspectual markers, is a relative strength, despite its alleged complexity and despite the widely proposed hypothesis that autistic individuals have difficulty integrating information from different sources (for example, the Weak Central Coherence Hypothesis). In most studies, autistic participants' performance on semantic computation has been found to be comparable to that of neurotypical controls, at least when language-matched to autistic participants. Several scholars have highlighted how weakness in semantic composition at the sentence level does not seem to be attributable to autism but rather to (morpho) syntactic difficulties, similar to those observed in individuals with DLD. This points to the necessity to carefully control for morphosyntactic ability, distinguishing between ALN and ALI, but also analyzing correlations between morphosyntactic abilities and performance on semantic tasks, something that is missing in many studies. Moreover, difficulties in the area of semantics are frequently interpreted not as a deficit but as a delay in emergence.

We emphasize, however, that research on semantics in autism is scarce, and that the studies discussed in this chapter have limitations. Many semantic phenomena have not yet been investigated in autism. One example is the interesting semantic contrast between gradable adjectives whose meaning is inherently lexical (such as *dirty*, which means "not clean," independent of context) and relative adjectives that can only be interpreted by making reference to a set (*tall child* vs. *tall man*) that often needs to be recovered from the context, a step that may be challenging for autistic people. Further investigations of this type are needed before conclusions about semantic abilities in autism can be made.

Among the limitations of existing studies is that of participant selection. The linguistic and cognitive profiles of individuals on the autism spectrum are very heterogeneous. Most studies on semantics in autism have included exclusively autistic participants with typical language ability (ALN). Semantic research on individuals with ALI, autistic people who are minimally verbal, and/or those who have intellectual disability, is still scarce. Moreover, the many different tests used to assess general language and/or other cognitive abilities make direct comparisons between studies impossible in most cases.

A second issue concerns the impact and limitations of the types of tasks used to test autistic participants. As pointed out by Naigles and Tovar (2012), implicit measures may provide a better tool to test the knowledge of autistic individuals, something that may be obscured in explicit tasks. Tasks such as preferential looking (IPL), in which eye movements or gazes are monitored while the participants listen to sentences, do not require any explicit action on the part of the participant. Therefore, they may be more suitable to detect what participants implicitly know about language. They also limit the interference of other factors that may affect performance on language tasks, such as the need for joint attention or social interaction, to supply an explicit answer (e.g. pointing) or to provide a metalinguistic judgment (e.g. say whether a sentence is true or not). Although implicit tools require more sophisticated technology, the many limitations of explicit tasks need to be taken into consideration when planning a linguistic assessment, especially in the case of neurodiverse populations (see Chapter 16).

What Do You Know Now?

Understanding language is not a result of merely knowing what words mean. The meaning of a sentence is derived by using combinatorial rules to combine the meaning of the words in the sentence.

- Sentence meaning is obtained by combining the meaning of the words in the sentence according to combinatorial rules.
- Knowing content words (nouns, verbs, adjectives, and adverbs) is not enough; word order and function word operations and interactions (syntax), and temporal and aspectual morphemes (morphology) also matter.
- Intuitively, the process of semantic composition, which involves also the integration of different linguistic cues, may be challenging for autistic individuals. However, this does not seem to be the case in general.
- Autistic individuals with typical structural language abilities do not seem to have particular problems with semantics, although their incremental processing of sentence meaning seems to be slower and a full mastery of complex semantic meaning may be delayed.
- Since semantics is tightly linked to syntactic and morphological operations, understanding the meaning of complex expressions may be challenging for autistic people with a structural language impairment (ALI; see also Chapter 3 and Chapter 16).

Suggestions for Further Reading

Unfortunately, there is no book or article that is specifically devoted to sentence-level semantics in autism. To learn more about semantics in general, a classic textbook is Chierchia and McConnell-Ginet 1990. A more recent textbook is Portner 2004. If you are interested in the acquisition of semantics, we suggest Syrett and Arunachalam 2018.

References

Bartolucci, G., Pierce, S.J., and Streiner, D. (1980). Cross-sectional studies of grammatical morphemes in autistic and mentally retarded children. *Journal of Autism and Developmental Disorders* 10 (1): 39–50.

Bavin, E.L., Prendergast, L.A., Kidd, E. et al. (2016). Online processing of sentences containing noun modification in young children with high-functioning autism. *International Journal of Language and Communication Disorders* 51 (2): 137–147.

Brock, J., Norbury, C., Einav, S. et al. (2008). Do individuals with autism process words in context? Evidence from language-mediated eye-movements. *Cognition* 108 (3): 896–904.

Candan, A., Kuntay, A.C., Yeh, Y.C. et al. (2012). Language and age effects in children's processing of word order. *Cognitive Development* 27 (3): 205–221.

Chen, L., An, S., Dai, H. et al. (2022). Use of aspect markers by Mandarin-speaking children with high-functioning autism plus language impairment and children with Developmental Language Disorder. *Journal of Communication Disorders* 99: 106245.

Chevallier, C., Wilson, D., Happé, F. et al. (2010). Scalar inferences in Autism Spectrum Disorders. *Journal of Autism and Developmental Disorders* 40 (9): 1104–1117.

Chierchia, G. and McConnell-Ginet, S. (1990). *Meaning and Grammar: An Introduction to Semantics*. Cambridge, MA: MIT Press.

Chierchia, G., Crain, S., Guasti, M.T. et al. (2001). The acquisition of disjunction: evidence for a grammatical view of scalar implicatures. In: *Proceedings of the 25th Boston University Conference on Language Development* (eds. A. Do, L. Domínguez, and A. Johansen), 157–168. Somerville, MA: Cascadilla Press.

Frith, U. (1989). *Autism: Explaining the Enigma*. Oxford, UK: Wiley Blackwell.

Gualmini, A. (2008). The rise and fall of Isomorphism. *Lingua* 118 (8): 1158–1176.

Hurewitz, F., Papafragou, A., Gleitman, L. et al. (2006). Asymmetries in the acquisition of numbers and quantifiers. *Language Learning and Development* 2 (2): 77–96.

Kambanaros, M., Christou, N., and Grohmann, K.K. (2019). Interpretation of compound words by Greek-speaking children with Autism Spectrum Disorder plus language impairment (ASD-LI). *Clinical Linguistics and Phonetics* 33 (1–2): 135–174.

Lidz, J. and Musolino, J. (2002). Children's command of quantification. *Cognition* 84 (2): 113–154.

Mani, N. and Huettig, F. (2012). Prediction during language processing is a piece of cake – but only for skilled producers. *Journal of Experimental Psychology: Human Perception and Performance* 38 (4): 843–847.

McGregor, K.K., Rost, G.C., Guo, L.Y. et al. (2010). What compound words mean to children with Specific Language Impairment. *Applied Psycholinguistics* 31 (3): 463–487.

Modyanova, N., Perovic, A., and Wexler, K. (2017). Grammar is differentially impaired in subgroups of Autism Spectrum Disorders: evidence from an investigation of tense marking and morphosyntax. *Frontiers in Psychology* 8: 320.

Naigles, L.R. and Tovar, A.T. (2012). Portable intermodal preferential looking (IPL): Investigating language comprehension in typically developing toddlers and young children with autism. *Journal of Visualized Experiments* 70: e4331.

Noveck, I.A., Guelminger, R., Georgieff, N. et al. (2007). What autism can reveal about every... not sentences. *Journal of Semantics* 24 (1): 73–90.

Pijnacker, J., Hagoort, P., Buitelaar, J. et al. (2009). Pragmatic inferences in high-functioning adults with autism and Asperger Syndrome. *Journal of Autism and Developmental Disorders* 39 (4): 607–618.

Portner, P.H. (2004). *What Is Meaning? Fundamentals of Formal Semantics*. Hoboken, NJ: Wiley.

Roberts, J.A., Rice, M.L., and Tager-Flusberg, H. (2004). Tense marking in children with autism. *Applied Psycholinguistics* 25 (3): 429–448.

Schaeken, W., Van Haeren, M., and Bambini, V. (2018). The understanding of scalar implicatures in children with Autism Spectrum Disorder: Dichotomized responses to violations of informativeness. *Frontiers in Psychology* 9: 1266.

Scontras, G. and Pearl, L.S. (2021). When pragmatics matters more for truth value judgements: an investigation of quantifier scope ambiguity. *Glossa: A Journal of General Linguistics* 6 (1): 110.

Su, Y.E. and Naigles, L.R. (2019). Online processing of subject-verb-object order in a diverse sample of Mandarin-exposed preschool children with Autism Spectrum Disorder. *Autism Research* 12 (12): 1829–1844.

Su, Y.E and Naigles, L.R. (2021). Comprehension of grammatical aspect markers *le* and *zai* in a diverse sample of Mandarin-exposed preschool children with Autism Spectrum Disorder. *Reading and Writing* 36: 1369–1392.

Su, Y.E. and Su, L.Y. (2015). Interpretation of logical words in Mandarin-speaking children with Autism Spectrum Disorders: uncovering knowledge of semantics and pragmatics. *Journal of Autism and Developmental Disorders* 45 (7): 1938–1950.

Swensen, L.D., Kelley, E., Fein, D. et al. (2007). Processes of language acquisition in children with autism: evidence from preferential looking. *Child Development* 78 (2): 542–557.

Syrett, K. and Arunachalam, S. (ed.) (2018). *Semantics in Language Acquisition* 24. Amsterdam: John Benjamins.

Tek, S., Mesite, L., Fein, D. et al. (2014). Longitudinal analyses of expressive language development reveal two distinct language profiles among young children with Autism Spectrum Disorders. *Journal of Autism and Developmental Disorders* 44: 75–89.

Tovar, A.T., Fein, D., and Naigles, L.R. (2015). Grammatical aspect is a strength in the language comprehension of young children with Autism Spectrum Disorder. *Journal of Speech, Language, and Hearing Research* 58 (2): 301–310.

Vicente, A., Barbarroja, N., and Castroviejo, E. (2023). Linguistic, concept and symbolic composition in adults with minimal receptive vocabulary. *Clinical Linguistics & Phonetics* 38 (2): 155–171.

Wagner, L., Swensen, L.D., and Naigles, L.R. (2009). Children's early productivity with verbal morphology. *Cognitive Development* 24 (3): 223–239.

Zhou, P., Zhan, L., and Ma, H. (2019). Predictive language processing in preschool children with Autism Spectrum Disorder: an eye-tracking study. *Journal of Psycholinguistic Research* 48: 431–452.

6

Implicit Meaning

Napoleon Katsos and Agustín Vicente

> **What Do You Think?**
> When a teacher gives the instruction "Open your books on page 37," an autistic student may do so but not also start doing the work on that page as the rest of the class does. Furthermore, when an autistic individual is told, "I'm so hungry I could eat a horse," they may respond that this is not a nice thing to do to a horse.
> Another – hypothetical – example is the following: Jack's mom asks if he would like to come along with her on her shopping trip. He happily agrees, but when she opens the door to go out, it is raining heavily. Jack's mom says, "Oh, what a great day to go shopping!" Jack stares at her in surprise.
> What kinds of language use may autistic people find difficult?

Introduction

This chapter discusses meaning that is implicitly communicated and the difficulties that many autistic individuals experience in order to understand nonliteral or figurative language. Implicit or pragmatic meaning includes cases in which a speaker means something in addition to what they say literally, and cases in which they mean something different from what they say literally. So, when teachers say, "Open your books on page 37," they usually mean that in addition to going to page 37 (the literal interpretation), the students should also engage in the activity described on page 37. And when Jack's mom says, "Oh, what a great day to go shopping!" she actually means the opposite.

Exploring the phenomenon of implicit meaning in autism, we address the following main questions:

- To what extent do autistic people have difficulties with implicit meaning?
- Do autistic people have difficulties with all kinds of implicit meaning?
- What is the underlying source of implicit meaning difficulties in autism?

Anchoring

Before discussing the strengths and difficulties of implicit meaning experienced by autistic people, we first introduce and discuss how implicit meaning can be expressed through language and how this is acquired and processed by neurotypicals.

Disciplines that study meaning in language, such as linguistics, cognitive science, and philosophy of language, usually draw a distinction between **explicit** and **implicit meaning**. The former is meaning that a speaker has communicated on record (what the words literally mean), while the latter is meaning that can be inferred by what the speaker has said but is not part of what has been communicated on record. Here, we use the terms **literal** for explicit meaning and **implicit** for meaning that is inferred but has not been said. Most cases of implicit meaning concern situations where there is an implicit addition or modification to what has been said. To work out what exact modification needs to be made, listeners need to take into consideration the context of the conversation and commonly assumed principles of conversational behavior, such as the fact that a speaker is cooperative and that they are aiming to be relevant, truthful, concise, and informative (Grice 1975).

Let us consider a few straightforward cases of implicit meaning that one would hardly notice in everyday conversation. When asked if the party was a success, Joan replies that *everyone loved it*. Here, in a phenomenon linguistically coined **quantifier domain restriction**, *everyone* should be modified to mean 'everyone who came to the party', rather than generally 'everyone in the world'.

Besides implicit meaning that involves modification of the literal meaning, there is **figurative** meaning. Figurative meaning includes exaggeration, irony, metaphor, and metonymy. These cases employ context and pragmatic principles of conversation to work out the speaker's intended meaning that may be quite distant from what has been literally said. The example we mentioned in the "What do you think?" section above (*I'm so hungry I could eat a horse*) is a case of exaggeration, in which the speaker is communicating the great extent and intensity of their hunger, but they do not literally mean what they say. The other example (*Oh, what a great day to go shopping!*) is a case of irony, in which the departure from the literal meaning is even more marked because it means the opposite of what is literally said.

The phenomenon of **implicature** is another instance of implicit meaning. It involves the addition of some inferred meaning to what the speaker has literally said in order to make sense of the unfolding conversation. As such, it is an enrichment of what is literally said. Imagine that speaker A asks *Did you meet your friend's parents?* and speaker B replies *I met the mother*. Intuitively, we understand that B is communicating that they met the mother but not the father (the latter being a pragmatic inference or "implicature"). Although this has not been said literally, the implicit meaning (*but not the father*) follows from an inference we make by assuming that speaker B is giving the most informative, truthful, and relevant answer. Once we assume that they do so, we can reason that had they met their friend's father, they would have said so (because saying so would be informative and relevant to the conversation). This kind of implicature is known as **quantity implicature** because it concerns the quantity of information that the speaker offers.

A specific sub-kind of quantity implicature is the **scalar implicature**. Consider speaker A saying: *I have invited some of my friends for dinner*. There is a so-called

---

Acronym and Terminology Reminder

ALI: Autism with language impairment.
ALN: Autism with normal language.
Figurative Language/Speech/Meaning: Departing from literal meaning.
Implicature: Meaning in conversation that is implied (but not literally stated).
Indirect Request: Request through a nonrequest speech act, e.g. question: *Can you pass me the salt?* for *Please pass me the salt*.
Irony: Stating the opposite of what is meant, e.g. it's raining heavily outside, and you say, *Oh, it's such nice weather!*
Implicit Meaning: Meaning that is conveyed but not explicitly stated.
Metaphor: Metaphor implicitly states resemblance between two things, e.g. *Time is money*.
Metonymy: Replacement of object/person name by term associated with object/person, e.g. *the Crown* to refer to a monarch.
Relevance Implicature: Implicature that makes a statement relevant, e.g. A says, *Do you want to join us for the trip?* and B replies, *I do not fly*. B does not literally say so, but B's answer implies "no."
Quantifier: Word/phrase expressing relations of quantity between sets of words, e.g. *all, some, each*.
Scalar Implicature: Type of Quantity Implicature involving an informativeness scale, e.g. <*some, all*>. Use of the first, less informative, member implies denial of the second, more informative, member: *Some students failed* implies that not all students failed.
Linguistic Pragmatics: Pragmatics that relies on structural language abilities and sensitivity to conversation principles, but crucially NOT on perspective-taking.
Speech Act: Statement, question, promise, request, etc.
Structural Language: Formal aspects of language related to phonology, morphology, syntax, and semantics.
ToM: Theory of Mind. Ability to infer and understand mental states (e.g. beliefs, true, or false) in oneself and others.

information scale at work here, namely <*some, all*>, in which *some* is the less informative member of the scale and *all* the more informative one. Based on this scale, we intuitively infer that speaker A has invited some but not all of their friends for dinner (otherwise speaker A would have used the more informative member of the scale, namely, *all*). Likewise, if we say *the coffee is warm*, we usually mean that it is just warm, not hot, even though being warm is compatible with being hot. Hearers assume that if the coffee had been hot (a more informative, stronger, member of the scale <*warm, hot*>), the speaker would have said so. What is common between quantity implicatures and scalar implicatures is that what is literally said is enriched with the negation of something more informative that was not said.

Relevance implicatures arise when what is literally said is not relevant enough. However, once an implicature is made, the literal answer combined with the implied one becomes sufficiently relevant, as in the following example: Question: *Will you come play football with us?* Response: *I've hurt my knee*. Here the literal answer does not provide a yes/no response, which is what is required. However, bearing in mind that when people have hurt their knee, they usually do not play football, the no response becomes easily available. Manner implicatures are based on whether something is said in a typical, brief, and stylistically-neutral way, or whether it is said in a marked, wordy, or unusual way. For example, if following a loud smashing sound someone would say *Will made the plates break* rather that *Will broke the plates*, we are likely to infer that Will did this either involuntarily or without direct causality (e.g. by pushing something else that made the plates fall down, by mistake). If Will had actively and with intention broken the plates, one would have said *Will broke the plates*.

The implicature examples given above demonstrate how pragmatic inferences are related to the ability to reason about the speaker's intentions. **Theory of Mind** (ToM) is the term used in linguistics, psychology, and cognitive science to refer to the ability to infer and understand mental states (e.g. beliefs) in oneself and others (see also Chapters 3, 8–10, 13, and 14). As such, the production and comprehension of implicatures seem to involve ToM and will be further discussed in the section "Implicit meaning in autism" below.

Typically developing children understand implicatures early on in development. For example, 3-year-olds can understand relevance implicatures, and most 5-year-olds can understand some kinds of quantity implicatures (Katsos 2014). Neurotypical adults infer implicatures, taking into consideration what the speaker knows and does not know (Breheny et al. 2013).

Another instance of implicit meaning is the production and comprehension of **speech acts**: the communicative function of sentences that goes beyond grammatical mood. That is, while languages such as English have grammatical means to indicate if a sentence is an assertion, a request, or a question, this grammatical mood does not fully determine the effect of the sentence in a conversational context. Consider a speaker who makes the assertion *It is cold in here* or *I am a little bit hungry*. Besides being assertions, these sentences (indirectly) ask for something to be done, namely, for the room temperature to be increased or for how to spend a short break. As such, these assertions serve the communicative function of a request. Such sentences are **indirect speech acts**, and they need to be understood in the context of a conversation with reference to conversation principles. There are also sentences that serve as indirect speech acts because they are conventionalized that way. For example, English questions such as *Could you [VERB]?* are usually conventionally polite requests, as they are often accompanied by politeness markers such as *please* or *if you don't mind*. Indirect requests are understood by age 3 (Ledbetter and Dent 1988). Interestingly, the more skilled children are with language in general, the more responsive they are to indirect requests, a point that becomes relevant in the section "Implicit meaning in autism" below.

Metaphors, such as *She has a heart of gold*, and other figurative tropes such as irony (as exemplified above by *Oh, what a great day to go shopping*), are also part of implicit communication in that they feel like actual departures from the literal meaning of a sentence. Performance on **metaphors** increases when the property that is attributed to the topic of the metaphor is visually (or otherwise perceptually) salient as opposed to a mental, abstract property. For instance, children aged 3 can understand that *the tower with the hat* can refer to a tower with a red pointy roof (Pouscoulous and Tomasello 2020) but have more difficulty understanding predicative metaphors such as *Lucy is a soldier*, referring to a girl who is very brave, which is not understood until they are 6. As for **irony**, some studies suggest that by age 6, typically developing children are able to identify and understand ironic utterances without much difficulty (Filippova 2014; Köder and Falkum 2021).

The summary above of implicit/pragmatic meaning phenomena and reports of their early acquisition by typically developing children is the outcome of relatively recent research. Earlier language acquisition and psycholinguistics research proposed that typically developing children first went through a literalist stage that could last until they were 10 years old. This understanding reflected certain theoretical approaches to linguistic theory that placed language use (pragmatics) outside the core of language competence (grammar, or structural language, including phonology, morphology, syntax, and semantics). Currently, however, children are considered "early birds" in terms of pragmatic development, i.e. in understanding what speakers mean despite not using language literally. When young children do not understand pragmatic inference or figurative use of language, it seems related to other relevant factors and not to the absence of pragmatic competence per se. For example, young children tend to have difficulty understanding abstract metaphors, but not more perceptually based ones, suggesting they are still developing the notion of abstractness but not that they cannot understand metaphors.

Implicit Meaning in Autism

To What Extent Do Autistic People Have Difficulties With Implicit Meaning?

The prevailing view in the 1980s-1990s was that all autistic individuals had a general pragmatic impairment that prevented them from producing and understanding implicit meaning. There were two general statements within this view, namely, that all autistic people were facing pragmatic challenges and that all aspects of pragmatics were impaired. Pragmatic difficulties could be improved with explicit training and educational interventions, but without them, autistic individuals were assumed to be literalists by default. Such views were linked to another influential idea about autism, namely, that autistic people had deficits in ToM (Baron-Cohen, Leslie, and Frith 1985). The assumption that implicit meaning involves pragmatic reasoning, which in turn involves reasoning about the mental states of speakers and listeners, resulted in the view that a pragmatic impairment was part of the symptomatology of autism itself.

This has led researchers to consider pragmatic difficulties as the hallmark of autism. It was claimed that autistic people frequently demonstrate unusual conversational behavior, including implicatures, figurative language, the use of context to disambiguate words with multiple meanings, topic maintenance and topic shift, the comprehension of humor, the drawing of inferences from narratives, and indirect requests (see Volden and Phillips 2010).

A particularly influential study in this respect was one by Happé (1993), investigating three figurative speech phenomena of increasing conceptual complexity, namely, **similes** (John was [clever] like a fox), metaphors (John was a fox), and irony (What a clever boy you are in a context in which the addressee has made a major mistake). Importantly, Happé grouped autistic participants according to their ability to attribute a false belief to another person (representing ToM); no-ToM, first-order ToM (the ability to attribute a false belief), and second-order ToM (the ability to attribute a false belief about a belief). The results revealed that overall, autistic people were challenged by metaphors and irony, i.e. the two phenomena without a linguistic marker to indicate that a figurative interpretation is needed (unlike for similes, in which like overtly indicates that John had some property that foxes have but is not a fox literally). Importantly, success with first-order ToM was associated with success with metaphors, and success with second-order ToM was associated with success with irony. This pattern of results suggested that irony is more conceptually complex than metaphors: irony expresses a belief about a belief, just as second-order ToM does.

We will see in the following paragraphs that all these assumptions have been revised and qualified to some extent. Since Happé's (1993) study, an increased interest in pragmatics and autism has revealed several new key findings. Let us take up some of the cases we discussed in the Anchoring section.

Scalar implicatures involve understanding *some* as *some but not all*, or *warm* as *warm but not hot*. It is important to realize that scalar implicatures can be derived by the knowledge that certain expressions can be ranked according to how informative they are (*<some, all>*; *<warm, hot>*), without necessarily considering the context of the conversation. Recent studies on autism report no pronounced difficulties with scalar implicatures, especially once structural language skills (in particular, morphosyntax, the structure of sentences – see Chapter 3) are taken into account. Indicatively, Andrés-Roqueta and Katsos (2020) presented autistic children with statements including the quantifier *some*, which were meant to describe visually depicted situations where the quantifier *all* would be more appropriate than *some* (see Figure 6.1). If autistic children were sensitive to the pragmatic maxim that requires speakers to be sufficiently informative, and if they understood that *some* implies *not all*, they should reject these statements.

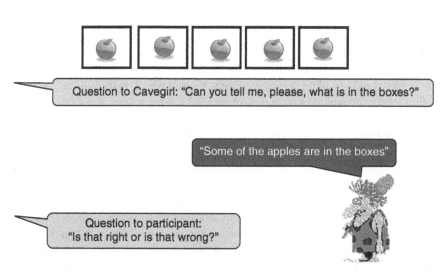

Figure 6.1 Sample display of trial from scalar implicature task. *Source:* Courtesy of Napoleon Katsos.

Autistic children rejected these statements at rates that were below those of age-matched typically developing children. However, the rate of rejection by the autistic children was similar to the rates of language-matched typically developing children (that is, children that were chronologically younger than their autistic peers but had the same scores in structural language, namely, receptive and expressive grammar and vocabulary tests). Importantly, regression analyses showed that it was the structural language score (the composite of the receptive and expressive grammar and vocabulary scores) that predicted success with informativeness and scalar implicature for the autistic children. Chronological age and ToM were not reliably predicting success.

Another area where autistic individuals may face difficulties is the ability to restrict the domain that is talked about into what is relevant for the conversation (de Villiers, Myers, and Stainton 2013). Recall that this is a case where language is implicitly modified in the context of use, e.g. when someone says, "No one even understood the test," this means that no student understood it, rather than no one in the world. However, whether this aspect of language use is particularly dependent on structural language skills is not yet known.

Wilson and Bishop (2022) investigated autistic adults' comprehension of relevance implicatures, which necessitate considering exactly the point of the conversation. They conducted an experiment with mini-dialogues such as the one below. The context is that Tom and Sally just walked into a restaurant and addresses a man (John) with a question:

SALLY: Can the two of us sit here?
JOHN: The children just went to find the toilet.

Participants were asked: "Do you think Tom and Sally can sit there?" Autistic individuals without language difficulties performed well on the task, even though they were twice as likely to choose a **nonnormative** or unusual interpretation of an implied meaning (a *yes* answer instead of a *no* answer in this case) and five times as likely to select an *I don't know answer* when asked about the presence of an implied meaning. A significant correlation in the autistic group was found between these difficulties with implicature derivation on the one hand and discomfort with uncertainty and self-reported communication challenges on the other hand. However, the authors did not find a relation with ToM abilities, suggesting that uncertainty concerning what is actually implied is unrelated to ToM issues.

Studies from the 1980s and 1990s report difficulties grasping indirect ways of speaking (Paul and Cohen 1985), for example, requests such as "I'll be happy if you color this circle blue." Kissine et al. (2015), however, suggest that there are no special difficulties in indirect requests either. Their study shows that autistic children perform the action that is appropriate when the experimenter requests Mr. Potato's hat by saying, "Oh! Mr. Potato has no hat on!" Kissine et al. argue that the difference between their results and Paul and Cohen's is due to the naturalness of their stimuli.

Metonymy consists of a meaning shift in which a word is substituted for another word that it is closely related to (e.g. *The White House has decided...*, where *The White House* refers to the president). Rundblad and Annaz (2010) report that autistic children exhibit a delay in metonymy comprehension as compared to typically developing peers. The delay was in line with the autistic children's vocabulary growth (which is often delayed as compared to typically developing children's vocabulary). This confirms that pragmatic meaning may be challenging for autistic individuals, but it casts doubt on the claim that underdeveloped ToM is the cause of all pragmatic difficulties. In fact, it suggests that autistic children with precocious vocabulary growth do not face such pragmatic difficulties.

Since the publication of Happé's (1993) study, Norbury (2005) and other studies (Gernsbacher and Pripas-Kapit 2012; Kalandadze et al. 2018; Kalandadze, Bambini, and Næss 2019) claim that autistic individuals do not necessarily experience difficulty understanding metaphors. Including general language assessment in their studies, they argue that if autism is accompanied by language delay, there are difficulties with metaphors, but that autistic participants without language delay perform as well as neurotypical controls. Nevertheless, other research teams do find literalist biases in autistic individuals even when they are matched on structural language to neurotypical individuals (Chahboun et al. 2017). Interestingly, the few studies done on metaphor production suggest that autistic individuals do not find it particularly difficult to express themselves using metaphors (Kasirer and Mashal 2016).

Findings are also mixed for studies on irony in autism. A systematic meta-analysis of autism and figurative language, including irony, reports that while many autistic people are challenged by irony, there are also autistic individuals who perform as well as neurotypical controls. The key predictor of difficulty with irony is a low score on structural language ability (Kalandadze et al. 2018). Nonetheless, other recent studies that examined irony report that irony can be challenging for autistic people even when language skills are taken into account (Deliens et al. 2018; Andrés-Roqueta and Katsos 2020; Panzeri et al. 2022).

In summary, older studies on implicit/pragmatic meaning in autism focused on the relationship with ToM and concluded that underdeveloped ToM led to difficulty understanding pragmatic meaning. As such, pragmatic difficulty was considered part of autism symptomatology itself. Recent studies take structural language skills into account and distinguish between autistic people with and without impairment in structural language (ALI vs. ALN, see Chapter 1). These studies often show that poorer structural language skills lead to difficulty understanding certain types of pragmatic meaning. This raises the question as to whether all pragmatic difficulties should be considered part of autism itself, given that some difficulties do not seem to relate to ToM or to any autistic characteristics, but just to the structural language difficulties that some autistic individuals exhibit.

Do Autistic People Have Difficulties With All Kinds of Implicit Meaning?

An influential line of research has been comparing autistic people's performance on various pragmatics phenomena, addressing the question of which types of pragmatics rely on structural language competence exclusively and which ones are (also) related to ToM. For example, Deliens et al. (2018) report that autistic adults with linguistic abilities within the typical range performed as well as neurotypical adults in a task that required comprehension of indirect speech acts but not in a task that required comprehension of irony. According to the authors, these results suggest that there is an area of pragmatic competence where autistic individuals whose structural language is good are not affected. They call such an area **egocentric** pragmatics (Kissine 2016) because it does not involve adopting the perspective of the speaker or thinking why speakers said what they said. In contrast, irony comprehension demands mind-reading (**allocentric** pragmatics) and is often difficult for autistic people.

In another study, Andrés-Roqueta and Katsos (2020) administered two pragmatics tasks to autistic children and language-matched typically developing children as well as language-matched children with Developmental Language Disorder (DLD) and age-matched neurotypical peers. They tested quantity implicatures, which did not require perspective-taking (see Figure 6.1), as well as a task on comprehension of high-order strategic speaking, such as pretending or telling a white lie, in order not to hurt a friend's feelings, which do require consideration of the speaker's nonobvious intentions. Indicatively, in a white lie situation, a child received a present from her friends for her birthday. She tells her friends: "That's exactly what I wanted" when opening the present and seeing it was a basketball, when in fact what she really wanted was roller skates. In this situation, the speaker and the addressee did not only have different knowledge about what the child really wanted, but the speaker also had conflicting desires and emotions (the private desire for roller skates and the emotion of disappointment, contrasting with the desire and emotion expressed publicly to her friends). In the first task, Andrés-Roqueta and Katsos found that success at deriving quantity implicatures was predicted by structural language skills only (and the autistic children performed as well as the two language-matched groups: the younger typically developing group and the DLD group). However, performance with the strategic speaking task was predicted by both structural language and ToM scores, with autistic children performing lower than the other two language-matched groups.

Taken together, this emerging body of research suggests that while structural language competence is an especially important factor for success in pragmatics, there are still some aspects of pragmatic skills that autistic people may find challenging to an extent that is beyond what one would anticipate from language competence alone.

What Is the Underlying Source of Implicit Meaning Difficulties in Autism?

As said, in the 1980s–1990s, it was believed that all kinds of pragmatic difficulties were widespread in the autistic spectrum. In part, such a belief rested on two assumptions: (i) that understanding pragmatic use of language implies reasoning about what speakers intend to communicate implicitly given what they have said explicitly; and (ii) that it is characteristic of autistic individuals to have difficulties understanding other people's behavior in terms of what they aim to do. The more recent research we reviewed above is very much embedded in this paradigm, but the emphasis is put on the variety of types of pragmatic meaning. Through this research, several distinctions within pragmatics have recently been made. These distinctions may help us further understand autistic people's challenges with implicit meaning.

As mentioned, Kissine (2016) argues for a distinction between egocentric and allocentric pragmatics. According to this distinction, autistic individuals are not expected to have difficulties understanding nonliteral uses of language that do not require adopting the perspective of the speaker (egocentric pragmatics). For example, understanding *some* as *some but not all* does not require adopting the perspective of the speaker, while understanding irony requires reasoning about whether the speaker can be talking seriously, being seriously mistaken, etc., which is reminiscent of ToM (allocentric pragmatics).

A related, but somewhat different, distinction is made by Andrés-Roqueta and Katsos (2017, 2020) and Katsos and Andrés-Roqueta (2021), who draw the line between **linguistic pragmatics** and **social pragmatics**. While linguistic pragmatics rests upon structural linguistic abilities and sensitivity to conversation principles, social pragmatics relates to the ability to entertain the interlocutor's point of view as well (ToM). The hypothesis is that autistic people are challenged only with social pragmatics, whereas with linguistic pragmatics they will perform as well as their structural language skills allow them to. As described above, Andrés-Roqueta and Katsos (2020) provide evidence for this hypothesis using different pragmatic phenomena and different situations. For linguistic pragmatics, they used scalar implicatures in situations where the speaker and the addressee share all the knowledge that is relevant. For social pragmatics, they used more complex situations, such as when the speaker was telling a white lie, in order not to hurt her friend's feelings.[1]

Importantly, the distinction between linguistic and social pragmatics does not apply to pragmatic meaning phenomena per se (such as implicatures on the one hand and lies or irony on the other); instead, it applies to communicative situations in which the mental states of the speaker and hearer are aligned (in which case linguistic pragmatics skills ought to suffice and ToM is not needed) or not aligned (in which case social pragmatics skills will be required and ToM is needed). For example, linguistic pragmatics skills may often suffice to understand scalar implicatures. However, some communicative situations in which the speaker's knowledge of the situation differs from that of the listener may require social pragmatic skills to infer a scalar implicature.

To pursue this suggestion, Katsos and Ostashchenko (2021) tested the distinction between linguistic and social pragmatics using quantity implicatures. They created situations where linguistic or social-pragmatic skills were needed for successful communication, for one and the same pragmatic phenomenon. Specifically, they presented autistic and neurotypical adults whose structural language and nonverbal IQ abilities were within the typical range, with four cards. Three of the cards were visible to both the speaker and the listener, but the fourth card was always hidden from the speaker and visible only to the listener. In some critical cases, the speaker described the card he wanted to get using an utterance, which was literally true for two cards that were visible to both the speaker and the listener. Importantly, the description was compatible with only one card, as long as the listener was informative and understood the description with a quantity implicature. See Figure 6.2a for such a situation where the speaker says, "Give me the card with pears" when there is a card with pears only and a card with pears and something else. In situations like these, the listener may draw the quantity implicature that *card with pears* implies 'card with only pears', because if the speaker wanted the card that had pears and bananas, he would have said so. Because the speaker and the listener share all the relevant knowledge and their mental states are aligned, this is a linguistic-pragmatic situation, and the

---

[1] Note that Andrés-Roqueta and Katsos (2020) propose a narrower definition of the term "linguistic pragmatics" than the one that is often used (see, for example, Chapter 8). The broader interpretation of "linguistic pragmatics" refers to all of the ways in which pragmatic meaning is encoded by linguistic elements. For example, a speaker can choose an indefinite article (*a*) over a definite article (*the*) to indicate information that is new to the listener, use a pronoun (*they*) rather than a full noun (*the students*) to indicate information that is familiar to the listener, use the quantifier *some* rather than *all* (from the scale <*some, all*>) to emphasize the meaning 'not all', use a metaphor (*kick the bucket*) to express another meaning ('die') or use a certain intonation (prosody) to indicate irony.

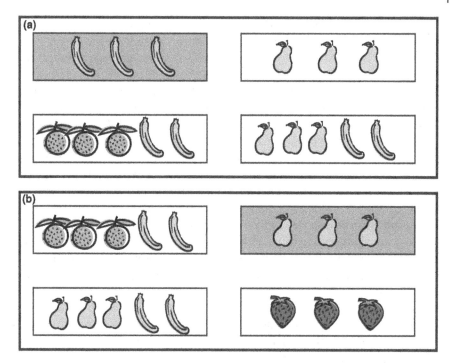

Figure 6.2 (a and b) Visual display for linguistic-pragmatic situation (a) and social-pragmatic situation (b), in which card in shaded background is visible to listener only, while other three cards are visible to both speaker and listener. In both (a) and (b) speaker says "Give me the card with pears." *Source:* Courtesy of Napoleon Katsos.

hypothesis is that autistic people whose linguistic abilities are within the typical range will do as well as their neurotypical peers.

In the social-pragmatics cases, the speaker again asked for *the card with pears*, but they did so in a situation where there was a mutually visible card with pears and something else. This was the only one of the mutually visible cards that showed pears, and therefore the description *the card with pears* was sufficient to identify this card among the other cards. However, the hidden card that was visible only to the listener displayed only pears (see Figure 6.2b). If the listener employed ToM and took into account the speaker's knowledge, who is not aware of what is shown on the hidden card, this time they ought to give the card with pears and bananas instead of the card with only pears. But if the listener did not employ ToM to consider what the speaker knows, they would select the card with just pears, as they did in the linguistic-pragmatic condition. Autistic participants performed as well as the neurotypical peers in the linguistic-pragmatics situations, but their performance with social pragmatics was significantly lower than that of their neurotypical peers. This finding is in line with the hypothesis that autistic people will find pragmatics challenging only in social-pragmatic situations when ToM is required. Importantly, it is not the type of pragmatic phenomenon that predicts whether ToM is required, but the communicative situation itself, as shown by the different performance with one and the same phenomenon, implicature, in linguistic- and social-pragmatic situations.

Turning to the broader picture concerning what such differences between autistic and nonautistic individuals may relate to, there are approaches that go beyond emphasizing structural language or ToM. An influential explanation of challenges with implicit/pragmatic meaning is **executive dysfunction**: the difficulty to inhibit literal meaning in order to get to the nonliteral interpretation (e.g. Mashal and Kasirer 2011). Another contender is the **weak central coherence processing** view, which explains literalism as an effect of the nonglobal or **local** processing characteristic of autism. This would make it difficult to integrate the contextual information required to properly understand nonliteral use of language (Happé and Frith 2006). Furthermore, a recent study by Vicente and Falkum (2023) proposes that understanding nonliteral meaning literally may relate to the **rigidity** observed in many autistic individuals. Note that such a literalist bias does not consist so much in experiencing difficulties interpreting nonliteral language as rather in interpreting it literally, which is what many autistic people experience, according to first personal accounts. Such a bias has not been explored in depth in the scientific literature, but it questions the idea that nonliteral uses of language that do not require perspective shifting only relate to structural language. Vicente and Falkum (2023) suggest that the literalist bias may relate to strict rule-following, but it may also be related to other rigidity symptoms that are characteristic of autism (see Petrolini, Jorba, and Vicente (2023) for a reflection about notions of rigidity), such as insistence on sameness (Kanner 1943) or a tendency to experience more uncertainty (Vicente, Michel, and Petrolini 2023).

Of course, it is possible that the differences in findings found between different research teams relate to the experimental paradigms employed. In one of the most comprehensive reviews on the topic, Kalandadze, Bambini, and Næss (2019) identify several dimensions that may affect performance in metaphor comprehension tasks. Among them, experimental design and setting appear to be the most relevant. For instance, while Norbury (2005) uses a forced choice task, where participants are asked to select a response out of several options, Chahboun et al. (2017) use a lexical priming task, which is based on quick associations. In the lexical priming paradigm, participants see a word on the screen, followed by either a word or a nonword (e.g. *dog* or *dax*). Participants are asked to respond as fast as possible, whether what they saw was a word or a nonword. Fast responses indicate strong priming, which in turn close association in the semantic network between both words (e.g. *doctor* and *nurse* would prime each other more strongly than *dog* and *vase*). In general, more differences are found using implicit measures such as reaction times or gaze following than using explicit tasks (see Chapter 5). Similarly, multiple-choice and nonverbal enactment tasks (i.e. acting out a metaphor with toys after having heard a story containing such metaphor) are less demanding than tasks centered around verbal explanation, such as answering open questions about metaphors heard in a story.

It is also probably the case that more structured tasks, like forced choice tasks, are more amiable to autistic participants. This could explain why many autistic people experience difficulties in the area of nonliteral uses of language in daily life conversations, which are paradigmatically more unpredictable and involve a greater number of variables. Such difficulties are reflected in first personal accounts, such as those analyzed by Morra (2016), who finds that only 37% of the autistic individuals participating in a forum found metaphor comprehension "unproblematic." Interestingly, in that same forum, 63% of respondents declared to use metaphors very often. All this suggests a picture according to which autistic individuals are far from having pragmatic impairment (excluding perhaps irony and sarcasm, which – in Andrés-Roqueta and Katsos' terminology – are often used in situations that require social pragmatic processing). Nevertheless, autistic individuals may still experience difficulties when nonliteral language occurs in an otherwise noisy environment.

Another intriguing possibility is that autistic people experience pragmatic challenges, especially when they are interacting with neurotypical people, who employ conceptual relations that are characteristic of their way of thinking. Morra (2016) reports that many autistic participants complain that neurotypicals do not understand their metaphors. It might be that the difficulties that autistic individuals experience with metaphors created by neurotypical individuals are on a par with the difficulties that neurotypical individuals exhibit in understanding metaphors generated by autistic individuals. This hypothesis is couched in the theoretical framework of the **Double Empathy Problem** (Milton 2012). This framework challenges the notion that a lack of ToM resides within the core of autistic cognition. Instead, it suggests that nonautistic people, including researchers, may have difficulty understanding the experiences of autistic individuals as well as the other way round. In further support of this line of investigation, Crompton et al. (2020a and 2020b) report that interactions between autistic and nonautistic people can be rated as having poor rapport and as leading to loss of information that is exchanged, but this is not the case when autistic people are interacting with other autistic people. This emerging view of autism places emphasis on the difference of autism, rather than the deficit or difficulty, and it calls for a characterization of how autistic people use language in their own right without asking whether autistic people have impaired or disordered pragmatics. However, it should be noted that in Crompton et al. (2020a and 2020b), the autistic or nonautistic status of each conversational partner was revealed to the participants. Some other studies suggest that when participants are not aware of the diagnostic status, autistic individuals are perceived as atypical by both autistic and nonautistic raters. This would suggest that there may not be an implicit neurotype convergence taking place but instead, participants may be affected by their assumptions about group membership (Morrison et al. 2020).

In our view, this is an important development in the study of autism. Without ignoring the fact that for many autistic people, comprehension and production of language in general and pragmatic language specifically is a major challenge, it is also important to approach the study of language and pragmatics through the lens of diversity in order to understand the full range of what communication means.

All in all, there are many abilities and factors that may contribute to pragmatic communication in autism. Figure 6.3 visually represents these.

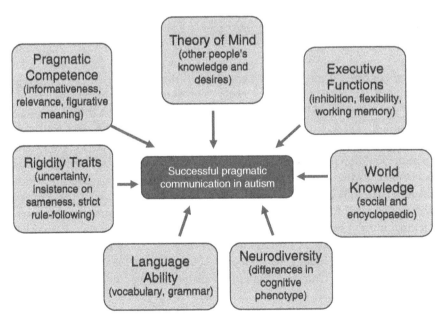

Figure 6.3 Abilities and factors that may contribute to pragmatic communication in autism. *Source:* Napoleon Katsos and Agustín Vicente.

Focus on a Specific Study

As mentioned, Norbury's (2005) study (together with her 2004 study on idioms) has been a turning point in studies on comprehension of implicit/pragmatic meaning by autistic individuals. It is worth focusing on this specific study both because of its findings on the crucial role of structural language in pragmatic success for autistic people and because of the matching paradigm that she used, whereby autistic children are grouped based on whether they also have a language impairment or not. Norbury evaluates the performance of autistic children with and without language impairment in a metaphor comprehension task very similar to the one used by Happé (1993), who claimed to have shown that autistic children's low performance in the metaphor comprehension task was related to their impairment in a ToM task. Norbury casts doubt on this account by arguing that core language skills (by which she means vocabulary and morphosyntax) need to be considered as part of the interpretation since they might be the actual responsible factor for the observed impairment in figurative language comprehension. In fact, neither ToM nor autistic features emerge as relevant predictors in Norbury's regression model, while core language skills do predict metaphor comprehension. Moreover, when matched on core language abilities, autistic children performed just as well as their typically developing younger peers on the metaphor comprehension task. Norbury therefore concludes that good vocabulary and morphosyntax are stronger predictors of good performance at the metaphor comprehension task than ToM.

Norbury's paper used a particularly suitable design for investigating the role of structural language on metaphor comprehension by building the presence of autism and language difficulties into the group design itself. She compared typically developing children (no language difficulty, no autism) to autistic children with no language difficulty (ALN), as well as autistic children with language difficulty (ALI), and children without autism but with language impairment (DLD). The metaphor comprehension task (a forced choice task) employed in Norbury's study requires participants to choose the most appropriate continuation of a sentence out of four possibilities. An example of an experimental item is given below:

> The heating had been left on overnight, and the room was very warm.
> It was:
> - an oven
> - a blanket
> - a grill
> - a spice

The metaphor to be chosen (i.e. the correct answer) is *oven*, since ovens and warm rooms are most similar. The two groups with language difficulties (either with or without autism) did not choose this as frequently as children without particular language difficulties. This is as follows: children with language difficulties do not have enough semantic knowledge to realize that the way in which a room is warm is more akin to the way an oven is warm than to the way a blanket is warm (in that both the oven and the room heat fill a space). In Norbury's words (2005, p. 384), "children must acquire sufficient world knowledge and have broad enough semantic representations to capture the comparison being made."

After Norbury's pioneering study, many authors have endorsed the importance of the **structural language** hypothesis (see references in Gernsbacher and Pripas-Kapit 2012; Kalandadze et al. 2018), whereby pragmatic difficulties in autism are neither universal to all autistic people nor primarily associated to ToM. Instead, the hypothesis is that the difficulties in understanding nonliteral language observed in many autistic people relate to delays in the development of structural linguistic abilities. In this respect, such difficulties should not be different from those experienced by individuals with language impairment (DLD) or from younger typically developing children with a similar level of linguistic development.

Conclusion

This chapter attempted to answer the following questions:

- To what extent do autistic people have difficulties with implicit meaning?
- Do autistic people have difficulties with all kinds of implicit meaning?
- What is the underlying source of implicit meaning difficulties in autism?

The early days of the study of language in autism propagated that all autistic people had exceptional difficulty producing and understanding implicitly communicated nonliteral and figurative language (as part of pragmatics). More recent key studies have, however, revealed that an important factor in challenges with implicit meaning in autism is structural language competence. Nevertheless, even for autistic people with strong structural language competence, there are recent reports that pragmatic meaning comprehension and production are not identical to that of neurotypicals, with multiple hypotheses being put forward, ranging from the role of ToM to Executive Functions (mental skills for planning, remembering, inhibiting, etc.). Moreover, it is possible that here there is an effect of neurodiversity and different thinking styles that goes both ways: autistic people may not fully appreciate the pragmatic use of language by neurotypicals and the other way around. Future research is likely to focus on understanding how autistic people comprehend and produce pragmatic meaning in their own right, in addition to exploring the differences with neurotypical peers.

> **What Do You Know Now?**
> Although the examples presented in the "What do you think?" box are difficult for many autistic individuals, they occur in the noisy environment of daily life conversations, in which uncertainty accumulates. Perhaps implicit/pragmatic meaning challenges also relate to differences between the pragmatic profiles of autistic and neurotypical people, leading to misalignment.
> - Autistic people often do not understand or produce implicit meaning in the way that neurotypical people do.
> - Not all autistic people demonstrate the same kind of challenges with regard to implicit meaning, and not all kinds of implicit meaning are difficult for autistic people.
> - Many of the challenges that autistic people face with implicit/pragmatic meaning are due to often unassessed and underestimated structural language difficulty in autism, rather than being a corollary of autism itself.
> - Nevertheless, ToM is still likely to play a role in explaining some pragmatic challenges in autism (see also Chapter 8).
> - "Difficulty" with implicit/pragmatic meaning in autism may also be considered "difference" in thinking style between autistic and neurotypical people.

Suggestions for Further Reading

If you want to know more about the role of structural language in pragmatics in autism, you could read Norbury, Gemmell, and Paul 2014, which reviews a number of relevant findings and also asks whether there are people who have difficulties specifically with pragmatic communication without having autism. If you would like to know more about why pragmatics may sometimes, but not always, be impaired in autism, Katsos and Andrés-Roqueta (2021) take stock of the findings and make predictions for further research. Finally, arguments on why pragmatics in autism may be best characterized by difference rather than deficiency can be found in Crompton et al. 2020a and 2020b. These studies report that there was substantial information loss when sharing a story between multiple participants, of whom some were autistic and some nonautistic. However, when the narration chain included only autistic or only neurotypical participants, there was no information loss. If you are interested in this line of work, also read Morrison et al. 2020, who raise some important challenges.

References

Andrés-Roqueta, C. and Katsos, N. (2017). The contribution of grammar, vocabulary and Theory of Mind in pragmatic language competence in children with Autistic Spectrum Disorders. *Frontiers in Psychology* 8: 996.

Andrés-Roqueta, C. and Katsos, N. (2020). A distinction between linguistic and social pragmatics helps the precise characterization of pragmatic challenges in children with Autism Spectrum Disorders and Developmental Language Disorder. *Journal of Speech Language and Hearing Research* 63 (5): 1494–1508.

Baron-Cohen, S., Leslie, A.M., and Frith, U. (1985). Does the autistic child have a "Theory of Mind"? *Cognition* 21 (1): 37–46.

Breheny, R., Ferguson, H.J., Katsos, N., et al. (2013). Taking the epistemic step: toward a model of on-line access to conversational implicatures. *Cognition* 126 (3): 423–440.

Chahboun, S., Vulchanov, V., Saldana, D. et al. (2017). Can you tell it by the prime? A study of metaphorical priming in high-functioning autism in comparison with matched controls. *International Journal of Language and Communication Disorders* 52 (6): 766–785.

Crompton, C.J., Ropar, D., Evans-Williams, C.V. et al. (2020a). Autistic peer-to-peer information transfer is highly effective. *Autism* 24 (7): 1704–1712.

Crompton, C.J., Sharp, M., Axbey, H. et al. (2020b). Neurotype-matching, but not being autistic, influences self and observer ratings of interpersonal rapport. *Frontiers in Psychology* 11: 586171.

de Villiers, J., Myers, B., and Stainton, R.J. (2013). Revisiting pragmatic abilities in Autism Spectrum Disorders: a follow-up study with controls. *Pragmatics and Cognition* 21 (2): 253–269.

Deliens, G., Papastamou, F., Ruytenbeek, N. et al. (2018). Selective pragmatic impairment in Autism Spectrum Disorder: indirect requests versus irony. *Journal of Autism and Developmental Disorders* 48 (9): 2938–2952.

Filippova, E. (2014). Irony production and comprehension. In: *Pragmatic Development in First Language Acquisition* (ed. D. Matthews), 261–278. Amsterdam: John Benjamins.

Gernsbacher, M.A. and Pripas-Kapit, S.R. (2012). Who's missing the point? A commentary on claims that autistic persons have a specific deficit in figurative language comprehension. *Metaphor and Symbol* 27 (1): 93–105.

Grice, H.P. (1975). Logic and conversation. In: *Syntax and Semantics* (eds. P. Cole and J. Morgan), 41–58. New York: Academic Press.

Happé, F. and Frith, U. (2006). The weak coherence account: detail-focused cognitive style in Autism Spectrum Disorders. *Journal of Autism and Developmental Disorders* 36 (1): 5–25.

Happé, F.G. (1993). Communicative competence and Theory of Mind in autism: a test of relevance theory. *Cognition* 48 (2): 101–119.

Kalandadze, T., Bambini, V., and Næss, K.A.B. (2019). A systematic review and meta-analysis of studies on metaphor comprehension in individuals with Autism Spectrum Disorder: do task properties matter? *Applied Psycholinguistics* 40 (6): 1421–1454.

Kalandadze, T., Norbury, C., Nærland, T. et al. (2018). Figurative language comprehension in individuals with Autism Spectrum Disorder: a meta-analytic review. *Autism* 22 (2): 99–117.

Kanner, L. (1943). Early infantile autism. *The Journal of Pediatrics* 25: 211–217.

Kasirer, A. and Mashal, N. (2016). Comprehension and generation of metaphors by children with Autism Spectrum Disorder. *Research in Autism Spectrum Disorders* 32: 53–63.

Katsos, N. (2014). Scalar implicature. In: *Pragmatic Development in First Language Acquisition* (ed. D. Matthews), 183–198. Amsterdam: John Benjamins.

Katsos, N. and Andrés-Roqueta, C. (2021). Where next for pragmatics and mind reading? A situation-based view (response to Kissine). *Language* 97 (3): 184–197.

Katsos, N. and Ostashchenko, E. (2021). The role of visual perspective-taking in pragmatic inferencing. Lightening talk presented at *MK40: Common Knowledge, Common Ground, and Context in Communication*. University College London (25–26 June 2021).

Kissine, M. (2016). Pragmatics as metacognitive control. *Frontiers in Psychology* 6: 1–11.

Kissine, M., Cano-Chervel, J., Carlier, S. et al. (2015). Children with autism understand indirect speech acts: evidence from a semi-structured act-out task. *PLoS One* 10 (11): e0142191.

Köder, F. and Falkum, I.L. (2021). Irony and perspective-taking in children: the roles of norm violations and tone of voice. *Frontiers in Psychology* 3 (12): 624604.

Ledbetter, P.J. and Dent, C.H. (1988). Young children's sensitivity to direct and indirect request structure. *First Language* 8 (24): 227–245.

Mashal, N. and Kasirer, A. (2011). Thinking maps enhance metaphoric competence in children with autism and learning disabilities. *Research in Developmental Disabilities* 32 (6): 2045–2054.

Milton, D.E. (2012). On the ontological status of autism: The 'double empathy problem'. *Disability & Society* 27 (6): 883–887.

Morra, L. (2016). Raising awareness of how Asperger persons perceive their capacity to use Metaphors. *Medicina e Storia XVI* (9–10): 129–146.

Morrison, K.E., DeBrabander, K.M., Jones, D.R. et al. (2020). Outcomes of real-world social interaction for autistic adults paired with autistic compared to typically developing partners. *Autism* 24 (5): 1067–1080.

Norbury, C.F. (2005). The relationship between Theory of Mind and metaphor: evidence from children with language impairment and Autistic Spectrum Disorder. *British Journal of Developmental Psychology* 23 (3): 383–399.

Norbury, C.F., Gemmell, T., and Paul, R. (2014). Pragmatics abilities in narrative production: a cross-disorder comparison. *Journal of Child Language* 41 (3): 485–510.

Panzeri, F., Mazzaggio, G., Giustolisi, B. et al. (2022). The atypical pattern of irony comprehension in autistic children. *Applied Psycholinguistics* 43 (4): 757–784.

Paul, R., & Cohen, D. J. (1985). Comprehension of indirect requests in adults with autistic disorders and mental retardation. *Journal of Speech, Language, and Hearing Research* 28 (4): 475–479.

Petrolini, V., Jorba, M., and Vicente, A. (2023). What does it take to be rigid? Reflections on the notion of rigidity in autism. *Frontiers in Psychiatry* 13 (14): 1072362.

Pouscoulous, N. and Tomasello, M. (2020). Early birds: Metaphor understanding in 3-year-olds. *Journal of Pragmatics* 156: 160–167.

Rundblad, G. and Annaz, D. (2010). The atypical development of metaphor and metonymy comprehension in children with autism. *Autism* 14 (1): 29–46.

Vicente, A. and Falkum, I.L. (2023). Accounting for the preference of literal meanings in ASC. *Mind & Language* 38 (1): 119–140.

Vicente, A., Michel, C., and Petrolini, V. (2023). Literalism in autistic people: a predictive processing proposal. *Review of Philosophy and Psychology*.

Volden, J. and Phillips, L. (2010). Measuring pragmatic language in speakers with Autism Spectrum Disorders: comparing the children's communication checklist—2 and the test of pragmatic language. *Journal of the American Journal of Speech-Language Pathology* 19 (3): 204–212.

Wilson, A.C. and Bishop, D.V. (2022). Stage 2 registered report: investigating a preference for certainty in conversation among autistic adults. *PeerJ* 10: e13110.

7

Narration

Elena Peristeri, Philippine Geelhand, and Ianthi Maria Tsimpli

> **What Do You Think?**
> Bob is an autistic boy aged 8. His mother has just read the Cinderella story to him. Upon finishing the story, she says: "Now, can you tell me the story in your own words?" Bob says: "At twelve o'clock midnight, the clock rang 'Dong, dong, dong, dong, dong, dong, dong, dong, dong, dong, dong!' twelve times, and Cinderella said goodbye to the prince. Cinderella ran away wearing a pair of blue, turquoise slippers. While running, she lost her left slipper. He found it the next day and went to her home. Cinderella was sitting next to her stepsister. He tried the slipper on her foot and gave it back to her. He didn't see the cinders in her hair or the ashes on her face." Bob's mother wonders why he retells the story in this particular way and how other children would do this. What do you think?

Introduction

The overall structure and organization of a story, or narrative, also known as **narrative macrostructure** or **narrative discourse structure**, plays a crucial role in creating and understanding an intelligible and meaningful story. Storytelling is an integral part of our lives and serves various communicative functions, including providing information about real or fictional events, including the relationships between them (temporal, causal, etc.), and the characters involved. The communicative value of a narrative mainly originates from its relevance, since the narrator wishes to convey information about a certain set of events that are somehow "worthy" of telling. Given its interactional nature, storytelling becomes a collaborative product of the narrator and the listener; the narrator needs to adjust their story based on what the listener already knows and understands, and the listener needs to make assumptions and predictions about how language in a story serves various purposes and functions. Thus, the ability

Language in Autism, First Edition. Edited by Jeannette Schaeffer et al.
© 2025 John Wiley & Sons Ltd. Published 2025 by John Wiley & Sons Ltd.

to tell and comprehend stories requires the simultaneous integration of linguistic, cognitive, and social cues. Since each of these factors may be atypical in autism, autistic people may display a different macrostructure in their storytelling and comprehend stories differently from nonautistic individuals. This chapter therefore addresses the following questions:

- What does narrative macrostructure look like in narratives produced by autistic individuals?
- What factors can explain differences in the narrative macrostructure of autistic and nonautistic individuals?
- Does comprehension of narratives differ between autistic and nonautistic individuals?

Anchoring

When people tell or retell a story, they need to organize their story in such a way that the listener(s) can follow and understand the story as easily as possible. To this end, the narrator must apply structure to the story, also referred to as narrative macrostructure. Efficient narrative macrostructure requires the integration of different types of linguistic (including pragmatic) knowledge (see Chapter 1) into the narration. The following sections introduce some of the most widely acknowledged elements of narrative macrostructure: (i) story structure components and structural complexity, which contribute to the global organization of the story's content; (ii) internal state terms, which are words that describe the internal feelings, emotions, thoughts, intentions, and perceptions of others; (iii) cohesive ties, which are words used to create links throughout the story, e.g. pronouns such as *she, he, they*, and connectives such as *because, after*; (iv) narrative comprehension, which includes deriving inferences from the narrative (see Chapter 6 on implicit meaning for more details).

Acronym and Terminology Reminder
Connective: Word or phrase that links words, phrases, or clauses (e.g. *and, or, because, after*).
Cohesive Ties: Words used to create links throughout a story, e.g. pronouns (referential ties) and connectives (relational ties).
EF: Executive Function – set of mental skills for planning, remembering, etc. (inhibition, flexibility, attentional control, Working Memory, etc.)
Internal State Terms: Words that describe internal feelings, emotions, thoughts, intentions, and perceptions.
Narrative Macrostructure: Overall structure and organization of a story.
Narration: Telling a story.
Pronouns: Words such as *she, he, they*.
SES: Socioeconomic status.
Structural Language: Formal aspects of language related to phonology, morphology, syntax, and semantics.
ToM: Theory of Mind – ability to infer and understand mental states (e.g. beliefs, true, or false) in oneself and others.

Several theories and models of macrostructure have been formulated to evaluate the organization of narratives at a global level. The **Story Grammar** framework is the most widely accepted model of macrostructure nowadays (Stein and Glenn 1979). It attempts to capture information that adults and children consider important to include in stories (Gagarina et al. 2016). This model characterizes and quantifies the macrostructure components presented by the narrator, including the setting (time and place), goals of the characters in the story, attempts made by the characters to reach their goals, outcomes, and reactions of the characters. Topic coverage is examined by determining how many episodes an individual has attempted to express. Episodes themselves are composed of goals, attempts, outcomes, and reactions of the characters. If episodes are consistently produced with at least two of the three necessary components (i.e. goal, attempt, and outcome), then the speaker is expressing partially or completely complex episodes. According to a number of studies, the **Goal-Attempt-Outcome** (GAO) sequence represents the highest level of structural complexity, since goals motivate attempts, which can, in turn, cause or motivate a series of outcomes (e.g. Westby 2012).

The use of **internal state language** in narratives requires understanding of the characters' feelings, thoughts, and perceptions and understanding that characters can have different perspectives on the same event. Internal state terms can be divided into subcategories, such as emotional (*happy, sad, feel*), cognitive (*think, remember, know*), or perceptive (*hear, see*) terms.

Creating **cohesive ties** throughout the narrative structure also contributes to narrative macrostructure. Ties between story events can be formed through **reference chains**, where different expressions are used to identify the story characters throughout the narrative (e.g. phrases such as *the boy* or pronouns such as *he*). To figure out the right expression to use, speakers consider various factors, such as what the listener already knows and what has been previously narrated. When we use words or phrases to refer to something, we are trying to convey certain aspects of the thing we have in mind, which the listener reconstructs by integrating what is said with what they already know and what they expect. As such, the referential form we choose depends on both our own thinking and what we think the listener knows/understands in the story we are telling. This is an unconscious process, taking place automatically and implicitly in neurotypical people.

The choice of **referential ties** in a narrative requires the narrator to consider the listener's knowledge and understanding in order to effectively communicate information to them. For instance, the introduction of characters is typically done using an indefinite noun phrase, a noun phrase with an indefinite article, such as *a(n)* (e.g. *Once upon a time, there was **an elephant-girl**...*). Maintaining reference can be accomplished through the use of pronouns, overt (e.g. ***She** packed her lunch*) and null (e.g. *She packed her lunch; ø put it in her bag and ø left the kitchen*), as well as definite noun phrases (a noun phrase with a definite article – *the*). The choice between these two depends on the degree of ambiguity created for the listener in the unfolding discourse. So, for example, the pronoun *they* clearly refer to *the elephant* and *the giraffe* in the following: *The elephant and the giraffe decided to race to the swimming pool.* **They** *started running*.

In contrast, using a pronoun to refer to the giraffe (*The elephant and the giraffe decided to race to the swimming pool.* **He** *started running first*) would be a source of ambiguity as the pronoun *it* could also refer to the elephant. In such cases, using a definite noun phrase is more appropriate (*The elephant and the giraffe decided to race to the swimming pool.* **The giraffe** *started running first*). Definite noun phrases can also be used to reintroduce characters following the mentioning of another character, as in the following: *The elephant started crying. A lifeguard arrived.* **The elephant** *explained what happened* (see also Chapter 8 on referential ties).

In addition to referential ties, cohesive ties in narration can be established using **relational ties,** or **connectives**, such as *then*, *after*, *because*, and *therefore*. Relational ties provide specific instructions to the listener on how to connect events or ideas together. Using fewer of them can affect **narrative coherence**, and how well a story makes sense. When a discourse relation, i.e. a relation between the ideas of two sentences/clauses/utterances, is left implicit, it places a burden on the listeners, who have to infer the connection by themselves, potentially affecting their understanding (e.g. *The floor is wet* **because** *the janitor just mopped it* vs. *The floor is wet. The janitor just mopped it*). Table 7.1 presents a summary of the macrostructure components and their definitions (with examples).

Various tools exist to elicit narratives for assessment or research purposes. One of the most popular narrative elicitation tools is the LITMUS Multilingual Assessment Instrument for Narratives (MAIN; Gagarina et al. 2019), which allows for comparable assessment of narrative skills and in different elicitation modes, including telling (production of an original story), retelling (reproduction of a story that has been previously read/heard), and model story (providing a framework for individuals to follow in their own storytelling), and, where relevant, in several languages in the same child. MAIN also includes a set of comprehension questions that allows for assessment of the child's ability to derive inferences from the narrative told or retold. Other narrative tools include the Bus Story (Renfrew 2010), wordless picture books such as *Frog, Where Are You?* (Mayer 2003), and the Edmonton Narrative Norms Instrument (ENNI; Schneider, Dubé, and Hayward 2005); see Figure 7.1. Although not a typical narrative tool, ADOS-2, a standard diagnostic assessment tool, is also commonly used to elicit narrative productions from autistic adolescents and adults with fluent speech. The ADOS-2 includes a narrative task based on the wordless picture book *Tuesday* (Wiesner 1991).

Table 7.1 Summary of macrostructure components.

Macrostructure components	Definition	Examples
Story grammar	Characterizes and quantifies macrostructure components presented by the narrator	*story setting, characters' goals, attempts, resolution*
Internal state language	Language used to express the thoughts, feelings, beliefs, desires, and perceptions of characters	*sad, happy, think, want*
Cohesive ties	Linguistic expressions used to tie story events together	
Referential ties	Expressions used to identify story characters throughout the narrative	*a dog, the boy, he, they*
Relational ties (connectives)	Words/expressions indicating the type of relationship between story events/ideas	*then, after, because, therefore*

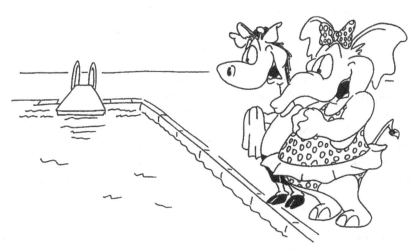

Figure 7.1 Example picture from the Diving Board story, Edmonton Narrative Norms Instrument (ENNI). *Source:* Schneider, Dubé, and Hayward (2005). Reproduced with permission from Terry Willis, Wooket Studios.

The responses and behaviors observed during a narrative task contribute to the overall assessment of social and communication skills, making this type of assessment especially relevant for study of language in autism.

Narration in Autism

What Does Narrative Macrostructure Look Like in Narratives Produced by Autistic Individuals?

Narrative production can be challenging for autistic individuals, even for those with average or above-average cognitive and language skills. When narrating a picture storybook, autistic individuals tend to tell stories that are under- or over-informative. Specifically, they may either skip pieces of information that rely on implied meaning, such as the story characters' emotions, beliefs, and intentions, or they may include irrelevant information and excessive details about the pictures in the storybook, with less engagement in figuring out the broader meaning and relations between the story's events and characters. These specificities in narrative production have implications for the macrostructure as they result in less coherent stories. Research has shown that autistic individuals struggle to link information to situations in a coherent way using sentences that encode causal, temporal, or spatial relations. They also seem to have difficulties verbalizing inferences about characters or situations in the stories. Limited **pragmatic inferencing skills**[1] (see Chapter 6) have also been shown to have negative effects on autistic individuals' ability to adequately explain the story characters' reactions in both narrative production and comprehension. The paragraphs below provide some further details on what narrative macrostructure looks like in autism.

Autistic children often seem to face significant challenges when it comes to the structural complexity of narratives, especially in understanding and expressing the motivations or goals of the characters within the story (Diehl, Bennetto, and Young 2006). Even when autistic children include story grammar components in their narrative episodes, they are more likely to use descriptive fragments (e.g. *The elephant-girl ran to the swimming pool. She slipped*) and less likely to represent the goals of the characters within a causal framework (e.g. *The elephant-girl started running, **because** she wanted to arrive first at the swimming pool, and she slipped*; Peristeri, Andreou, and Tsimpli 2017).

---

1 Pragmatic inferencing skills refer to the ability to draw conclusions about meaning based on contextual cues and background knowledge within a given communication situation. It is like figuring out the "hidden" message by paying attention to how people talk and the context they are in.

Note, in this respect, that current scoring schemes in instruments used for elicitation of narratives may not be suitable for defining particular features of narratives specific to autism, such as irrelevant or noninstrumental pieces of information that autistic individuals tend to include in their narratives. Negative score metrics could shed light on autistic individuals' preference for and valuation of off-topic information as well as on their ability to focus on meaningful information during narrative production. This proposal is supported by the results of the study by Geelhand et al. (2020). Specifically, these authors found that compared to the narratives of their nonautistic peers, those produced by the autistic adults included more features highlighting the development of the participants' own evaluation of the story and of the narrative task itself (e.g. more discourse markers, such as *well*, *you see*, and irrelevant comments), and fewer features to develop the story characters and establish a relationship between the story events (e.g. fewer internal state terms and connectives).

Zooming in on internal state terms, several other narrative studies in autism have also found that individuals on the autism spectrum tend to use fewer internal state terms than their peers. This may stem from their difficulty in monitoring and reasoning about the story characters' mental states. For instance, autistic children and adolescents have been found to score particularly poorly on the Strange Stories test (Happé 1994). In this test, some stories require attributing mental states to characters in complex and ambiguous social scenarios (i.e. scenarios depicting different components of ToM, such as white lies or sarcasm), in comparison to stories that require causal reasoning about physical states only (i.e. the stories are not social in nature and do not involve mental states). Rumpf et al. (2012) also found that school-aged autistic children without cognitive and language delays used fewer cognitive internal state terms during storytelling compared to nonautistic children.

Like children and adolescents, autistic adults also include fewer mental state terms than nonautistic adults in their narratives. Geelhand et al. (2020) found that autistic adults produced fewer cognitive (e.g. *believe*, *question*), emotional (e.g. *to be happy/sad*), and physiological (e.g. *see*, *hear*) terms than their nonautistic peers, but there were no group differences in modal (*want*, *desire*) and evaluative terms (*apparently*, *obviously*), suggesting that autistic adults provided less information about the mental reasoning and emotional and sensorial experiences of the story characters.

Narratives produced by autistic people tend to reveal difficulties with elements that tie the story together – both relational ties and referential ties, which provide cohesion to the story. With regards to relational ties, several studies have found that autistic children and adults use fewer connectives such as *then*, *after*, *because*, and *therefore*, to establish ties between story events in their narratives (e.g. Diehl, Bennetto, and Young 2006; Colle et al. 2008; Geelhand et al. 2020).

As for referential ties, choosing the appropriate expressions to refer to things, animals, and people relies on the interaction between language and perspective-taking abilities, which are known to be altered in autistic individuals (see Chapter 8 for more details about referential forms and use in autism). Indeed, both autistic children and adults have been shown to have difficulties using pronouns. Colle et al.'s (2008) narrative study was among the first to show that autistic adults produce more ambiguous references when referring to characters other than the main characters of the story. Referential ambiguity occurs in language when pronouns have several possible antecedents (words or phrases that a pronoun refers back to for its meaning). For example, consider the sentence: *The elephant and the giraffe saw the diving board.* ***He*** *wanted to dive in.* In this sentence, the pronoun *he* is ambiguous: it could refer to either *the elephant* or *the giraffe*, making it unclear which animal wants to dive in. An equivocal relationship between a pronoun and its antecedent can make it challenging to keep track of the presence, recency, and prominence of referents in previous discourse.

Referential ambiguity can also occur when a pronoun is used without a clear antecedent (e.g. *Once upon a time, she…*), which indicates difficulties in recognizing the need to introduce the referent before using the pronoun. Studies have found that autistic children tend to produce more ambiguous and underinformative pronouns (underspecified) compared to nonautistic peers (Novogrodsky and Edelson 2016). Conversely, it has also been found that autistic children and adolescents use more explicit and overinformative (overspecified) expressions, such as noun phrases or proper names, e.g. *Cinderella*, and fewer pronouns in narrative production than their nonautistic peers.

While difficulties in narrative production are well documented in autistic individuals, relatively less is known about their narrative comprehension skills. Autistic children have been shown to perform significantly lower in inferential comprehension than their nonautistic peers (Norbury and Bishop 2002; Westerveld and Roberts 2017) or children with Developmental Language Disorder (DLD) (Norbury and Bishop 2002). Also, Nuske and Bavin (2011) found that autistic children showed specific difficulties answering questions that required script inferencing, i.e. making inferences based on expected patterns of socially relevant, daily events, such as going to the supermarket or visiting a museum, as opposed to factual questions that required deductive logical reasoning. (Here, "script" refers to a mental representation of a sequence of actions or behaviors that are typically expected to occur in a particular situation.) More specifically, autistic children experience greater difficulty than their nonautistic peers in bridging a causal inference between two activities in a social event script (e.g. going to the swimming pool). For example, autistic children had difficulties figuring out why a person would want to go to a swimming pool and then being angry about not being allowed to swim due to forgetting their swimsuit at home (Dennis, Lazenby, and Lockyer 2001).

Summarizing, narrative macrostructure seems to present a major challenge for autistic people. Autistic individuals tend to tell stories that are under- or overinformative. In comparison to neurotypical people, they may use fewer story grammar components expressing information about the story setting, characters' goals, attempts, and resolutions, fewer internal state terms, and fewer cohesive (referential and relational) ties expressing referential, temporal, or causal relations between events and characters in the story.

What Factors Can Explain Differences in the Narrative Macrostructure of Autistic and Nonautistic Individuals?

Several underlying mechanisms for the differences in narrative macrostructure between autistic and nonautistic people have been suggested. Differences in expressing complex episodes in narrative production seem to reflect general narrative impairment in autistic individuals rather than difficulties with expressive language (language production) (e.g. Manolitsi and Botting 2011; Baixauli et al. 2016). Norbury, Gemmell, and Paul (2014) found that mastery of structural language (which, in this study, included lexical/vocabulary skills – see Chapter 2, morphosyntax – see Chapter 3, and phonology – see Chapter 4) in a group of autistic children was negatively correlated with the number of relevant information units in their narratives. This suggests that structural language abilities do not facilitate the use of central "gist" episode components in autistic children's storytelling.

In their study on narrative comprehension, Westerveld and Roberts (2017) also examined the role of autistic children's structural language skills. They found that while autistic children, both those with and those without language difficulties, struggled more to infer information than their nonautistic peers, the autistic children with no language difficulties performed equally well compared to their nonautistic peers on factual narrative comprehension. Their findings suggest that autistic children are prone to experiencing inferential comprehension difficulties regardless of their structural language abilities. While there are not many narrative studies with autistic children that have taken into account structural language skills (vocabulary, grammar) and/or included participants with different levels of language abilities, the overall emerging research indicates challenges in inferential comprehension for all autistic individuals relative to other nonautistic individuals.

Core extralinguistic cognitive factors seem to play a particularly important role in narrative macrostructure in autistic individuals. A prominent example is **Theory of Mind (ToM)**. ToM refers to the ability to infer and understand mental states (e.g. beliefs, true, or false) in oneself and others. Difficulties in using ToM to interpret behavior as well as to simulate a perspective that is counter to one's own make it hard for people with autism to adopt the story characters' emotional and cognitive viewpoints in order to explain their motivations and reactions.

For example, differences in ToM abilities are proposed to be one of the main factors underlying the reduced use of internal state terms in autistic individuals' narratives. Boorse et al. (2019) showed that autistic children tended to produce considerably fewer emotional and cognitive terms (e.g. *to want, to feel*) in their narratives as compared to nonautistic peers, while cognitive terms were positively correlated with the autistic children's ToM skills. Different ToM abilities in autistic children have also been suggested to explain referential ambiguity in their narrations. That is, the production of more ambiguous and underinformative pronouns (pronouns without a clear antecedent, e.g. *Once upon a time, she...*) by autistic children as compared to nonautistic peers has been attributed to their mentalizing (ToM) difficulties (Novogrodsky and Edelson 2016).

Difficulties with **Executive Function (EF)**, the set of mental skills used for planning, remembering, etc. (inhibition, flexibility, attentional control, Working Memory, etc.), may also impact narration. Recall that, besides producing ambiguous and underinformative pronouns, autistic children and adolescents also use more explicit and overinformative (overspecified) expressions, such as noun phrases or proper names, e.g. *Cinderella*, and fewer pronouns in narrative production than their nonautistic peers. It has been suggested that this is due to their EF difficulties (Arnold, Bennetto, and Diehl 2009) (see Chapter 8). Although both proposed explanations, i.e. differences in ToM and differences in EF, have been invoked in studies of reference use in autistic individuals' narrative macrostructure, it is still unclear if and how ToM and EF challenges have distinct impacts on the way autistic individuals make referential choices during narrative production.

Another extralinguistic cognitive factor that may affect narrative macrostructure in both autistic and nonautistic individuals is related to remarkable attention to detail and difficulty in seeing the "big picture" (i.e. generalization and integration of local details into a global entity), which have been previously linked to autism in what is known as the **central coherence** account. Along with ToM and EF, central coherence has been associated with autistic individuals' performance in various macrostructural measures, including story structure, structural complexity, and narrative comprehension (Beaumont and Newcombe 2006; Peristeri et al. 2020).

In addition to difficulties with cognitive functions, sociodemographic factors, such as experience with dual or multiple languages (**multilingualism**) and the person's **socioeconomic status (SES)**, have also been found to influence the cognitive patterns underlying narrative macrostructure in autistic people. Some research suggests that multilingualism boosts various cognitive functions relevant for narrative macrostructure, such as social cognition, in particular, ToM and EF. For neurotypical people, it has been suggested that multilingualism enhances awareness of the perspectives of others (boosting ToM development), due to the fact that multilingual people need to first consider their interlocutor's language before deciding which language to use. Enhanced skills due to bilingualism have also been reported for autism: by Durrleman, Peristeri, and Tsimpli (2022) for ToM, and by Gonzalez-Barrero and Nadig (2019) and Peristeri, Vogelzang, and Tsimpli (2021) for EF, such as cognitive flexibility and attention shifting, which are often areas of difficulty in autism. However, see Lehtonen, Fyndanis, and Jylkkä (2023) for a different perspective on the extent of multilingual advantages in executive functioning.

Some studies on bilingual autistic individuals have shown that they produce more fully developed episodes in narrative production than their monolingual autistic peers (Peristeri et al. 2020). If multilinguals indeed have more developed EF skills, and if EF skills play a mediating role in narrative macrostructure, this may explain the more fully developed episodes in the narrative production of autistic bilinguals as compared to autistic monolinguals. However, more research is needed to firmly establish this.

Also, note that in the studies by Peristeri and colleagues investigating narratives in bilingual children, these children were born to families where one parent spoke the societal language, Greek, and the other another language, so they were exposed to two languages since birth, though they were Greek-dominant. Future research needs to include other types of bilingualism (e.g. sequential bilingualism) (see Chapter 13) as well as different languages (and language combinations for bilingual autistic individuals) focusing on the way languages express (or not) macrostructural properties. For example, it would be interesting to explore whether typologically diverse languages, such as Russian and Greek that express definiteness on nouns differently (Russian through word order, Greek with a definite article), would have different effects on the referential ambiguity of the narratives of Russian–Greek bilingual autistic children, depending on whether they would produce the narrative in Greek or Russian (see Chapter 13).

Turning now to SES, this is often measured in terms of the number of years of education of the mother. SES has been found to enhance both verbal and nonverbal intelligence indices (including EF) in a group of bilingual autistic children, especially in those coming from low-SES households (Peristeri, Silleresi, and Tsimpli 2022). However, there is scant research on how sociodemographic factors, such as bilingualism (see Chapter 13 for more details) or SES, affect narrative macrostructure in autism, so more research is needed to establish SES influence on storytelling skills.

In sum, narrative macrostructure abilities in autistic people differ from those of nonautistic people, irrespective of autistic people's nonverbal intelligence and language skills. Even autistic individuals whose IQ, and lexical, morphosyntactic, and phonological skills fall within the normal range seem to experience narration challenges (Baixauli et al. 2016). Core extralinguistic cognitive functions such as ToM and EF, which are often vulnerable in autism, do seem to be associated with narrative skills. If sociodemographic factors such as multilingualism and high SES boost ToM and EF, as has been suggested by some, it is worth further exploring the question as to whether multilingualism and high SES may enhance narrative skills in (some) autistic people.

Focus on a Specific Study

A big question in narrative studies in autism is whether lexical skills play a role in shaping autistic individuals' narrative performance. The study by Peristeri, Andreou, and Tsimpli (2017) addressed this question by stratifying 30 Greek-speaking autistic children aged 6–12 (mean age: 9) into low and high vocabulary ability groups based on their expressive vocabulary scores. All of the autistic children had Full Scale IQs over 80 and thus no intellectual disability. The children's expressive vocabulary was tested through the Greek adaptation of the Renfrew Word Finding test (Vogindroukas, Protopapas, and Sideridis 2009). The two groups, along with age-matched nonautistic peers, were tested on oral retelling using a picture story from the Edmonton Narrative Norms Instrument (ENNI) that includes eight pictures and three complete episodes. One of the study's aims was to investigate how different levels of vocabulary ability (low vs. high) influence three key aspects of narrative macrostructure, namely, cohesion, internal state language, and story grammar.

Cohesion was measured by the use of two types of embedded clauses (clauses that cannot stand alone as a sentence, also known as subordinate, or dependent clauses): adverbial clauses and relative clauses. Adverbial clauses, e.g. the bold-faced part in *My grandma bought me a bicycle* **when I was 7**, starting with the connective *when*, contribute to cohesion by providing temporal information. Adverbial clauses can also express causal information, as illustrated by the bold-faced part starting with the connective *because* in *I was happy* **because I could cycle to school**. Relative clauses, for example, the bold-faced part in *The book* **that I bought** *was torn*, contribute to cohesion by providing referential information: the relative clause *that I bought* grounds the noun phrase *the book* (the head of the relative clause) with respect to discourse information and elaborates on the referential properties of *the book*. Second, the study looked at internal state language, by analyzing lexical expressions that encode the story characters' internal states. Internal state terms also often feature in another type of embedded clause: the complement clause *Susan was happy* **that she came by train** – see also Chapter 3. Lastly, the study investigated the story's macrostructure by analyzing story grammar components (e.g. story setting, characters' goals, attempts, and outcomes).

Regarding cohesion, the study found that autistic children across the board were less competent than a comparison group of nonautistic children at using adverbial and relative clauses to encode causal, temporal, and referential relations between the events and characters of a story. Furthermore, although the autistic children with high vocabulary skills tended to do better at expressing temporal and causal relations (through the use of adverbial clauses) than the autistic children with low vocabulary skills, this difference between the two autistic groups was not statistically significant.

As for the use of internal state language, the study revealed that both the high vocabulary and the low vocabulary autistic groups used fewer internal state terms than their nonautistic peers. Nevertheless, there were some differences between the two autistic groups. The autistic children with high vocabulary skills tended to use significantly more lexical markers that encoded the characters' emotional states (e.g. *sad, angry, happy*) and cognitive viewpoints (e.g. *think, wonder*), possibly related to ToM, than the low vocabulary group. The low vocabulary group seemed to rely more on the use of lexical items that encoded perceptual states (e.g. *see, hear*), unrelated to ToM, to make sense of the inner world of the story characters. These findings align with the developmental literature showing that perception verbs (*see, hear*) are generally acquired before cognitive verbs (*think, wonder*) (Davis and Landau 2020), and that the use of internal state terms denoting the thoughts and emotions of the characters of a story is related to sociocognitive skills, such as empathy and ToM (Mar and Oatley 2008). Furthermore, there was a significant difference concerning the use of verb complement clauses (often making use of internal state terms), whereby the autistic children with low vocabulary skills performed significantly lower than the autistic children with higher vocabulary skills. Interestingly, the rate of complement clause use was positively correlated with the use of internal state terms encoding emotional states and cognitive viewpoints (i.e. ToM-related internal state terms).

The findings by Peristeri, Andreou, and Tsimpli (2017) regarding internal state language underline the promising role of narration in the study of the sociocognitive skills (such as empathy and ToM) of autistic individuals and the way these skills are related to these individuals' lexical ability. Nevertheless, more research is needed to shed light on the causal mechanisms behind the relation between vocabulary skills and internal state term use in autistic children's narrative macrostructure performance.

The results pertaining to story grammar showed that story grammar elements were equally low across the high and low vocabulary autistic children and, in fact, fell far below the story grammar units produced by their nonautistic peers. This particular finding suggests that the autistic children with high vocabulary skills failed to leverage their intact lexical resources to cope with the demands of producing complete episodes in their narration.

Interestingly, the authors reported a strong link between the scores for story grammar complexity and use of adverbial and relative clauses (containing cohesive ties) for all children. In contrast, there was no link between story grammar complexity scores and use of other types of embedded clauses, such as verb complement clauses (e.g. *Susan was happy **that she came by train***). This suggests that being able to produce complex morphosyntactic structures (such as sentences with embedded clauses) in general is not enough to produce coherent stories. Instead, being able to produce sentences that include causal or temporal information (as in adverbial clauses) or referential information (as in relative clauses) is a major contributor to the organization of events in storytelling by autistic children.

Overall, the study by Peristeri, Andreou, and Tsimpli (2017) reveals intriguing asymmetries in the role that lexical skills play in autistic children's narrative macrostructure, depending on the narrational demands of the various macrostructural dimensions. Higher vocabulary skills appear to positively influence the use of ToM-related internal state language. However, more demanding macrostructural components such as cohesion and story grammar seem to weaken the compensatory effect of the autistic children's lexical skills. In other words, stronger vocabulary skills do not appear to boost cohesion or story grammar complexity. As an alternative strategy, the autistic children in this study tended to use coordination (connecting two sentences by using *and*, *or*, *but*), rather than embedding. This suggests that autistic children tend to retell stories by means of linear (i.e. coordination), rather than hierarchical (i.e. subordination, embedding) structures to communicate the core part of a story.

The result that even the high-vocabulary autistic group performed more poorly than the nonautistic comparison group on all three measures of macrostructure in Peristeri et al.'s study speaks against the idea that autistic children without language and cognitive delay are able to efficiently organize their narrative macrostructure, at least in the same way(s) that nonautistic children do (e.g. Landa 2000). Another takeaway message from this study is that narrative macrostructure is not a monolithic process, in that cohesion devices, internal state terms, and story grammar elements are differentially affected by the lexical skills of autistic children.

The part of the study by Peristeri, Andreou, and Tsimpli (2017) discussed above is one of the few studies that have investigated the impact of autistic children's lexical skills on narrative macrostructure. The authors also looked at the effect of particular aspects of morphosyntax on story grammar (specifically, use of adverbial, relative, and complement clauses). However, the impact of language skills beyond the lexicon (including structural language) on narrative performance in autism needs much further exploration. For example, more research is needed to examine the effect of global morphosyntactic skills on autistic children's narrative macrostructure.

Conclusion

This chapter set out to address the following questions:

- What does narrative macrostructure look like in narratives produced by autistic individuals?
- What factors can explain differences in the narrative macrostructure of autistic and nonautistic individuals?
- Does comprehension of narratives differ between autistic and nonautistic individuals?

Studies on narrative macrostructure in autism show that autistic individuals have selective difficulties in narrative macrostructure and aspects of narrative comprehension, compared to their nonautistic peers, even if they have IQ and language skills that fall within the normal range. Although autistic individuals can create some aspects of narrative structure, they tend to use fewer story grammar components, less internal state language, and fewer cohesive ties, which makes it more difficult for the listener to piece together a coherent and meaningful story. The impact of general language (including structural language) skills on narration in autism remains underexplored. Future research needs to address the effect of, for example, morphosyntax on autistic people's narrative performance.

It is important to note that the magnitude of narrative difficulties seems to vary depending on core aspects of an autistic individual's language, social, and cognitive profiles. Furthermore, sociodemographic factors such as bilingualism and SES may play a role. Although there are indications that multilingualism may enhance autistic children's ToM and EF skills, and therefore macrostructural narration abilities, more research is needed to establish the impact of bilingualism, ToM, and EF (e.g. memory, attention, cognitive flexibility) on narrative macrostructure in autism.

There is also a need for investigation of other, e.g. sentence-level semantic factors, that may contribute to macrostructural narration. For example, evidential contexts, i.e. expressing direct knowledge of an event through perception (*I **see** that Kim is at home; she's sitting on the couch*) or indirect knowledge of an event through inferencing (*Kim **seems** to be at home; the door is open*), may have an effect on the way autistic individuals are able to utilize their linguistic and extralinguistic cognitive resources to cope with macrostructural demands in their narratives.

In sum, research is beginning to explore the relationship between narrative macrostructure, skills in each linguistic domain (see Chapter 1), extralinguistic cognitive skills such as EF and ToM, and sociodemographic factors including multilingualism and SES in autism. Further research is crucial, as knowledge of the mechanisms underlying narrative performance in autism may foster understanding among non-autistic people of the characteristics of narrations produced by autistic people.

> **What Do You Know Now?**
> Now that you have a better overview of how autistic individuals typically construct the macrostructure of their narratives, you can better understand why it was difficult to follow Bob's narrative given at the beginning of the chapter.
> - Bob's narrative does not contain many references to the internal states of the characters in his story. As we have seen, autistic individuals may have difficulties expressing the internal mental states of the story's characters.
> - Bob's narrative also lacks connectives and contains ambiguous references. As we have seen, cohesive ties, such as referential expressions and connectives, may be an area of difficulty for autistic individuals.
> - Macrostructural skills in autistic individuals appear to vary depending on the specific resources (language, social, and cognitive) required by each aspect of macrostructure, as well as their sociodemographic profile (bilingual experience and socioeconomic status).

Suggestion for Further Reading

If you are interested in learning more about narration in autism, we recommend the meta-analysis by Baixauli et al. 2016, as they provide a comprehensive overview of articles on this topic, highlighting common findings and patterns across studies.

References

Arnold, J.E., Bennetto, L., and Diehl, J.J. (2009). Reference production in young speakers with and without autism: effects of discourse status and processing constraints. *Cognition* 110 (2): 131–146.

Baixauli, I., Colomer, C., Roselló, B. et al. (2016). Narratives of children with high-functioning Autism Spectrum Disorder: a meta-analysis. *Research in Developmental Disabilities* 59: 234–254.

Beaumont, R. and Newcombe, P. (2006). Theory of Mind and central coherence in adults with high-functioning autism or Asperger Syndrome. *Autism* 10 (4): 365–382.

Boorse, J., Cola, M., Plate, S. et al. (2019). Linguistic markers of autism in girls: evidence of a "blended phenotype" during storytelling. *Molecular Autism* 10: 14.

Colle, L., Baron-Cohen, S., Wheelwright, S. et al. (2008). Narrative discourse in adults with high-functioning autism or Asperger Syndrome. *Journal of Autism and Developmental Disorders* 38 (1): 28–40.

Davis, E. and Landau, B. (2020). Seeing and believing: the relationship between perception and mental verbs in acquisition. *Language Learning and Development* 17 (1): 26–47.

Dennis, M. Lazenby, A.L., and Lockyer, L. (2001). Inferential language in high-function children with autism. *Journal of Autism and Developmental Disorders* 31 (1): 47–54.

Diehl, J.J., Bennetto, L., and Young, E.C. (2006). Story recall and narrative coherence of high-functioning children with Autism Spectrum Disorders. *Journal of Abnormal Child Psychology* 34 (1): 87–102.

Durrleman, S., Peristeri, E., and Tsimpli, I.M. (2022). The language-communication divide: evidence from bilingual children with atypical development. *Evolutionary Linguistic Theory* 4 (1): 5–51.

Gagarina N., Klop D., Tsimpli I. M. et al. (2016). Narrative abilities in bilingual children. *Applied Psycholinguistics* 37 (1): 11–17.

Gagarina, N.V., Klop, D., Kunnari, S. et al. (2019). MAIN: Multilingual Assessment Instrument for Narratives. *ZAS Papers in Linguistics* 56: 155.

Geelhand, P., Papastamou, F., Deliens, G. et al. (2020). Narrative production in autistic adults: a systematic analysis of the microstructure, macrostructure and internal state language. *Journal of Pragmatics* 164: 57–81.

Gonzalez-Barrero, A.M. and Nadig, A.S. (2019). Can bilingualism mitigate set-shifting difficulties in children with Autism Spectrum Disorders? *Child Development* 90 (4): 1043–1060.

Happé, F.G.E. (1994). An advanced test of Theory of Mind: understanding of story characters' thoughts and feelings by able autistic, mentally handicapped, and normal children and adults. *Journal of Autism and Developmental Disorders* 24 (2): 129–154.

Landa, R. (2000). Social language use in Asperger Syndrome and high-functioning autism. In: *Asperger Syndrome* (eds. A. Klin, F.R. Volkmar, and S.S. Sparrow), 125–155. The Guilford Press.

Lehtonen, M., Fyndanis, V., and Jylkkä, J. (2023). The relationship between bilingual language use and Executive Functions. *Nature Reviews Psychology* 2: 360–373.

Manolitsi, M. and Botting, N. (2011). Language abilities in children with autism and language impairment: using narrative as an additional source of clinical information. *Child Language Teaching and Therapy* 27 (1): 39–55.

Mar, R.A. and Oatley, K. (2008). The function of fiction is the abstraction and simulation of social experience. *Perspectives on Psychological Science* 3 (3): 173–192.

Mayer, M. (2003). *Frog, Where Are You?* New York: Penguin.

Norbury, C.F. and Bishop, D.V.M. (2002). Inferential processing and story recall in children with communication problems: a comparison of Specific Language Impairment, pragmatic language impairment and high-functioning autism. *International Journal of Language and Communication Disorders* 37 (3): 227–251.

Norbury, C.F., Gemmell, T., and Paul, R. (2014). Pragmatics abilities in narrative production: a cross-disorder comparison. *Journal of Child Language* 41 (3): 485–510.

Novogrodsky, R. and Edelson, L.R. (2016). Ambiguous pronoun use in narratives of children with Autism Spectrum Disorders. *Child Language Teaching and Therapy* 32 (2): 241–252.

Nuske, H.J. and Bavin, E.L. (2011). Narrative comprehension in 4–7-year-old children with autism: testing the Weak Central Coherence account. *International Journal of Language and Communication Disorders* 46 (1): 108–119.

Peristeri, E., Andreou, M., and Tsimpli, I.M. (2017). Syntactic and story structure complexity in the narratives of high- and low-language ability children with Autism Spectrum Disorder. *Frontiers in Psychology* 8: 2027.

Peristeri, E., Baldimtsi, E., Andreou, M. et al. (2020). The impact of bilingualism on the narrative ability and the Executive Functions of children with Autism Spectrum Disorders. *Journal of Communication Disorders* 85: 105999.

Peristeri, E., Silleresi, S., and Tsimpli, I.M. (2022). Bilingualism effects on cognition in autistic children are not all-or-nothing: the role of socioeconomic status in intellectual skills in bilingual autistic children. *Autism: The International Journal of Research and Practice* 26 (8): 2084–2097.

Peristeri, E., Vogelzang, M., and Tsimpli, I.M. (2021). Bilingualism effects on the cognitive flexibility of autistic children: evidence from verbal dual-task paradigms. *Neurobiology of Language* 2 (4): 558–585.

Renfrew, C.E. (2010). *Bus Story Test, Revised Edition*. Speechmark.

Rumpf, A.-L., Kamp-Becker, I., Becker, K. et al. (2012). Narrative competence and internal state language of children with Asperger Syndrome and ADHD. *Research in Developmental Disabilities* 33 (5): 1395–1407.

Schneider, P., Dubé, R.V., and Hayward, D. (2005). *The Edmonton Narrative Norms Instrument*. Available at: www.rehabresearch.ualberta.ca/enni (accessed 15 March 2024).

Stein, N. and Glenn, C. (1979). An analysis of story comprehension in elementary school children. *New Directions in Discourse Processing* 2: 53–120.

Vogindroukas, I., Protopapas, A., and Sideridis, G. (2009). *Expressive Vocabulary Assessment* (Greek version of Renfrew Word Finding Vocabulary Test). Crete: Glafki.

Westby, C. (2012). Teaching students to make inferences. *Word of Mouth* 23 (4): 6–8.

Westerveld, M.F. and Roberts, J.M.A. (2017). The oral narrative comprehension and production abilities of verbal preschoolers on the autism spectrum. *Language, Speech, and Hearing Services in Schools* 48 (4): 260–272.

Wiesner, D. (1991). *Tuesday*. Houghton.

8

Discourse

Flavia Adani, Petra Hendriks, and Arhonto Terzi

> **What Do You Think?**
> You and Sue met at a siblings' support group: you each have an autistic brother. One day, you are discussing how your brothers use language. Sue says that sometimes she can't follow what her brother is talking about when he uses pronouns, like *she* and *them*, and Sue has no idea to whom or what they are referring (e.g. *I don't like him!* said in a context where no male person has been mentioned yet). You recognize that your brother does this, too, but say that other times he keeps repeating the name of the person or thing he is talking about, and this also sounds very odd (e.g. *I saw this boy yesterday. I don't know this boy, but this boy came up to me, and…*). Sue hadn't noticed this with her brother. You and Sue wonder what could be causing these strange uses of language and how common they are in autism.

Introduction

Speakers use language in order to express their thoughts, intentions, and desires. Ideally, they take into consideration the setting of the conversation: the point of view of the person(s) they are speaking with and what has been said before. Language consists of sounds, words, and sentences, but also of **discourse**, which consists of larger chunks of language and how they flow together in a conversation. Discourse includes conversational skills such as turn-taking, timing, and topic management, which are often impacted in autism (see "Suggestions for Further Reading" at the end of the chapter). Such conversational skills are said to be part of social pragmatics. Discourse also includes how competent speakers and hearers adapt and interpret the form and meaning of a sentence according to the surrounding discourse. This is often referred to as **linguistic pragmatics**[1]: how the form or meaning of a sentence relates to its surrounding linguistic discourse. This chapter focuses on the latter: how autistic people deal with language between sentence and discourse.

Two quintessential domains in which discourse meets and interacts with sentence structure are **Information Structure** and **Reference** (to be defined in the Anchoring section below). These both involve being able to track, encode, and interpret information in the flow of a conversation or a text. This ability entails knowing what has already been mentioned, what the interlocutors already know, and what is new to them, or what is contrasted with something else. This chapter discusses how autistic individuals use and understand language in discourse by focusing on the following two questions:

- How do autistic individuals manage Information Structure in conversational exchanges?
- How do autistic individuals manage Reference in conversational exchanges?

Anchoring

Communicating with other people includes talking about the world, but also expressing desires and intentions. To this end, speakers combine sounds into words (**phonology**, see Chapter 4) and words into sentences (**morphosyntax**, see Chapter 3), from which meaning is derived (**semantics**, see Chapter 5). However, to efficiently get their message across, speakers do not just need to construct well-formed sentences. They also need to take into consideration their interlocutor(s), as well as the context in which they communicate their intentions, desires, etc. One of the issues that the field of **pragmatics** (see also Chapters 6 and 7) is concerned with is how sentences are constructed and interpreted when context and interlocutor perspective are taken into consideration. This is likely to be influenced by discourse properties, perspective-taking abilities, Theory of Mind (ToM), and memory resources of the speaker and the listener.

As mentioned in the Introduction, two key concepts in the area of discourse pragmatics are **Information Structure** and **Reference**. Information Structure is the way information is organized in a sentence in order to take the context and the conversation partners into consideration. It involves the linguistic concepts of **Topic** and **Focus**, which, roughly, are associated with phrases that denote old information (Topic), i.e. information already known to the hearer, and new information (Focus), i.e. information that is new to the hearer.

---

1 But see Chapter 6 for slightly different definitions of linguistic pragmatics and social pragmatics.

Reference is the relationship between linguistic expressions (e.g. noun phrases, pronouns) and entities in the world. It concerns how **pronouns** (words such as I, me, you, she, they) but also **noun phrases**, such as *the cat, a house, my cousin*, and proper names, such as *Tweety* and *Albert Einstein*, are used and interpreted in discourse. Note that a noun phrase with a definite article (*the* in English), such as *the cat*, refers to information that is already known by the hearer (old information), and a noun phrase with an indefinite article (*a/an* in English), such as *a house*, refers to information that is not known by the hearer (new information). As such, definite noun phrases often express Topic, and indefinite noun phrases often express Focus. In other words, the choices between definite and indefinite articles and between nouns and pronouns are also linked to Information Structure.

Languages use a number of strategies to encode Topic and Focus. Use of definite/indefinite articles is one way, intonation is another way. Let us consider first Focus, which is typically associated with new information, indicated simply by changing the intonation, for example, by placing stress on a particular word in the sentence. This is illustrated in the dialogue in (1). Speaker B, who answers Speaker A's question, stresses the **subject** (in this case the person that is performing the action expressed by the verb) *John*, to convey new information (the small capitals indicate stress).

> **Acronym and Terminology Reminder**
> **Ambiguous Pronoun:** Pronoun without a clear referent, for example, when no referent or more than one potential referent was mentioned in the preceding discourse.
> **Definite Article:** Words such as the in English.
> **Discourse:** Chunks of language, and how they flow together in a conversation.
> **Focus:** Information that is new to the hearer.
> **Indefinite Article:** Words such as a/an in English.
> **Information Structure:** How information is organized in a sentence in order to take the context and the conversation partners into consideration.
> **Linguistic Pragmatics:** How the form or meaning of a sentence relates to its surrounding linguistic discourse.
> **Object (Direct Object):** In an active sentence, the person or thing undergoing the action expressed by the verb.
> **Pronoun (Pronominal):** Words such as I, me, you, she, they.
> **Prosody:** Melodic structure, including stress, intonation, and rhythm organization.
> **Reference:** Relationship between linguistic expressions (e.g. noun phrases, pronouns) and entities in the world or in discourse. For example, the bottle refers to some particular bottle in the context, and her refers to some particular female individual in the context.
> **Subject:** In an active sentence, the person, place, or thing performing the action expressed by the verb.
> **ToM:** Theory of Mind. Ability to infer and understand mental states (e.g. beliefs, true, or false) in oneself and others.
> **Topic:** Information that is already known to the hearer.
> **Working Memory:** Ability to hold information for a short time while performing a cognitive task.

(1) a. Speaker A: Who read *The Terracotta Dog*?
b. Speaker B: JOHN read *The Terracotta Dog*.

Stress is part of what is called **prosody**. In this case, prosody has a grammatical function: it indicates the information status (Focus) of the subject (see also Chapter 9). Now, note that in (1b), the default subject–verb–object word order of English does not change: *John*, the subject, appears first, and *The Terracotta Dog*, the **object** (the person or thing undergoing the action expressed by the verb), appears after the verb. However, word order change can also be employed as a strategy to highlight Focus. An example is contrastive (or corrective) Focus, as in (2).

(2) a. Speaker A: John read *The Shape of Water*.
b. Speaker B: No, you're wrong. *The Terracotta Dog* he read.

Speaker B corrects speaker A on which book of the Italian mystery author Andrea Camilleri John read. This is accomplished by placing the noun phrase to be corrected, in this case, the object *The Terracotta Dog*, at the very beginning of the sentence, contrasting this noun phrase with the noun phrase *The Shape of Water*. This changes the default subject–verb–object order of English. Using this marked word order highlights the contrastive Focus status of the fronted object (*The Terracotta Dog*). At the same time, the intonation changes: the fronted object, *The Terracotta Dog* in (2b), is stressed and sounds different from the object, *The Shape of Water* in (2a).

Likewise, speakers may highlight information that has already been talked about in the conversation or that their interlocutor already knows, i.e. old information or Topic. This can be done by introducing the relevant phrase by expressions, such as *as for...*, *regarding...*, etc., illustrated in (3).

(3) As for John, he already left for the office.

Here, the proper name *John* is the Topic of the sentence, to which the pronoun *he* refers.

Languages such as Greek, Spanish, and Italian have additional, **syntactic** options for highlighting Topics. For example, they can place an object at the beginning of the sentence, with a pronoun later on in the sentence, to refer to the fronted object. This is exemplified in (4).

(4) Marta, Giovanni *la* invita sicuramente alla festa.
Marta, Giovanni *her* invite surely to the party.
'As for Marta, Giovanni is surely inviting her to the party.'

The Topic status of the object *Marta* is expressed both by fronting it and by inserting the pronoun *la* (corresponding to *Marta*) in the sentence. Note that intonation in the above examples is part of the speaker's grammar (for emotional intonation, see Chapter 9).

Another domain in which speakers' syntax interacts with discourse is the domain of Reference. A type of referring expression that has been studied extensively is pronouns, as already illustrated in (4). Pronouns are small words that do not have a reference of their own but acquire it by being associated with some other word or phrase, their **referent**. So, in (4), the pronoun *la* 'her' does not refer to anyone by itself; its reference is identified by *Marta*. The referent for the pronoun in (4) is thus found within the same sentence. The interpretation of pronouns requires morphosyntactic information. Depending on the language, this information can be related to gender (e.g. masculine, feminine, neuter), number (e.g. singular, plural), and/or syntactic structure. Chapter 11 discusses the syntactic conditions on the use of pronouns. The interpretation of pronouns also requires knowledge of contextual information, the subject of this chapter. We illustrate how pronouns are related to context in (5) and (6), two sentences, and one following the other, in a discourse. Consider who the pronouns *he* and *her* in (6) refer to.

(5) Mario met an intelligent and interesting girl at the party last week.

(6) I heard yesterday that *he* is actually in love with *her*.

The most natural interpretation of *he* in (6) is *Mario* in (5), and the most natural interpretation of *her* in (6) is the *intelligent and interesting girl* in (5). As (5) and (6) show, personal pronouns tend to refer to referents that are prominent in the linguistic discourse, for example, because they were mentioned in the previous sentence. This is called **discourse prominence**, and it is an important aspect of contextual information. Summarizing, the examples in (1)–(6) illustrate how speakers express subtle differences in meaning by integrating syntax, intonation (e.g. stress), context, and the knowledge they assume their interlocutors have.

In addition to the structure of the sentence, intonation, and the discourse prominence of referents, the perspectives of speaker and listener are relevant for determining the Information Structure of sentences or the intended interpretation of referring expressions. As such, the cognitive mechanism of **Theory of Mind** (ToM) (see Chapter 1) may play an important role here. ToM is the ability to infer and understand mental states (e.g. beliefs, true or false) in oneself and others.

Furthermore, **Working Memory**, the ability to hold information for a short time while performing a cognitive task, may prove important for the appropriate use of referring expressions: when referring to the referent (*Mario* in (5)) with a pronoun (*he* in (6)), the referent needs to be held active in Working Memory to interpret the pronoun. As both ToM and Working Memory are sometimes reported to be compromised in autistic individuals, Information Structure and Reference may present difficulties to them.

As we have noted, the Information Structure concepts of Topic and Focus are encoded by means of prosody (intonation) and/or morphosyntax. Earlier studies on their acquisition by neurotypical children investigated the prosodic marking of Focus, mainly because they were concerned with English where prosody is the predominant means of marking Focus (Hornby 1971). In addition, Chen (2011) examined accent placement and accent type to encode Topic and Focus in Dutch-speaking children aged 4–8 years, using pictures to elicit naturally spoken declarative sentences. She claimed that the younger group had not fully attained adult preferences for Topic marking, in contrast to the older children. Szendrői et al. (2018) investigated the acquisition of prosodic Focus marking in 3-to-6-year-old English, French, and German-speaking children, showing that even the youngest children understood prosodically marked Focus. The study also supported an older observation that if a language employs more means to encode Information Structure, e.g. morphosyntax, less attention is paid to prosody. This is why French-speaking children provided fewer Focus corrections for focused subjects than English-speaking children. Fewer studies have investigated the morphosyntactic means of marking Information Structure. De Cat (2011) investigated Topic and Focus in French-speaking preschoolers (ages 2;6–5;6) with a story-telling task and concluded that they used definite and indefinite noun phrases rather successfully. When they erred, they used indefinites rather than definites to encode old information (Topic).

Regarding the acquisition of Reference, the first words neurotypical children produce when they are between roughly 12 and 18 months old are often already referential in nature, for example, nouns like *Daddy*, *kitty*, or *ball*. The first pronouns emerging in child language are demonstrative pronouns (*that*). Children already use demonstrative pronouns in their spontaneous speech before age 2 to refer to things that are present in the situational context. Personal pronouns (*I, you, he, she*) typically appear slightly later, around age 2. In general, it is assumed that neurotypical English- or French-speaking children master the pronoun system and most of its referential properties around 30 months of age, although this may differ for other languages (see Orvig 2019, for an overview). However, neurotypical development of the use of pronouns and other referring expressions in a discourse context is only completed by around age 9 (Berman 2009). Two remarks are in order here. First, there is considerable individual variation among neurotypical children in the speed and order of acquisition of referential abilities. Second, some aspects of the use and understanding of referring expressions remain challenging until a later age (for example, reference in narratives). This is why language experiments with autistic children usually include a control group of neurotypical children of the same age. This allows researchers to determine whether and how autism affects performance on a particular referential task using a specific discourse context.

Discourse in Autism

Language abilities in social interaction, also referred to as social pragmatics (including conversational skills such as turn-taking, timing, and topic management), are generally regarded as an area of weakness in autism. An important question is whether the interaction of sentence structure and discourse (linguistic pragmatics) is also affected in autism. In what follows, we discuss how autistic individuals manage Information Structure and Reference, two domains that are part of linguistic pragmatics. Since there is virtually no literature on this topic in autistic adults, we concentrate on autistic children and adolescents. We note that in most studies on discourse in autistic children, the children reported on do not have co-occurring intellectual disability (but see Chapter 10).

How do Autistic Individuals Manage Information Structure in Conversational Exchanges?

Research on how autistic individuals encode and interpret focused and topicalized expressions is not abundant, despite the fact that autism symptomatology could be expected to have an effect on this. This is because Information Structure is concerned with how the message is structured when the speaker takes into account what their interlocutor knows and does not know, which may be different from the speaker's knowledge. In other words, an autistic individual with ToM challenges (i.e. restricted ability to take into account others' mental states) may have trouble tracking Topic and Focus. A couple of studies have investigated Information Structure from the vantage point of prosody and showed that autistic individuals do better at understanding prosody than on using it appropriately themselves (see Chapter 9). Filipe et al. (2014) found that Portuguese-speaking autistic children with unimpaired structural language abilities had no trouble distinguishing statements from questions but differed from neurotypical children in aspects of their own prosody (duration and pitch) when they produced such utterances. Moreover, Rapin et al. (2015) found that autistic children distinguished focused from nonfocused nouns in terms of pitch, sound intensity, and duration of their interlocutor's speech. In contrast, in their own speech, they marked the focused variant less prominently than neurotypical children.

As mentioned in the Anchoring Section, Focus and Topic may also involve distinct syntactic structures. Terzi, Marinis, and Francis (2016) studied such aspects of Focus and Topic structures in Greek-speaking children with autism using a task with pictures in which a contrast between several protagonists was created (see Figure 8.1). The experimenter provided an incomplete sentence beginning with a focused object, as in (7). Children were asked to complete the sentence that the experimenter started (see (8)).

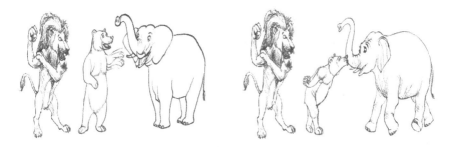

Figure 8.1 Example of pictures from the Focus/Topic experiment. *Source:* Courtesy of Theodoros Marinis and Arhonto Terzi.

(7) Experimenter:
Edho echume ena liondari, mia arkuda ke enan elefanda. Pion filai i arkuda? TON ELEFANDA ...
here have-2-plural a lion-neuter, a bear-feminine, and an elephant-masculine. whom kiss-3-singular the bear-feminine? the elephant-masculine...
'Here (we) have a lion, a bear, and an elephant. Who does the bear kiss? The elephant ...'

(8) Target answer: ... filai i arkuda
... kisses the bear
'... the bear kisses.'

Autistic children, but not neurotypical children, often incorrectly added pronouns following focused constituents, as in (9) (where the pronoun *ton* 'him' refers to the focused object "the elephant"), resulting in an ungrammatical response.

(9) Autistic child: ... **ton** filai i arkuda.
... **him** kisses the bear.
'...the bear kisses him [= the elephant].'

These ungrammatical responses involved use of the syntax for **topicalized** nouns (which get an additional pronoun in adult Greek) in structures in which the noun was not topicalized, but rather **focalized**, resulting in an Information Structure mix-up. Terzi and colleagues (2016) attributed this behavior to problems autistic children may have in simultaneously integrating the rules from the different linguistic components involved, namely syntax (movement of the focused constituent to the beginning of the sentence), linguistic pragmatics (selecting which noun phrase corresponds to the focused part in the Information Structure of the sentence), and prosody (specific stress pattern on the fronted noun phrase). As Terzi, Marinis, and Francis (2016) measured grammatical abilities independently, and there was no significant difference between the two groups, language impairment, which affects a subgroup in autism[2], cannot be an explanation for the autistic children's ungrammatical responses in this study.

Difficulty integrating information from different linguistic components may also be responsible for a particular difficulty observed in Dutch-speaking autistic children. These children fail to place the direct object before an adverb of negation (such as *niet* 'not') in appropriate contexts, as in (10a). This special word order in Dutch is called the **scrambled** word order. It tends to be used for definite or indefinite direct objects that refer to an entity that can be uniquely identified. For example, the indefinite noun phrase *twee boeken* 'two books' in (10a), which appears in the scrambled position, must refer to two specific books that were already mentioned in the preceding discourse. Direct objects that do not refer to a specific entity must remain in the nonscrambled position in Dutch, which is reserved for focus-marked (stressed) phrases. This is illustrated in (10b), where the same indefinite noun phrase as in (10a) *twee boeken* 'two books,' now does not refer to two specific books, since it appears in the nonscrambled position following the adverb of negation.

(10) a. Elmo gaat **twee boeken** niet lezen. (scrambled word order)
Elmo goes two books not read
'Elmo is not going to read the two books'
b. Elmo gaat niet **twee boeken** lezen. (nonscrambled word order)
Elmo goes not two books read
'Elmo is not going to read any two books'

In an elicited production task, Schaeffer (2017) found that Dutch-speaking autistic children aged 5–14 used scrambled word order with specific entities less often than their neurotypical peers. This could not be attributed to their difficulties with ToM or grammar, as the autistic children did not differ from their neurotypical peers in their ToM scores and did not show grammatical impairment either. Hence, Schaeffer argued that the autistic children in this study had problems integrating the relevant information regarding Information Structure (topic and focus), reference, and word order.

Another area in which autistic children may differ from their neurotypical peers is their use of articles. In languages such as English and Dutch, definite articles such as *the* are used when the referent is familiar to the hearer (i.e. known), and indefinite articles such as *a* are used when the referent is new. In an elicited production task used with the same group of Dutch-speaking children between ages 5 and 14 years, Schaeffer, van Witteloostuijn, and Creemers (2018) found that autistic children overused indefinite articles compared to neurotypical children;

---

[2] This language-impaired subgroup in autism is often referred to as ALI – Autism with Language Impairment (see Chapter 1).

that is, they also used indefinite articles when the referent had already been introduced in the discourse and a definite article would have been appropriate. For example, they would say, "The puppet rolled a ball" after they had just mentioned the ball. At the same time, these autistic children did not overuse definite articles in contexts in which the referent was new, a pattern that is often associated with underdeveloped ToM in the literature. Since ToM abilities in these autistic children did not differ from those of their neurotypical peers, their correct use of definite articles was not surprising. Since their overuse of indefinite articles was found to correlate with their phonological memory skills, which were weaker than those of neurotypical children, Schaeffer et al. suggested that autistic children may have difficulty storing the preceding discourse in phonological memory. This difficulty, in turn, could make it hard for them to determine whether the context required the use of the more informative definite article. Unable to sort out the context due to memory limitations, these children apparently simply resort to the default option that is semantically correct in all contexts, namely the indefinite article.

Summarizing, while grammatical impairment may potentially provide an explanation for autistic children's difficulties with Information Structure, most studies discussed here controlled for grammatical impairment and attribute the difficulties to the problems autistic people may have with the integration of information from different sources. Discourse management, and in particular, Information Structure, requires the integration of information from syntax, discourse, and prosody, and also memory skills to process this information.

How Do Autistic Individuals Manage Reference in Conversational Exchanges?

Speakers can use a variety of expressions, such as noun phrases and pronouns, to refer to people, things, and events. To ensure successful communication, these expressions must be interpreted by listeners in the same way the speaker intended. Autistic children seem to perform similarly to neurotypical children in their interpretation of pronouns (Perovic, Modyanova, and Wexler 2013; Terzi et al. 2014; Kuijper, Hartman, and Hendriks 2021; Chapter 11; but see Overweg, Hartman, and Hendriks 2018, for the finding that autistic children have difficulty interpreting the pronouns *I* and *you* that usually refer to the speaker and the addressee in a conversation). However, findings regarding the production of pronouns and other referring expressions are mixed.

Many studies have investigated reference in production using a narrative production (storytelling) task or narrative retelling (story-retelling) task. Some of these studies have reported that autistic children differed from their neurotypical peers in that they were **over-informative** (too explicit), using a noun phrase where a pronoun would have been more appropriate (see the example in the "What Do You Think?" box above).

Some studies have also reported the opposite, namely, that autistic children were less explicit and frequently used a pronoun when actually a noun phrase was needed. For example, Novogrodsky (2013) tested English-speaking autistic children and neurotypical children (age range: 6–14 years). In this study, 24 autistic children and 17 controls matched on verbal abilities and age, retold a story that was told to them by the researcher and, as a second task, told a story themselves based on a wordless picture book (Frog, where are you?, Mayer 1969). No difference between the groups was found in pronoun production in the story-retelling task, but in the storytelling task, the autistic children produced more ambiguous third-person subject pronouns (e.g. *he, she, him*) than their neurotypical peers. Ambiguous pronouns are pronouns without a clear referent, for example, when no referent or more than one potential referent was mentioned in the preceding discourse. In Novogrodsky's experiment, the autistic children produced more pronouns that had no referent in the preceding linguistic discourse. One autistic child said: "Once upon a time there was a frog and **he** said 'Frog, where are you?'." Here, the pronoun *he* referred to a boy in the picture that was not yet introduced verbally. As an explanation for the gap between the two narrative tasks (storytelling and story-retelling), Novogrodsky suggested that storytelling is cognitively more demanding than story-retelling since it requires narrative planning. Furthermore, Novogrodsky and Edelson (2016) showed that this difficulty in pronoun use was observed for different types of pronouns (e.g. subject pronouns such as *he/she* and possessive pronouns such as *his*) – in other words, it was a problem with pronouns, and not a problem with, for example, subjects.

However, other narrative production studies have not found substantial differences between autistic children and their neurotypical peers. To illustrate this, we discuss two narrative production studies, one on Dutch, and the other one on Greek. A further illustration is provided by two studies investigating German and Hebrew using a different task, namely an elicitation task. We begin with Kuijper, Hartman, and Hendriks (2015), a study using a narrative production task with Dutch-speaking children with and without autism, aged 6–12 years. Children told narratives such as the one in (11) on the basis of picture stories as in Figure 8.2.

(11) Example of a narrative by an autistic 6-year-old child from Kuijper, Hartman, and Hendriks (2015), translated from Dutch:
[1] The ballet dancer has a watering can. [2] She opens the tap and puts water in the watering can. [3] She waters the plants. [4] And the doctor picks them. [5] The doctor gives the flower to the ballet dancer. [6] The ballet dancer puts the flower on her head.

The 46 autistic children did not differ from their 38 age-matched, typically developing peers in their use of pronouns and noun phrases for introducing new referents, maintaining reference, and reintroducing earlier mentioned referents in

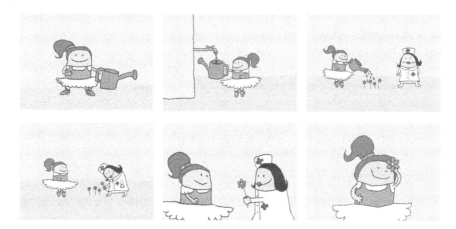

Figure 8.2 Example of a picture story in a narrative production task. *Source:* Courtesy of Petra Hendriks.

their narratives. The lack of a difference between the two groups may be attributed to the fact that the picture stories were simple and short and did not contain many details (Malkin, Abbot-Smith, and Williams 2018); notably, they contained only two characters. In other words, autistic children may be able to produce referring expressions in an appropriate manner in simple tasks. Crucially, the autistic children in Kuijper, Hartman, and Hendriks's (2015) study were as explicit as their neurotypical peers when reintroducing a referent that was not the discourse topic at that point in the story (e.g. *the ballet dancer* in the final sentence of the example narrative in (11)). Across groups, the use of a noun phrase instead of a pronoun was associated with better ToM abilities and higher Working Memory capacity, indicating the importance for speakers to take into account their listener's perspective in their production of referring expressions.

In another study, Terzi et al. (2019) explored the reference of both subject and object pronouns in Greek. Greek is a **null subject** language, which means that subject pronouns can be either overtly expressed or may remain unexpressed (e.g. the Greek rendition of "we" in sentence (7) above). Therefore, Terzi et al. assessed the reference of both overt and unexpressed (null) pronoun subjects and pronouns in object position. Twenty children with autism (ages 5–8 years) were individually matched on their verbal abilities with 20 neurotypical children of a similar age. The two groups did not differ in their production of pronouns for which the reference was not clear (ambiguous pronouns). However, neurotypical children used proportionally more pronouns than noun phrases in subject position, while children with autism used equal proportions, despite the fact that the two groups did not differ on Working Memory. The authors concluded that the autistic children's performance was not markedly different from neurotypical children's because they were at an age (5–8 years old) in which referential abilities are not fully established (Berman 2009).

In contrast to the studies discussed above, which used storytelling and story-retelling tasks, Stegenwallner-Schütz and Adani (2020) used a sentence elicitation task in which participants watched short picture sequences (e.g. Baseline and (a) in Figure 8.3), heard descriptions of pictures, and were then asked a related question. The target response involved producing a referring expression modified by a **relative clause** (e.g. the bold-faced part in *The boy **who is petting a horse***). The degree of contrast between competing noun referents in this task was manipulated. For instance, a low degree of contrast was instantiated by a visual display such as (a) in Figure 8.3, in which two boys were presented, one petting a cow and the other boy petting a horse, followed by the question *Which boy is Max photographing?*, where Max refers to the little mouse holding a camera in (a). The target response for picture (a) is *Max is photographing the boy who is petting a horse*. Conversely, the two boys would be highly contrasted if, in addition to petting different animals as in Baseline, they are each being photographed by a different animal, as in (b): one boy (petting a cow) is being photographed by a little mouse (Max, see previous example), and the other boy (petting a horse) is being photographed by a little bird, who was previously introduced as Tom. Picture (b) was then followed by the question, *Which boy is Max photographing, and which boy is Tom photographing?* The target responses are provided in (12) and (13). The relative clause *that is petting a cow* (in 12) or *that is petting a horse* (in 13) tells us something about the boy.

(12) Max is photographing the boy that is petting a cow [Max = mouse]

(13) Tom is photographing the boy that is petting a horse [Tom = bird]

Stegenwallner-Schütz and Adani analyzed the various referring expressions that the participants used in their responses: *the boy/the one that is petting a cow/a horse* (see 12). Seventeen German-speaking autistic children aged between 8 and 16 were compared to a group of age-matched neurotypical children. All

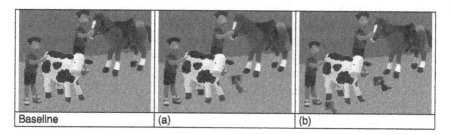

Figure 8.3 Example of visual displays in a sentence elicitation task. *Source:* Courtesy of Andrea Zukowski.

participants were more likely to produce answers containing a noun phrase when its referent was highly contrasted (as in the (b) picture in Figure 8.3). However, when the noun was the subject of the preceding sentence, children from both groups more frequently produced answers with pronouns (e.g. *the one that is petting a cow*, where *the one* in German would be realized as a pronoun, e.g. *der*) or without a noun or a pronoun (e.g. *ø that is petting the cow*, where ø indicates an unexpressed constituent). These different types of answers provide evidence that the autistic children were sensitive to the discourse status of referents (such as being contrastive) to a similar extent as neurotypical children. Furthermore, low Working Memory capacity was associated with a greater likelihood of producing pronouns or zero forms, suggesting that Working Memory, in addition to ToM, contributes to the adequate production of referring expressions in discourse (as in Kuijper, Hartman, and Hendriks 2015).

In another study using an elicitation task, Hebrew-speaking autistic children, aged 4–9 years, without Disorder of Intellectual Development (DID, see also Chapters 1 and 10) produced a lower rate of pronouns compared to neurotypical controls (Meir and Novogrodsky 2019). For example, autistic children omitted pronouns (producing *The father is lifting* for the target sentence *The father is lifting him*, where *him* refers to a child mentioned in the prompt sentence). Importantly, the use of both subject and object pronouns by the children with autism was predicted by their morphosyntactic abilities, and the use of subject pronouns was additionally predicted by their Working Memory capacity and ToM skills. Meir and Novogrodsky concluded that pronoun production in autism is affected by features directly related to autism (such as Working Memory and ToM) as well as by co-occurring language impairment that characterized some of the participants. Note that in this study, in contrast to Stegenwallner-Schütz and Adani's (2020) study, the elicitation task did not involve visual contrast in the picture stimuli. This difference could explain why autistic children differed from neurotypical children only in the study by Meir and Novogrodsky.

In sum, some studies suggest that autistic children have difficulties with references in conversational exchanges, while others indicate they do not. A possible explanation for these mixed results could be differences in task complexity. It seems that retelling a story is less complex than telling a story, as telling a story involves the demanding task of narrative planning. Also, when the story includes fewer characters, it is easier, as there are fewer referents one can confuse. Moreover, an unconstrained sentence production task is more challenging for children with autism than a picture-supported task. In addition, an association between ToM and Working Memory was found in several studies on the production of referring expressions. These findings suggest that difficulties with ToM or Working Memory could cause difficulties with referring expressions such as pronouns. Finally, among autistic children, those having co-occurring language impairment may show more difficulties in the production of referring expressions. This underscores the importance of considering task complexity and administering independent tests of structural language, ToM, and Working Memory when investigating linguistic-pragmatic discourse abilities in autistic individuals.

Focus on a Specific Study

So far, we discussed the question as to how the preceding discourse and the child's cognitive resources (such as ToM and Working Memory capacity) can modulate the production of referring expressions and whether divergences in the performance of autistic versus neurotypical individuals are detectable. Much of this line of work was inspired by a pioneering study by Arnold and her colleagues that was published in 2009. This study is one of the first to investigate the elicited production of referring expressions in autistic individuals by providing a fine-grained analysis of the linguistic discourse, rather than merely presenting a general count of pronouns or full noun phrases. Moreover, Arnold, Bennetto, and Diehl (2009) used an experimentally controlled setup (as opposed to an analysis of spontaneously produced language samples), which allowed them to determine the referents for most pronouns. Also, they are among the few researchers to date who provided a detailed analysis of autistic adolescents' abilities to produce referring expressions. Given that much of the neurotypical development of referring expressions continues up to at least age 9 years (Berman 2009), investigating how autistic adolescents master referring expressions in general as well as in comparison to neurotypical individuals is fundamental. However, to date, autistic adolescents' language remains an understudied domain. The strengths of the study by Arnold and colleagues also brought along some pitfalls. The autistic participants, who were only 23 in number, were subdivided into two even smaller age groups of unequal size, and the age cut-off between these groups was not developmentally justified. Furthermore, some of the theoretical assumptions put forward by the authors contrast with other literature on children's development of referential abilities. For instance, Arnold and colleagues assume that full noun phrases are "easy" forms that are produced under cognitive load when pronouns are avoided. In contrast, other studies (e.g. Kuijper, Hartman, and Hendriks 2015; Stegenwallner-Schütz and Adani 2020) assumed the opposite, namely that noun phrases are "challenging" forms that children only produce in particular contexts when they have sufficient cognitive resources (e.g. ToM abilities, Working Memory capacity). While taking all these limitations into account, given the central role that it has played for research on referring expressions in the past decades, we focus on this study. Arnold, Bennetto, and Diehl (2009) conducted a systematic analysis of the use of referring expressions by carrying out a narrative elicitation task. Their goal was to investigate the influence of the discourse on speakers' referential choices and assess the effects of memory load.

Participants were 23 English-speaking autistic children and adolescents (age range: 9–17 years) and a similar group of neurotypical controls, who were matched with the autistic group on age, (non)verbal IQ, receptive vocabulary, and gender. In order to investigate developmental trends, both groups were divided into younger ($n=10$; age range: 9–12 years) and older ($n=13$; age range: 13–17 years) subgroups. Each participant watched a 7.5-minute-long Sylvester and Tweety Bird cartoon, subdivided into three segments. After each segment, the video was paused, and the participants were asked to tell the story to another person using their own words. All unambiguous referring expressions were included in the analysis: zero (unexpressed) pronouns, overt (expressed) pronouns, definite noun phrases, and proper names. Table 8.1 presents these categories together with examples from the original article (Arnold, Bennetto, and Diehl 2009, p. 136).

The distance between each pronoun and its referent was calculated (i.e. from one clause back up to three clauses back; see examples in Table 8.2). Moreover, Arnold and colleagues looked at the grammatical function of the pronoun in the current clause with respect to the last utterance in which its referent was mentioned: subject in both utterances and subject versus nonsubject (i.e. direct or indirect object or object of prepositions) in the following utterance. Table 8.2 illustrates the coding categories and provides examples of utterances produced by the participants from the original article (Arnold, Bennetto, and Diehl 2009, p. 136).

Table 8.1 Coding categories for referential forms, with examples of referring expressions produced by participants.

Referential form	Example in child production (relevant referring expression underlined)
Zero pronoun*	he grabbed it; ø ran out the back alley; ø opened it up (Autistic participant, age 15)
Overt pronoun	after that **he** got kicked out (Autistic participant, age 10)
Definite noun phrase	while um **the bird** was singing (Neurotypical participant, age 12)
Proper name	**Tweety** flew out yelling help me help me (Autistic participant, age 15)

*The unexpressed pronoun indicated by ø refers to the pronoun *he* in the preceding clause.

Table 8.2 Coding of discourse status categories for Recency of mention and Grammatical function for pronouns.

Discourse status		Example in child production (relevant referring expression underlined)
Recency of mention (i.e. distance between the pronoun and its referent)	One clause back	while **Sylvester** was in a different one and **he** just ran into the building (Autistic participant, age 10)
	Two clauses back	and he's start **he's** running away with Tweety bird down the street and um the weight comes back down and hits **him** on the head (Neurotypical participant, age 17)
Grammatical function of the pronoun and its referent	Subject:Subject	and **he** runs and ø gets zapped again (Autistic participant, age 11)
	Subject:Nonsubject	and ø got the old lady and the old lady whacked **him** (Neurotypical participant, age 15)

Processing load was operationalized in terms of disfluency rate (e.g. hesitations like *uh* or *um*, see an example in Table 8.2) and utterance length, quantified in terms of number of words. Disfluencies were expected to be related to circumstances in which the speaker was having some difficulty in planning or producing their utterance.

The findings revealed that productions of referring expressions by autistic children and neurotypical controls were remarkably similar, despite the fact that the autistic participants tended to produce fewer referring expressions overall than controls because they produced shorter narratives. For both groups, zero and overt pronouns were more likely to be produced when their referent had been mentioned in the recent discourse (i.e. one clause back). As the distance between the pronoun and its referent increased (i.e. two clauses back), the occurrence of zero and overt pronouns decreased and, conversely, the occurrence of full noun phrases increased. This effect was triggered by the younger autistic group, while the other three groups (younger and older controls, older autistic group) did not differ from each other. As the distance between the pronoun and its referent further increased (i.e. three clauses back), the occurrence of pronouns steadily decreased, showing no differences among the groups.

Turning to the effect of the grammatical function of the referring expression and its referent mentioned in the previous clause (see Table 8.2), both autistic participants and neurotypical controls used more pronouns for entities that were previously mentioned in subject position than in object position. Moreover, there was a grammatical function effect, with most zero and overt pronouns being used when the referring expression and its referent were produced in subject position in the current as well as preceding sentence. As for the effect of cognitive load, both groups were more likely to produce zero and overt pronouns in fluent and shorter utterances (one to six words) and produced more full noun phrases in disfluent longer utterances.

These results show similarities as well as differences in the way children and adolescents with and without autism use referring expressions while telling a story. Both groups were sensitive to the same discourse properties. Yet, younger autistic participants were more likely to use noun phrases in contexts in which neurotypical controls used pronouns, especially when the referent was mentioned in the nonimmediately preceding discourse (i.e. two clauses back). Arnold and colleagues explained this pattern of overuse of noun phrases as the result of insufficient cognitive resources during utterance planning in this group. This led to a reduction in the activation of the referent in Working Memory, which they argued resulted in a higher rate of produced noun phrases. Thus, the autistic adolescents' use of noun phrases instead of pronouns is explained as an effect of the speaker's limited Working Memory capacity.

Arnold and colleagues concluded that speakers do not need to consider their interlocutor's mental state for reference production. Rather, the discourse provides enough information for them to produce the appropriate expression. This view contrasts with other studies on reference production with younger autistic children, such as Kuijper, Hartman, and Hendriks (2015), who found an association between the use of noun phrases in specific discourse contexts (namely after a topic shift) and better ToM skills, not tested in Arnold, Bennetto, and Diehl (2009). They argued that the speaker's use of noun phrases in these contexts is the result of successfully considering the interlocutor's mental state. Arnold, Bennetto, and Diehl's (2009) main conclusion was that perspective-taking and considering the interlocutor's mental state do not always, or even typically do not, play a role in reference production. We note that this study did not distinguish between discourse contexts that require perspective-taking (e.g. situations in which the speaker shifts to a new topic) and discourse contexts that do not. Furthermore, no ToM task was included to establish the role of perspective-taking in reference production, and digit span memory scores were not included in the analyses of referring expressions. Hence, the author's conclusions regarding the lack of a need for considering the interlocutor's mental state and the role of memory capacity are difficult to evaluate. Furthermore, as mentioned in the Anchoring Section, typical development of referring expressions is assumed to be largely completed by the end of elementary school years. However, most of the participants in the Arnold et al. study, aged 9–17 years, were older than this. It is therefore conceivable that the deviant pattern of overuse of noun phrases in the younger group of 9- to 12-year-olds is the result of a communicative strategy to avoid using pronouns because they have difficulty deciding when to use a pronoun or not, rather than because of reduced cognitive resources, as Arnold and colleagues suggest.

To conclude, Arnold, Bennetto, and Diehl (2009) were among the first studies to show that autistic children and adolescents (aged 9–17 years) are sensitive to discourse properties (such as recency of mention, and grammatical function of the referring expression and its referent) and to internal processing constraints (such as Working Memory).

Conclusion

This chapter considered whether discourse abilities are affected in autism and tried to answer the following questions:

- How do autistic individuals manage Information Structure in conversational exchanges?
- How do autistic individuals manage Reference in conversational exchanges?

We first examined the domain of Information Structure, noting the dearth of studies in autism investigating this area, despite its clear relevance for understanding language in autism (notably because of the interaction between syntax, prosody, discourse, and possibly ToM and Working Memory). The few existing studies indicated some difficulties with the production of prosody and incorrect use of some syntactic structures. We then concentrated on reference in autistic children, an area on which more research has been carried out because the dominant view is that reference management requires ToM abilities, which are assumed to be an area of weakness in autism. However, the findings regarding the production of referring expressions seem inconclusive, as it is not clear whether autistic children are just as capable as neurotypical children to produce appropriate referring expressions in discourse. Note that autistic children generally do not seem to differ from neurotypical children in their understanding of referring expressions. The reasons for these disparate results in production may be quite diverse. We suggested that the level of task complexity and the children's general language abilities may affect the different results between studies. The more complex the task, or the lower the language abilities of the autistic child, the greater the likelihood that the child will display deviant use of referring expressions as compared to neurotypical peers. Also relevant are the children's cognitive abilities: the better their ToM abilities or memory capacity, the more adultlike their production of referring expressions. A potentially fruitful future direction of research could be to investigate autistic children's reference production and comprehension in eye-tracking tasks: by tracking their eye gaze when they look at visual scenes, it can be determined which referents they consider at any given moment while producing or comprehending a referring expression. This may allow us to find out which aspects of the sentence or discourse cause particular difficulty for autistic children during sentence production or comprehension.

> **What Do You Know Now?**
> Information Structure and Reference are two domains in which discourse meets and interacts with sentence structure, and which may be different in autistic individuals because they involve perspective-taking and tracking old and new information in the context.
> - When referring, speakers not only need to pay attention to features of the discourse but must also consider their conversational partner's perspective. Both of these aspects of language use can be challenging for autistic children.
> - Information Structure is an area of language that may be particularly vulnerable for autistic individuals as a result of difficulties they seem to have with integrating information from syntax, linguistic pragmatics, and prosody into their discourse.
> - Some autistic children in some situations seem to have difficulty using pronouns and other referring expressions appropriately: they sometimes use full noun phrases or proper names when a pronoun would be more appropriate, and they sometimes use pronouns in cases in which a full noun phrase or a proper name would avoid ambiguity of reference.
> - Factors that relate to the task, such as task complexity, affect autistic children's use of referring expressions. In addition, cognitive factors, such as ToM abilities and memory capacity, affect their ability to produce and interpret successfully pronouns and other referring expressions.

Suggestions for Further Reading

If you want to know more about the use and interpretation of referring expressions in autism, the following readings are suggested: Malkin, Abbot-Smith, and Williams 2018 and Finnegan, Asaro-Saddler, and Zajic 2021. The former reviews the literature on reference in autism, and the latter provides a meta-analysis and systematic review of the use and interpretation of pronouns in autism. If you want to know more about Information Structure and prosody, you can read Filipe et al. 2014, Mann and Karsten 2021, and de Pape et al. 2012. If you want to expand your knowledge on other conversational skills, that are not discussed in this chapter (e.g. turn-taking, timing, and topic management), we recommend reading Tager-Flusberg et al. 2009.

References

Arnold, J.E., Bennetto, L., and Diehl, J.J. (2009). Reference production in young speakers with and without autism: effects of discourse status and processing constraints. *Cognition* 110 (2): 131–146.

Berman, R. (2009). Language development in narrative contexts. In: *Cambridge Handbook of Child Language* (ed. E.L. Bavin), 355–376. Cambridge, UK: Cambridge University Press.

Chen, A. (2011). Tuning information packaging: intonational realization of topic and focus in child Dutch. *Journal of Child Language* 38 (5): 1055–1083.

De Cat, C. (2011). Information tracking and encoding in early L1: linguistic competence vs. cognitive limitations. *Journal of Child Language* 38 (4): 828–860.

de Pape A.-M.R., Chen, A., Hall, G.B.C et al. (2012). Use of prosody and information structure in high functioning adults with Autism in relation to language ability. *Frontiers in Psychology* 3: article 72.

Filipe, M.G., Frota, S., Castro, S.L. et al. (2014). Atypical prosody in Asperger Syndrome: perceptual and acoustic measurements. *Journal of Autism and Developmental Disorders* 44 (8): 1972–1981.

Finnegan, E.G., Asaro-Saddler, K., and Zajic, M.C. (2021). Production and comprehension of pronouns in individuals with autism: a meta-analysis and systematic review. *Autism* 25 (1): 3–17.

Hornby, P.A. (1971). Surface structure and the topic–comment distinction: a developmental study. *Child Development* 42: 1975–1988.

Kuijper, S.J., Hartman, C.A., and Hendriks, P. (2015). Who is he? Children with ASD and ADHD take the listener into account in their production of ambiguous pronouns. *PLoS One* 10 (7): e0132408.

Kuijper, S.J., Hartman, C.A., and Hendriks, P. (2021). Children's pronoun interpretation problems are related to ToM and inhibition, but not working memory. *Frontiers in Psychology* 12: 610401.

Malkin, L., Abbot-Smith, K., and Williams, D. (2018). Is verbal reference impaired in Autism Spectrum Disorder? A systematic review. *Autism & Developmental Language Impairments* 3: 2396941518763166.

Mann, C.C. and Karsten, A.M. (2021). Assessment and treatment of prosody behavior in individuals with level 1 autism: a review and call for research. *The Analysis of Verbal Behavior* 37 (2): 171–193.

Mayer, M. (1969). *Frog, Where Are You?* New York: Dial Books for Young Readers.

Meir, N. and Novogrodsky, R. (2019). Prerequisites of third-person pronoun use in monolingual and bilingual children with autism and typical language development. *Frontiers in Psychology* 10: 452177.

Novogrodsky, R. (2013). Subject pronoun use by children with Autism Spectrum Disorders (ASD). *Clinical Linguistics & Phonetics* 27 (2): 85–93.

Novogrodsky, R. and Edelson, L.R. (2016). Ambiguous pronoun use in narratives of children with Autism Spectrum Disorders. *Child Language Teaching and Therapy* 32 (2): 241–252.

Orvig, A.S. (2019). Reference and referring in first language acquisition. In: *The Oxford Handbook of Reference* (eds. J. Gundel and B. Abbot), 283–308. Oxford: Oxford University Press.

Overweg, J., Hartman, C.A., and Hendriks, P. (2018). Children with Autism Spectrum Disorder show pronoun reversals in interpretation. *Journal of Abnormal Psychology* 127 (2): 228.

Perovic, A., Modyanova, N., and Wexler, K. (2013). Comprehension of reflexive and personal pronouns in children with autism: a syntactic or pragmatic deficit? *Applied Psycholinguistics* 34 (4): 813–835.

Rapin, L., Trudeau-Fisette, P., Bellavance-Courtemanche, M. et al. (2015). Production of contrastive focus in children with Autistic Spectrum Disorder. *Journal of the Acoustic Society of America* 137 (4): 2431.

Schaeffer, J. (2017). Unravelling the complexity of Direct Object Scrambling. *Language Sciences* 60: 173–198.

Schaeffer, J., van Witteloostuijn, M., and Creemers, A. (2018). Article choice, Theory of Mind, and memory in children with high-functioning autism and children with Specific Language Impairment. *Applied Psycholinguistics* 9 (1): 89–115.

Stegenwallner-Schütz, M. and Adani, F. (2020). Production of referring expressions by children with ASD: effects of referent accessibility and working memory capacity. *Language Acquisition* 27 (3): 276–305.

Szendrői, K., Bernard, C., Berger, F. et al. (2018). Acquisition of prosodic focus marking by English, French, and German three-, four-, five- and six-year-olds. *Journal of Child Language* 45 (1): 219–241.

Tager-Flusberg, H., Rogers, S., Cooper, J. et al. (2009). Defining spoken language benchmarks and selecting measures of expressive language development for young children with Autism Spectrum Disorders. *Journal of Speech Language and Hearing Research* 52 (3): 643–652.

Terzi, A., Marinis, T., and Francis, K. (2016). The interface of syntax with pragmatics and prosody in children with Autism Spectrum Disorders. *Journal of Autism and Developmental Disorders* 46: 2692–2706.

Terzi, A., Marinis, T., Kotsopoulou, A. et al. (2014). Grammatical abilities of Greek-speaking children with autism. *Language Acquisition* 21 (1): 4–44.

Terzi, A., Marinis, T., Zafeiri, A. et al. (2019). Subject and object pronouns in high-functioning children with ASD of a null-subject language. *Frontiers in Psychology* 10: 451534.

9

Prosody

Sandrine Ferré and Rhea Paul

> **What Do You Think?**
> When entering university, you want to make new friends and you start talking to your neighbor at the university restaurant. It appears that you are in almost all the same psychology classes! Although you are very excited, this guy does not seem to express any emotions when talking about this. His voice sounds flat and nasal to you, as if he does not care much about what he is saying. You are a bit disappointed, although he does seem to have some interesting ideas about human psychology. In the afternoon, you learn that he has autism. Would you revise your first impression?
>
> In a neuropsychology class, the professor plays a video of two people who self-identify as autistic conversing about friendship. One has a monotonic, robotic-sounding kind of speech that you have heard described as a characteristic of people with ASD. The other does not; his speech sounds pretty typical, although he has difficulty talking about what he thinks a friend is, and is somewhat literal in his understanding of friendship ("My friends are the people I play video games with online"). Do both speakers really have ASD?

Introduction

Because communication disorder is one of the primary characteristics required for a diagnosis of Autism Spectrum Disorder (ASD), prosody as an aspect of communication has long been a topic of interest in research on autism. Since the first identification of the autistic syndrome, abnormal prosody has been identified as a central feature of autism for individuals who speak, regardless of their language (Bonneh et al. 2011). Differences noted in early, observational reports included monotonic or robotic intonation, deficits in the use of pitch and control of volume, and deficiencies in voice quality. When prosodic atypicalities are present, they are one of the most recognizable and stigmatizing elements of ASD (Paul et al. 2005). They constitute one of the most significant obstacles to social integration and vocational acceptance, as they almost immediately create an impression of oddness. Nonetheless, one fact that begs for explanation stands out: if prosodic perception and production are central to affective and pragmatic communication, which are often impaired in speakers with ASD, why do only about half of speakers with ASD demonstrate readily identifiable expressive prosodic deficits? There are several reasons why this mystery matters. In this chapter, we will explore two main questions:

- How do individuals with autism perceive prosody?
- How do individuals with autism produce prosody?

Anchoring

Before we answer the questions, we provide some background on prosody and its role in language development. Speech, the expression of language by means of articulating sounds, can be divided into two domains: the **segmental** and the **suprasegmental**. Segmental aspects of speech include the organization, sequencing, and production of the sounds, or phonemes, which result in the articulation of speech (see Chapter 4). The suprasegmental level refers to all other aspects of the speech signal that accompany the segmentals, modulate meaning, and give each speaker a unique identity. We use the word **prosody** here to refer generally to the suprasegmental aspects of the speech signal that serve essential communication functions at the social/pragmatic level and also include accentual facts, rhythm, and intonation. These are expressed by measurable acoustic correlates, such as variations in duration, intensity (amplitude), and pitch (**fundamental frequency**, or F_0).

Prosody serves a variety of critical functions for communication: it is (i) extralinguistic in that it identifies characteristics of the speaker (gender, age, dialect), (ii) paralinguistic in that it conveys emotion alongside the conceptual meaning conveyed, and (iii) linguistic in that it signals pragmatic aspects, such as the communication situation and the speaker's state of mind (irony, sarcasm, neutrality), as well as structural language aspects, such as part-of-speech classification of lexical items (*CONvict* vs. *conVICT*), partitioning of sentence parts into phrases, and the identification of focus within sentences. The functions of prosody are generally divided into affective and linguistic domains. **Affective prosody** (AP) includes changes conveyed by modulations in pitch, intonation, rate, intensity, and rhythm used for varying social functions, such as marking differences among the ways an individual talks to peers, to young children, and to people of higher social status. AP is also involved in conveying a speaker's general emotional state, including excitement, anxiety, sadness, enthusiasm, etc. For example, a father would produce the utterance *My son's plane hasn't landed yet* with different suprasegmental characteristics, depending on whether he was feeling relaxed about having time before he had to leave for the airport or anxious because the plane hadn't landed on time. Similarly, prosody may contribute to the expression of intentional states such as irony and sarcasm. Saying *That was brilliant* would change in meaning from a compliment to a criticism, depending on the suprasegmental information (literal or sarcastic) conveyed along with the identical words.

Linguistic prosody comprises both grammatical and pragmatic elements. **Grammatical prosody** includes suprasegmental cues that are used to signal syntactic information within words or sentences. **Stress/accent** can be used grammatically within words in English to signal, for example, whether a token is used as a noun (*CONvict*) or a verb (*con-VICT*). **Pitch** contours signal the ends of utterances and denote, in English, for example, whether they are questions (rising pitch) or statements (falling pitch). In addition, the use of prosodic stress/accent and pauses often helps clarify potentially ambiguous syntax by defining **phrasal boundaries** (*dragonfly and carrot* vs. *dragon, fly, and carrot*; Chevallier et al. 2009).

> **Acronym and Terminology Reminder**
> **Acoustics (Acoustic):** The physical properties of speech sounds, such as amplitude, frequency, and duration.
> **Affective/Emotional Prosody:** The way emotion is expressed in speech, via modulations in pitch, rate, intensity, and rhythm.
> F_0: Fundamental frequency – the frequency at which the entire sound wave vibrates (due to vibration of vocal folds/cords) when a sound is produced. It is measured in Hertz (Hz).
> **Intonation:** Pitch variation across a phrase or a sentence, creating a specific melody or a contour for a given language and expressing a statement, a question, an order, and so on.
> **Lexical Stress:** Stress on a particular syllable within a word that causes a difference in word meaning (e.g. *PREsent* vs. *preSENT*, in English).
> **Linguistic Prosody:** The way speech is modulated to convey linguistic information (e.g. rising intonation to indicate a question or word stress to indicate whether a word is a noun or a verb, as in *PREsent* vs. *preSENT*) and pragmatic information (e.g. irony, sarcasm).
> **Pitch:** How high or how low a speech sound is produced or perceived.
> **Prosody:** Melodic structure, including stress, intonation, and rhythm organization.
> **Shifting:** The ability to move/shift one's attention from one task to another task.
> **Stress/Accent:** Prosodic variation (variation in intensity, frequency, and/or duration) with which a vowel is produced in order to provide grammatical information about a word or highlight an element of information in the speech.
> **Suprasegmental Aspects of Speech:** The melody of the speech signal that accompanies the production of speech sounds and modulates meaning.

A second function of linguistic prosody is pragmatic. **Pragmatic prosody** is used to carry social information beyond that conveyed by the syntax of the sentence. It communicates the speaker's intentions (beyond the expression of emotions) or the hierarchy of information within the utterance and results in optional changes in the way an utterance is expressed (see Chapter 8). Stress/accent, as one example, can be used to highlight an element of information within a sentence as the focus of attention. This pragmatic use of stress/accent, usually referred to as "emphatic" or "contrastive" stress, calls the listener's attention to information that is new to the conversation, unfamiliar, or unexpected. **Emphatic stress** is used to highlight the comment, or predicate, of an utterance, the portion that elaborates on the topic established within the discourse, as in *John went to Paris* where *Paris*, which is part of the predicate, receives emphatic stress compared to *John*, which is the topic. **Contrastive stress** is used when an element in the first speaker's utterance needs to be refuted by the new information presented by the second speaker, as in, *Will the red tie be OK? No, I need the blue one.*

In summary, while some aspects of grammatical prosody are obligatory elements in speech production, others convey information about salience, pragmatic intention, and affect that result through a range of additional modulations in the speech signal. These aspects of prosody are critical components of **communicative competence**. Deficits in the ability to produce or perceive them can lead to significant difficulties in social communication.

Regarding language development, prosodic use can be observed as early as the first year of life. Gratier and Devouche (2011), for example, report that mother–infant vocal interactions show infants' imitation and repetition of intonational contours by 3 months of age. During **babbling**, a language development phase during which children produce meaningless sequences of syllables, the duration, intensity, and frequency of syllables vary, presenting adult-like stress/accent patterns (at 7–14 months). There is a significant increase in the complex intonational structure of infant vocalizations at the same age. This increase is seen only in canonical babbling (strings of repetitive syllables such as /babababa/), but not in the less mature babbling that may persist, suggesting that in the second half of the first year, infants begin to apply melodic intonation only to their most speech-like productions. This vocal stage has been called **jargon babble**. It typically occurs between 9 and 18 months and overlaps with the baby's first words. Jargon vocalizations include complex, nonrepetitive syllables within a prosodic envelope that mimics the rhythm and melodies of the language being learned. This babble often sounds as if the child is speaking the ambient language, but the listener is mysteriously unable to understand the words. Jargon babble usually co-occurs with first word use.

In terms of perception, infants start picking up on the prosodic features of stress, intonation, and rhythm long before they begin to categorize the sounds of their language or grasp the meaning of its words. Babies as young as 7;6 months have been found to be sensitive to the alternating stress/accent patterns of words in English, and 14-month-olds can recognize novel words based on their stress/accent configuration. Thorson (2018) discusses how toddlers' ability to process prosody during this stage facilitates word learning.

Prosodic productions in the second to third year of life also demonstrate the central role of prosody in language development. Children between 1;9 and 2;5 use stress/accent to mark new, as opposed to given information in their two-word utterances. Significant effects of mothers and their 12- to 30-month-old children's influencing each other's pitch in conversational exchanges are seen, a process referred to as **entrainment**, the influence on one speaker's prosody by the prosody of the interlocutor.

Toddlers have also been shown to demonstrate growth in the processing of prosody. Research groups using different methodologies have shown that toddlers as young as 19 months are able to use prosodic information to access the syntactic structure of sentences. Lammertink et al. (2015) found that 2-year-olds from both English- and Dutch-speaking environments were already almost adult-like in their ability to use prosodic cues to anticipate upcoming turn endings in interactions with adults. In general, this research demonstrates that by the age of 2, infants are able to spontaneously produce pragmatically appropriate prosody for basic speech acts. These are utterances meant to serve a function, such as requesting, commanding, complaining, greeting, etc. (see Chapter 6). Infants also make use of prosodic information in processing the speech directed to them.

Research has also examined the extent to which preschool-aged children expand their understanding and use of prosody. For example, prosody plays a crucial role in mediating interactions among preschoolers and in fostering cooperation in play. Hupp et al. (2021) found that preschool children can use prosodic cues to determine the intended referent among words, and 4- to 6-year-olds were able to resolve ambiguous prepositional-phrase attachments (*You can feel the frog with the feather* [feel frog who is wearing a feather vs. use available feather to touch frog]).

Hübscher, Garufi, and Prieto (2019) and Pronina et al. (2021) reported that 3- to 5-year-olds use prosody before they use syntax or lexical choice to convey politeness as well as to encode basic speech acts such as information-seeking questions. Children this young, though, still have trouble using prosodic cues to devine speakers' beliefs, suggesting a limitation based on incomplete development of **Theory of Mind**, the mental ability to infer and understand mental states in oneself and others (see Chapter 6). Receptively, children aged between 3.5 and 4.5 years use prosodic information in both French (de Carvalho, Dautriche, and Christophe 2016) and English (de Carvalho, Dautriche, and Christophe 2016) to disambiguate homonymous words in sentences (e.g. *The baby flies//hide in the shadows* vs. *The baby//flies his kite*).

Despite these findings of relatively rapidly developing prosodic skills in preschoolers, the ability of children under 5 years of age to demonstrate these skills in unfamiliar test situations outside of natural communicative contexts has been found to be quite limited (Gibbon and Smyth 2013). In general, the acquisition by preschoolers of increasingly complex prosodic skills proceeds in parallel with their other linguistic developments. However, assessing these abilities with decontextualized, unnatural methods appears to underestimate the prosodic skills preschoolers show in everyday interactions, making it difficult to identify prosodic deficits at this developmental level.

By school age, though, children appear able to demonstrate a range of adult-like prosodic capacities. Foley, Gibbon, and Peppé (2011) found that 5- to 6-year-old children were able to demonstrate some functional prosodic skills on the Profiling Elements of Prosody in Speech-Children (PEPS-C; Peppé and McCann 2003), a nonnaturalistic assessment measure. There were, in addition, further developments between the ages of 5;9 and 9;5, and some aspects of prosody continued to develop up to 11 years, at least in this relatively contrived format.

Much of the research on prosody in school-aged children has focused on lexical stress. Smith and Robb (2006) asked children aged 5 through 7 years to repeat novel two-syllable words with stress/accent either on the first or second syllable to examine word duration in the two conditions (e.g. *poPI* vs. *POpi* within the phrase *This is the __*). Words with second-syllable stress were, overall, longer than those with first-syllable stress. The same words produced by preschoolers were more equal in duration. Thus, although many prosodic capacities are present early in life, their refinement extends into the school years.

One other aspect of prosody that has been examined in typical older children is the understanding of prosodic cues to nonliteral intentions, such as **irony**. Ballard et al. (2012) observed that preschool children with typical development show little comprehension of this intent and tend to interpret language literally, regardless of its intonation contour. They report that children start understanding irony around 6 years of age, but that irony comprehension is an ability that develops over a long period of time, into the teen years (see Chapter 6 on implicit meaning).

In sum, prosody is one of the earliest aspects of communicative competence to emerge in typical development, with several prosodic elements present in vocal interactions from the first year of life. In the toddler and preschool periods, children expand prosodic elements in both production and perception, and early school-age children can demonstrate many of these features. However, many of these elements continue undergoing refinement, in terms of acoustic precision and functional scope, particularly in the area of nonliteral intentions, at least until adolescence.

Prosody in Autism

While there is a consensus that individuals with autism have difficulties with the aspects of prosody that support social communication (i.e. pragmatics, see Chapter 6) due to the very characteristics of their disorder, there is also evidence of reduced performance in both production and comprehension of the linguistic functions of prosody (Paul et al. 2005; Peppé et al. 2011). As prosodic differences, with respect to typically developing (TD) speakers, are expressed through acoustic variations (such as duration, intensity, and pitch) some characteristics of prosody in speakers with ASD may be identifiable through acoustic analysis even when they sound like TD speakers. Several factors may contribute to this finding, including the diversity of the methodologies used, the heterogeneity of the syndrome, as well as a "lumping" of prosody into an undifferentiated concept that ignores the broad range of both acoustic and functional aspects of prosody. Moreover, a meta-analysis of studies of receptive prosody (Zhang et al. 2022) suggested that there is a tendency for research to focus on deficits in autism rather than strengths, as well as a bias toward publishing results in which differences are found, which may inflate the reported prevalence of prosodic disorders. Still, questions remain: What does our understanding of the neural processes supporting prosodic perception and production tell us about potential underlying sources of the autistic syndrome? Can understanding the way prosody and its deficits affect speakers with ASD contribute to our concept of the neurobiology of the autism spectrum? We will attempt to examine these issues in the following sections.

How Do Individuals with Autism Perceive Prosody?

As we saw earlier, prosody is based on a range of acoustic modulations. Thus, if we want to understand why prosody malfunctions, we must begin by investigating the perception of the various aspects of the auditory signal when they accompany language, as well as when they do not. In this section, we first review what we know about the perception of **acoustic features** that support prosody outside any language support (through what is called pure tones). We also take a look at perception of emotions through prosody and perception of the voice. These aspects are important to consider because impaired perception of these cues could lead, or be linked, to impaired perception of prosody during linguistic processing.

Perception of **pure tones** (sounds consisting entirely of a single pitch, heard as "beeps") has been examined to assess neurological mechanisms underlying nonverbal auditory perception of pitch, as a possible deficit in ASD. Some

electrophysiology studies measured the electrical activity of the brain while participants were listening to pure tones. They report that autistic subjects' responses to pure tone changes (for example, differentiating between a 216 and 299 Hz tone) are highly variable, ranging from within the norm to reduced amplitude or shorter latency of response compared to neurotypical individuals. In brain imaging studies of autistic individuals presented with pure tones, normal timing of auditory response, but atypical functioning of the left prefrontal cortex, were observed (Gomot et al. 2006).

Emotional prosody has often been identified as atypical in individuals with autism who develop language. When emotional valence is involved in the processing of nonverbal auditory stimuli (for example, perceiving the difference between stimuli with a neutral vs. an angry prosody), the results are again diverse, showing reduced, increased, or identical cerebral activations compared to those of neurotypical people. However, it appears that brain activity is modulated by salience and emotion in speakers with autism, even when they have difficulty understanding and producing emotional prosody themselves.

The involvement of **attention** may also contribute to explaining the diversity of results in nonlinguistic perception of prosodic elements, including in electrophysiology studies. For example, using an oddball paradigm where participants were exposed to sequences of similar sounds that were interrupted by a novel sound (e.g. /a/ /a/ /a/ /a/ **/u/** /a/ /a/), Gomot et al. (2006) observed reduced activation, in autistic subjects, in the brain areas involved in attention. This was obtained when the participants were listening to the stimulus without being asked to react upon detecting the novel sound. Crucially, no difference regarding brain activation between the autistic and neurotypical groups was found when the participants had to actively react (by pressing a button) to any novel sound detection.

As prosody is, in part, based on variations in frequency, it is of interest to ask how people with autism perceive the **voice** carrying this information. A reduced preference for the human voice compared to a synthetic voice has been found in children with autism (Kuriki et al. 2016). In adults with ASD, results vary, showing comparable or lower response to voice than in neurotypical adults while no difference between autistic and neurotypical adults has been found for nonspeech sounds. In children with ASD, human voice processing generates less activation in particular areas of the brain compared to neurotypical children. This varies with the age and verbal development of the children and with the degree to which they communicate by voice themselves (Latinus et al. 2019).

Although we know that some autistic individuals have difficulties interpreting prosodic cues, these difficulties are not universal in ASD. Studies have been conducted on populations of differing ages, nonverbal skills, severity of autism, language spoken, comorbid disorders, and so on. It is therefore difficult to generalize beyond the nonspecific observation of heterogeneity. For example, autistic adolescents were reported to process lexical stress less well than their neurotypical peers in one study (Paul et al. 2005), but not in another study (Lyons et al. 2014). However, in the first study, the participants presented a broad range of **autism severity**, whereas in the second study, the autistic group was much more homogenous. Similarly, children with a range of autistic severity show more phrasing errors (infelicitous placement of pauses within sentences) than either children with more circumscribed "High Functioning Autism" or those with typical development (Shriberg et al. 2001; Lyons et al. 2014). However, in contexts where prosody has a more strictly linguistic function, children with varying degrees of autism severity perceive prosody similarly to neurotypical children. This has been found in studies looking at the way syntactic units are **chunked**. One example involves investigating the ability to distinguish between a sequence of two individual words and a compound combining the same two words (as in *dragon, fly* vs. *dragonfly*). In the two-word sequence, an accent is carried by each word compared to only one in the compound. There is also less coarticulation (see Chapter 4) between two words occurring one after the other than between the segments of a single word (including compounds). The pitch curve (overall melody) also differs in two-word sequences compared to compounds. Finally, it is possible to find a very short pause between the words in two-word sequences, which is not the case in compounds. Studies investigating syntactic chunking often ask participants whether audio stimuli displaying different phrasal boundaries correspond to pictures that are shown to them (see Figure 9.1 for an example of a test item). In such studies, picture-matching accuracy has been shown

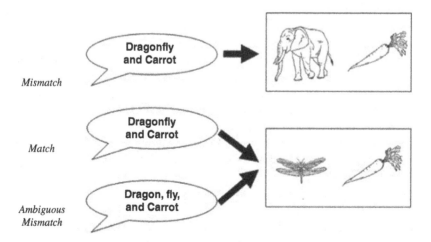

Figure 9.1 Example from a picture matching task used for investigating chunking abilities based on perception of prosodic cues. *Source:* Chevallier et al. (2009). Reproduced with permission of Elsevier.

not to differ between autistic and neurotypical children (Chevallier et al. 2009). In particular, in Figure 9.1, autistic children do not associate the stimulus *Dragon, fly, and Carrot* with a picture displaying a dragonfly and a carrot.

In terms of processing prosodic variation, individuals with autism perceive **rhythmic patterns** well, including when these patterns are meaningless (i.e. they are built with nonlinguistic stimuli) (Järvinen-Pasley et al. 2008). In this study, individuals with autism and neurotypical children were asked to judge the pitch contour information of sentences (e.g. *Let's go for a walk, Stella often dances, Sue always feels lonely*, and *Annabel is from Italy*; the linguistic perceptual condition) and strings of vowels (e.g. *A-A-A-A-A, AA-AAAA, A-AA-A-AA*, and *AAA-A-A-AAA*; the nonlinguistic perceptual condition) that matched the rhythm of the sentences. Participants were also asked simple comprehension questions to test access to meaning. The autistic children did better than the neurotypical children in the linguistic perceptual condition, whereas no difference was observed between the two groups in the nonlinguistic perceptual condition. The fact that the autistic children had high performance in both conditions suggests that meaning does not interfere with perception capacities in this population. This differs from neurotypical children, who despite lower performance in the linguistic perceptual condition, did better than the autistic children in comprehension. Ability to perceive rhythm in autism is also shown by the fact that autistic individuals do not differ from typically developing individuals in being able to follow the general rhythm of a spoken string (Key and D'Ambrose Slaboch 2021). Even autistic children with language impairment seem to have efficient perception of rhythm, as shown by a study based on musical stimuli (Heaton et al. 2018). In this study, these children were also shown to have INCREASED perception of F_0 variations relative to typically developing children. In contrast, autistic children are less sensitive to specific prosodic cues that mark linguistic (such as lexical stress) or affective information in the speech signal. They also have difficulties understanding the communication intent expressed by **intonational patterns** (Fine et al. 1991). In other words, they appear to benefit less from cues such as intonation and lexical stress in conversation. This being said, in structured tasks that involve active participation and focused attention, differences between subjects with and without autism often disappear (Heaton et al. 2018). Regarding underlying brain mechanisms, when prosody, especially emotional prosody, occurs on words, reduced brain activity in the right hemisphere (where much prosodic processing typically occurs) is identified in ASD relative to non-ASD control participants.

Some authors hypothesize that low-level information processing systems are hyper-developed in individuals with autism. This means that they are able to finely distinguish acoustic details and variation in auditory stimuli, but they fail to transform this information into high-level linguistic intent (that is to say, use it for language processing). The **Enhanced Perceptual Functioning Hypothesis**

(Mottron et al. 2006) suggests that the perceptual difficulties experienced by autistic individuals do not stem from basic processing demands but rather from having to integrate complex information across several brain areas. This process could cause system overload if additional aspects of processing are involved, as is the case with prosody (i.e. its meaning goes alongside, and is closely related to, the linguistic, cognitive, and social information processing necessary to understand everyday speech). The load of processing input at these multiple levels could therefore be too heavy, making the joint analysis of prosodic and linguistic cues difficult. This hypothesis could help explain why perception of prosody can be difficult for subjects with autism in somewhat unpredictable ways, based on the relative processing load demands rather than reaction to specific prosodic elements. As suggested by Fine et al. (1991), one way of further investigating this hypothesis would be to combine the study of the direction of pitch movement (pitch rise or pitch fall) and that of the communicative value of F_0 variations in autistic individuals. This would provide more insightful information regarding their prosodic capacities compared to only looking at simple deviations from standard intonational patterns.

How Do Individuals with Autism Produce Prosody?

This section first explores the acoustic characteristics of the voice of autistic individuals. One important element is the Fundamental frequency (F_0) of the voice. It corresponds to the frequency of movements of vocal folds/cords, which are located in the larynx and are caused to open and close very quickly by air rising from the lungs. As F_0 is also at the root of prosodic variations used in language, it is important to try to characterize the specific nature of the voice of autistic individuals. In an attempt to do so, we first discuss autistic voice characteristics, then go on to relate these characteristics to what is known about the production of linguistic prosody.

The voices of people with autism are often described as odd, exhibiting hypernasality and hoarseness (Shriberg et al. 2001). The search for sources of these differences has extended into the period of infancy. Studies in newborns have been carried out to look for a biomarker of autism in the cry vocalizations of toddlers with an increased risk of ASD (due to the presence of an older sibling diagnosed with ASD). Sheinkopf et al. (2012) observed higher F_0 values for pain-related cries, cries that are more poorly voiced, and a lower amplitude range from 6 months of age on in these toddlers compared to babies at low risk for ASD. In addition to these acoustic differences, parents identified the cries of these high-risk babies as being more negative and appearing to come from younger children. At 10 months of age, a number of acoustic characteristics (54 out of 88 characteristics extracted) of preverbal vocalizations allowed for the identification of children later diagnosed with autism (Pokorny et al. 2017). The vocal qualities of infants with autistic siblings may eventually contribute to provisional diagnosis of autism in the first year of life before other associated language disorders can be detected, enabling earlier intervention.

This notwithstanding, there is no single vocal profile of verbal individuals with autism. Generally, the voices of people with autism can be characterized by a higher pitch, longer pauses, increased hoarseness, nasality, and creakiness of voice. However, this profile varies according to age, sex, autism severity, and from individual to individual (Fusaroli et al. 2022). Thus, although it seems possible to use vocal behavior in the first year of life as a potential risk marker of ASD, it remains difficult to specify the exact vocal characteristics of speakers with ASD or predict them from early vocal behavior.

Measuring prosody as an undifferentiated phenomenon is difficult for several reasons. For one, prosody can manifest itself in various ways. Moreover, there is wide individual variation in typical speakers, and researchers have a very limited set of transcription and analytic tools at their disposal beyond basic acoustic measurements to characterize prosodic output. In addition to modulations related to emotion, age, gender, style, and voice, we need to identify modulations specific to purely acoustic aspects, including frequency, amplitude, and duration. A meta-analysis of prosodic production (Asghari et al. 2021) reported that some acoustic features (including mean pitch, pitch range, and vocal duration) appear to discriminate speakers with ASD from TD speakers, at least in adults, although findings are somewhat task-dependent. Other prosodic features, including vocal intensity, pitch variability, and speech rate, did not significantly discriminate between the groups. Focusing on F_0, for instance, a wide range of indices of prosodic modulation can be identified: average, median, minimum, and maximum F_0 at the level of the vowel, the syllable, the word, the phrase, the sentence, the utterance, and the speaker, to name just a few. In the literature on prosody in autism, each of these variables has been analyzed in the quest for a reliable marker of autism. But this effort has bumped up against the heterogeneity of the syndrome, as well as the multifactorial nature of prosody. For example, while F_0 is often characterized by lower values in ASD (whether in average, minimum, or maximum), the formant values of vowels[1] have often been found to be higher than normal (Velleman et al. 2009).

Likewise, results on **intensity** mirror those reported for frequency, in that between-group differences can occur in any direction or be absent. Thus, when

---

[1] Formant values are acoustic features that make it possible to distinguish between vowels. The first formant is influenced by the degree of the aperture of the mouth, and the second formant is influenced by the place of articulation of the vowel (indicated by the position of the tongue).

measuring the range of intensity across individuals, whether for vowels or utterances, significant variations appear in autism (Olivati, Assumpção, and Misquiatti 2017). However, when the average intensity is measured, no differences between the productions of individuals with and without autism have been found (Van Santen et al. 2010).

Similarly, neither duration nor rate of speech appears to be a dependable marker of prosodic deficit. The speech rate in ASD can be slower or equivalent to that of speakers with typical development (Patel et al. 2020). However, longer sentence duration has been observed, which has been attributed, primarily, to the presence of more numerous, longer pauses (Diehl and Paul 2013). Atypical pause production appears to be associated with a different rhythmic organization in autistic speech, at least for some individuals.

Stress/accent remains an area of difficulty in the speech production of autistic individuals, whether it is contrastive, emphatic, syntactic, or lexical. While it may be produced correctly in its lexical function (*CONvict* vs. *conVICT*) by adolescents with autism and no Developmental Intellectual Disorder, it tends to have greater duration than in the productions of individuals without autism. Adolescents with ASD thus appear to be able to rely on their underlying linguistic representations (i.e. what they know about how prosody works in their language) and to manipulate distinctiveness[2] with stress/accent in simple lexical contexts, but their modulations for the purpose of emphasis or contrast remain impaired (Grossman et al. 2010). Large variability in production ratios of lexical stress (which have a distinctive/linguistic value), with a tendency for them to be higher than average, is present in the speech of some people with ASD, but an absence of final sentence lengthening (which marks the end of a sentence and has a demarcation value) was observed in others (Velleman et al. 2009). Thus, it seems that when lengthening has a distinctive function, it tends to be more marked than when it only has a demarcative function, with less communicative value.

To sum up, it appears that we know little about the prosodic skills in production of people with autism and that, once again, heterogeneity prevails. Their voices are generally atypical, with deviant F_0 and formants, but this profile varies according to many criteria. Regarding the variables supporting prosody, a wide range of measurements have been made without leading to a solid conclusion that would be consistent for all. Finally, the manipulation of linguistic prosody seems to be effective only when it is very salient (such as the use of lexical accent).

---

[2] Distinctiveness is used in linguistics for any speech feature that enables a contrast to be made and allows for a distinction between two meaningful units (i.e. words).

Focus on a Specific Study

Diehl et al. (2015) provide data that can help explain the often unexpected, conflicting, and incoherent results of studies on prosody in autism. It accomplishes this using **eye-tracking**, a technology that monitors the eye positions and eye movements of the participants and that does not require explicit responses. This method allowed the researchers to conclude that, although speakers with ASD process prosody in much the same way as their peers without autism, the context and demands of the task have more marked effects on the performance of speakers with autism. This paper is also significant because the authors paid close attention to the methodology they used so that they could ensure that no other cognitive skills interfered with the measures tested. The review of the preceding literature is thus very important in their analysis.

This paper first reports results concerning the prosodic processing of syntactic ambiguities by children and adolescents with autism and no intellectual disability, which had been reported in a previous study (Diehl et al. 2008). By asking participants to move objects from one location to another, this study looked at whether participants with autism could use prosody as well as peers without autism to disambiguate sentences that differed only in prosodic cues (e.g. *[Put the dog in the basket] [on the star]*), only in syntactic cues (e.g. *[Put the dog that's in the basket on the star]*), or both (*[Put the dog that's in the basket] [on the star]*) (see Figure 9.2). Results showed poorer performance by the participants with autism when they had to rely only on prosody. In contrast, they performed on par with their peers when the syntax was unambiguous, regardless of whether the prosodic structure of the stimulus was congruent or not with syntax.

These results can be compared to those of Paul et al. (2005) and Chevallier et al. (2009), which showed that participants with autism used prosody in the same way as their peers without autism to chunk sentences in prosody-focused judgment tasks (see Figure 9.1). In Paul et al.'s (2005) task, the participants received the following instructions:

"Listen to each sentence on the recording, then circle the correct answer to the question that follows it on your paper. For example, if you hear 'Ellen, the dentist, is here' and the question reads 'Is she talking to Ellen?' you would circle 'no.' But if you hear 'Ellen, the dentist is here,' and the question reads 'Is she talking to Ellen?' you would circle 'yes'."

Diehl et al. (2015) hypothesized that in the Paul et al. (2005) and Chevallier et al. (2009) studies the way the stimuli were presented, with a clear focus on their prosody, may have helped participants to direct their attention to the prosodic cues. Focusing attention and foregrounding relevant aspects of stimuli may allow

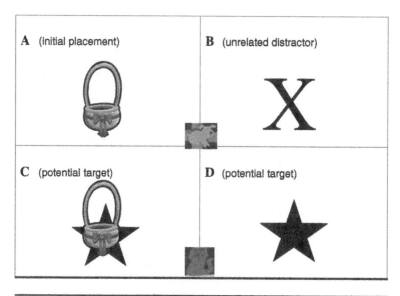

Figure 9.2 Syntactic ambiguity task layout and design. *Source:* Diehl et al. (2008). Reproduced with permission of Elsevier.

for more effective processing for people with autism, who nonetheless may have difficulty identifying the socially relevant aspects of stimuli (Hanley et al. 2014). Following the results of Snedeker and Yuan (2008) on young typically-children, Diehl et al. (2015) hypothesized that performance on their task by participants with ASD could be related to difficulty, not so much with prosody per se but

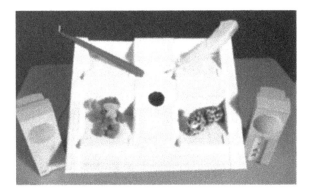

Figure 9.3 Sample trial in experimental setup. Here, the setup is related to the utterance *You can feel the frog with the feather*. The feather represents the target instrument, the frog (holding a feather) is the target animal, the feather that the frog is holding is the mini-instrument, and the candle and the leopard (holding a candle) are the distractor instrument and the distractor animal, respectively. *Source:* Diehl et al. (2015). Reproduced with permission of Cambridge University Press.

with **Executive Functions** such as shifting. Under this approach, subjects with ASD are considered to be unable to revise their initial interpretation in light of information appearing later in sentences.

Diehl et al.'s (2015) study used eye-tracking. The task, which is similar to the task used by Snedeker and Yuan (2008), was divided into two blocks of sentences, which required children to shift between two response types across trials. Thus, to perform above chance, participants had to change the interpretation they used for the first sentence type to succeed in the second block. Examples of the two sentence types are given in (1) and (2) (from Diehl et al. 2015), with the corresponding experimental setup appearing in Figure 9.3.

(1) You can feel the frog ... with the feather. (Use the barrette to feel)

(2) You can feel ... the frog with the feather. (Feel the one that has a feather)

In the first block, half of the participants were administered the first sentence type, as in (1), and the second half was administered the second sentence type, as in (2). In the second block, the conditions switched, and participants were administered sentences with the other prosody. The results showed that children and adolescents with autism with no intellectual disability do perceive changes in prosody, as shown by their ability to change their initial interpretation of the ambiguity. This shifting ability seems to occur from the age of 12 in children with autism and by age 7–8 in children without autism.

This conclusion opens up a wide field of investigation for understanding prosodic characteristics in ASD. It suggests that since participants with autism may use prosody to determine syntactic structure, the prosodic difficulties described in the literature are likely to stem from something other than a global deficit in prosodic processing. The authors entertain three hypotheses: (i) perception is intact, but deficits appear when prosodic information is used by another construct that is itself deficient (such as pragmatics); (ii) people with autism have prosodic disorders, but these disorders affect paralinguistic features that are not used for syntactic analysis; (iii) true prosodic deficits appear only in people who have a language delay: as prosody structures language acquisition, a person with a prosodic deficit should present with a delay in language acquisition, particularly in oral comprehension. It is difficult, though, to choose among these options without having a multifaceted view of prosody. As we have seen, prosody is at the interface of many mental faculties and calls upon a range of cognitive resources. Understanding prosodic disorders more deeply will require observation of their specific features, where the potential influence of other cognitive resources is controlled and manipulated.

Conclusion

This chapter set out to address the following questions:
- How do individuals with autism perceive prosody?
- How do individuals with autism produce prosody?

We showed that prosody is a multifaceted, multifunctional set of acoustic cues that accompany and modulate the meaning of the speech signal. Although elements of prosodic processing and expression appear in the first years of life, it takes until well into the school-aged period for all its elements to be acquired and mastered. Moreover, efficient use and understanding of prosody requires the integration of its acoustic characteristics with information from different cognitive functions, including social cognition, linguistic structure, Executive Function, and various motor and perceptual processes. Although unusual prosody was among the first characteristics noted in initial studies of autistic children, deficits in prosody are not universal in autism. When they are present, however, they are stubbornly persistent and strongly influential in producing negative attributions in listeners. Studies of prosodic performance in autism have produced conflicting, heterogeneous results that are difficult to interpret. Several factors may contribute to this confusion, including the diversity of the methodologies used, the heterogeneity of the syndrome, as well as a tendency to "lumping" prosody into an undifferentiated concept that ignores its broad range of both acoustic and functional aspects.

In an attempt to bring some small degree of order to this complex state of affairs, one hypothesis, following Diehl et al. (2015), is that what makes prosody hard for people with ASD is its intertwining with many other elements, which themselves may be sources of difficulty for this population, such as understanding the intentions of others, shifting attention, recognizing emotional influences, flexible processing, etc. It is the inextricable nature of prosody's connection with weak processing of a variety of information streams in autism that may lead to both inconsistent research findings and prevalent, yet nonspecific, deficits in use and understanding of prosody in natural contexts by speakers with ASD.

> **What Do You Know Now?**
> Prosody is a complex construct closely linked to several aspects of cognition, with important implications for autism:
> - Prosody is the suprasegmental aspect of the speech signal that uses pitch, stress/accent, amplitude, rhythm, timing, rate, and pauses to modulate meaning.
> - Prosody serves a range of functions, including identifying the part of speech of certain words, highlighting salient elements within a phrase or sentence, grouping words within the sentence, signaling speakers' intentions, and expressing a broad range of emotions through paralinguistic or suprasegmental information in the speech signal.
> - Prosody is intimately connected to many other domains and cognitive processes, such as social cognition, linguistic structure, emotional understanding, Executive Function, and auditory perception.
> - Prosodic skills emerge early in development, but they take until at least adolescence to be complete and fully elaborated.
> - Prosodic deficits have been noted since the first definition of the autistic syndrome, but they are not universal in all speakers with ASD.
> - When present, prosodic deficits are difficult to overcome and have significant, negative effects on social interactions.
> - Despite a range of studies, findings on prosodic understanding and use in autism are conflicting.
> - Difficulties with prosody in autism may result from the inextricable interrelationships between prosody and other aspects of psychological function, which overtax a range of vulnerable capacities in people with autism.

Suggestions for Further Reading

If you want to read more about auditory abilities in autism, we recommend you read Heaton et al. 2018. It will give you insights about brain imagery and help you understand how cognitive domains are intertwined with language. If you want to read more about perception and production of prosody in autism, we recommend you read Paul et al. 2005. It will give you an overview of how prosody can be assessed in perception and production in speakers with autism. If you want to read more about affective prosody, we recommend you read the recent overview by Zhang et al. 2022. It will increase your understanding of how affective prosody is assessed in the literature and how individuals with autism perceive it. If you want to learn about interventions for prosody in ASD, we recommend Holbrook and Israelsen 2020. It reviews a range of studies aimed at improving prosody in speakers with ASD and suggests which kinds of interventions appear to be most effective for decreasing atypical prosodic patterns in autistic speakers. Readers with an interest in clinical work on prosody in ASD will find the report of interest.

References

Asghari, S.Z., Farashi, S., Bashirian, S. et al. (2021). Distinctive prosodic features of people with: a systematic review and meta-analysis study. *Scientific Reports* 11: 23093.

Ballard, K.J., Djaja, D., Arciuli, J. et al. (2012). Developmental trajectory for production of prosody: lexical stress contrastivity in children ages 3 to 7 years and in adults. *Journal of Speech, Language, and Hearing Research* 55 (6): 1822–1835.

Bonneh, Y.S., Levanon, Y., Dean-Pardo, O. et al. (2011). Abnormal speech spectrum and increased pitch variability in young autistic children. *Frontiers in Human Neuroscience* 4: 237.

Chevallier, C., Noveck, I., Happé, F. et al. (2009). From acoustics to grammar: perceiving and interpreting grammatical prosody in adolescents with Asperger Syndrome. *Research In Autism Spectrum Disorders* 3 (2): 502–516.

de Carvalho, A., Dautriche, I., and Christophe, A. (2016). Preschoolers use phrasal prosody online to constrain syntactic analysis. *Developmental Science* 19: 235–250.

Diehl, J.J. and Paul, R. (2013). Acoustic and perceptual measurements of prosody production on the profiling elements of prosodic systems in children by children with Autism Spectrum Disorders. *Applied Psycholinguistics* 34 (1): 135–161.

Diehl, J.J., Bennetto, L., Watson, D. et al. (2008). Resolving ambiguity: a psycholinguistic approach to understanding prosody processing in high-functioning autism. *Brain and Language* 106 (2): 144–152.

Diehl, J.J., Friedberg, C., Paul, R. et al. (2015). The use of prosody during syntactic processing in children and adolescents with Autism Spectrum Disorders. *Development and Psychopathology* 27 (3): 867–884.

Fine, J., Bartolucci, G., Ginsberg, G. et al. (1991). The use of intonation to communicate in pervasive developmental disorders. *Journal of Child Psychology and Psychiatry* 32 (5): 771–782.

Foley, M., Gibbon, F.E., and Peppé, S. (2011). Benchmarking typically developing children's prosodic performance on the Irish-English version of the Profiling Elements of Prosody in Speech-Communication (PEPS-C). *Journal of Clinical Speech and Language Studies* 18 (1): 19–40.

Fusaroli, R., Grossman, R., Bilenberg, N. et al. (2022). Toward a cumulative science of vocal markers of autism: a crosslinguistic meta-analysis-based investigation of acoustic markers in American and Danish autistic children. *Autism Research* 15: 653–664.

Gibbon, F.E. and Smyth, H. (2013). Preschool children's performance on profiling elements of Prosody in Speech-Communication (PEPS-C). *Clinical Linguistics and Phonetics* 27: 428–434.

Gomot, M., Bernard, F.A., Davis, M.H. et al. (2006). Change detection in children with autism: an auditory event-related fMRI study. *Neuroimage* 29: 475–484.

Gratier, M. and Devouche, E. (2011). Imitation and repetition of prosodic contour in vocal interaction at 3 months. *Developmental Psychology* 47 (1): 67–76.

Grossman, R.B., Bemis, R.H., Skwerer, D.P. et al. (2010). Lexical and affective prosody in children with high-functioning autism. *Journal of Speech, Language, and Hearing Research* 53: 778–793.

Hanley, M., Riby, D.M., McCormack, T. et al. (2014). Attention during social interaction in children with autism: comparison to Specific Language Impairment, typical development, and links to social cognition. *Research in Autism Spectrum Disorders* 8 (7): 908–924.

Heaton, P., Tsang, W.F., Jakubowski, K. et al. (2018). Discriminating autism and language impairment and Specific Language Impairment through acuity of musical imager. *Research in Developmental Disabilities* 80: 52–63.

Holbrook, S. and Israelsen, M. (2020). Speech prosody interventions for persons with Autism Spectrum Disorders: a systematic review. *American Journal of Speech-Language Pathology* 29 (4): 2189–2205.

Hübscher, I., Garufi, M., and Prieto, P. (2019). The Development of polite stance in preschoolers: how prosody, gesture, and body cues pave the way. *Journal of Child Language* 46: 825–862.

Hupp, J.M., Jungers, M.K., Hinerman, C.M. et al. (2021). Cup! Cup? Cup: comprehension of intentional prosody in adults and children. *Cognitive Development* 57: 100971.

Järvinen-Pasley, A., Wallace, G.L., Ramus, F. et al. (2008). Enhanced perceptual processing of speech in autism. *Developmental Science* 11: 109–121.

Key, A.P. and D'Ambrose Slaboch, K. (2021). Speech processing in Autism Spectrum Disorder: an integrative review of auditory neurophysiology findings. *Journal of Speech, Language, and Hearing Research* 64 (11): 4192–4212.

Kuriki, S., Tamura, Y., Igarashi, M. et al. (2016). Similar impressions of humanness for human and artificial singing voices in Autism Spectrum Disorders. *Cognition* 153: 1–5.

Lammertink, I., Casillas, M., Benders, T. et al. (2015). Dutch and English toddlers' use of linguistic cues in predicting upcoming turn transitions. *Frontiers in Psychology* 6 (495): 274–291.

Latinus, M., Mofid, Y., Kovarski, K. et al. (2019). Atypical sound perception in ASD explained by inter-trial (in) consistency in EEG. *Frontiers in Psychology* 10: 1177.

Lyons, M., Schoen Simmons, E., and Paul, R. (2014). Prosodic development in middle childhood and adolescence in high-functioning autism. *Autism Research* 7 (2): 181–196.

Mottron, L., Dawson, M., Soulières, I. et al. (2006). Enhanced perceptual functioning in autism: an update, and eight principles of autistic perception. *Journal of Autism and Developmental Disorders* 36: 27–43.

Olivati, A.G., Assumpção, F.B.J., and Misquiatti, A.R. (2017). Acoustic analysis of speech intonation pattern of individuals with Autism Spectrum Disorders. *CoDAS* 29: e20160081.

Patel, S.P., Nayar, K., Martin, G.E. et al. (2020). An acoustic characterization of prosodic differences in Autism Spectrum Disorder and first-degree relatives. *Journal of Autism and Developmental Disorders* 50: 3032–3045.

Paul, R., Augustyn, A., Klin, A. et al. (2005). Perception and production of prosody by speakers with Autism Spectrum Disorders. *Journal of Autism Developmental Disorders* 35: 205–220.

Peppé, S. and Mccann, J. (2003). Assessing intonation and prosody in children with atypical language development: the PEPS-C test and the revised version. *Clinical Linguistics and Phonetics* 17: 345–354.

Peppé, S., Cleland, J., Gibbon, F. et al. (2011). Expressive prosody in children with autism spectrum conditions. *Journal of Neurolinguistics* 24: 41–53.

Pokorny, F.B., Schuller, B., Marschik, P.B. et al. (2017). Earlier identification of children with Autism Spectrum Disorder: an automatic vocalisation-based approach. *Proceedings of Interspeech*, 309–313.

Pronina, M., Hübscher, I., Vilà-Giménez, I. et al. (2021). Bridging the gap between prosody and pragmatics: the acquisition of pragmatic prosody in the preschool years and its relation with Theory of Mind. *Frontiers in Psychology* 12: 662124.

Sheinkopf, S.J., Iverson, J.M., Rinaldi, M.L. et al. (2012). Atypical cry acoustics in 6-month-old infants at risk for Autism Spectrum Disorder. *Autism Research* 5: 331–339.

Shriberg, L.D., Paul, R., Mcsweeny, J.L. et al. (2001). Speech and prosody characteristics of adolescents and adults with high-functioning autism and Asperger Syndrome. *Journal of Speech, Language, and Hearing Research* 44: 1097–1115.

Smith, A.B. and Robb, M.P. (2006). The influence of utterance position on children's production of lexical stress. *Folia Phoniatrica et Logopaedica* 58 (3): 199–206.

Snedeker, J. and Yuan, S. (2008). Effects of prosodic and lexical constraints on parsing in young children (and adults). *Journal of Memory and Language* 58: 574–608.

Thorson, J.C. and Morgan, J.L. (2021). Prosodic realizations of new, given, and corrective referents in the spontaneous speech of toddlers. *Journal of Child Language* 48: 541–568.

Van Santen, J.P., Prud'hommeaux, E.T., Black, L.M. et al. (2010). Computational prosodic markers for autism. *Autism* 14: 215–236.

Velleman, S.L., Andrianopoulos, M.V., Boucher, M. et al. (2009). Motor speech disorders in children with autism. In: *Speech Sound Disorders in Children: In Honor of Lawrence D. Shriberg* (eds. R. Paul and P. Flipsen), 141–180. San Diego: Plural Publishing Inc.

Zhang, M., Xu, S., Chen, Y. et al. (2022). Recognition of affective prosody in autism spectrum conditions: a systematic review and meta-analysis. *Autism* 26 (4): 798–813.

Part 2

Language in Autism: The View Across Language Domains

10

Language Development Across the Autism Spectrum

Silvia Silleresi and Laurice Tuller

> **What Do You Think?**
> A famous case of an autistic individual with a special talent for language is Christopher, who can read, write, speak, understand, and translate, in addition to his mother tongue, in more than twenty other languages (Smith and Tsimpli 1995). Christopher's tested IQ is extremely low, a level hinting at ineducability. What do you think of this combination of skill levels? Is it the exception that proves the rule?
>
> L. is a boy who was diagnosed on the autism spectrum at age 11. The diagnosis indicated that L. has very significant social-communication impairment. What would you expect regarding L.'s functional language abilities? What if L. were a girl?
>
> M. is a boy with autism who produced his first sentence at age 4. What do you think M.'s language skills will be like at age 10? And, what if, in addition, M. has received a diagnosis for ADHD or for epilepsy?

Introduction

It is commonly said that no two individuals on the autism spectrum appear the same way or present the same combination of difficulties and strengths. Autism **heterogeneity** represents one of the major challenges to understanding this condition, raising significant theoretical and clinical questions, especially when we consider how all primary and co-occurring factors might interact with each other. Focusing on language adds to the complexity of this enterprise. Language abilities range from absence of verbal ability or very little functional communication, together about 30% of individuals, to functional speech capabilities, in the remaining 70%. Among speaking children (70%), a significant number display **language impairment** (**LI**) beyond pragmatics. LI may selectively affect one or more different linguistic components, as well as either receptive and/or expressive modalities. Likewise, as seen in Chapter 6, different aspects of pragmatics may be affected or not. How are language abilities related to other factors in autistic children? We propose to break this question down into questions that touch upon important topics concerning language development across the autism spectrum: (i) severity of **diagnostic criteria** features (i.e. social communication and interaction, the **First dimension** of the diagnosis, and restricted and repetitive behaviors, the **Second Dimension** of the diagnosis), and presence of Disorder of Intellectual Development (**DID**)[1] (one of the primary descriptive specifiers), (ii) longitudinal changes, (iii) gender, and (iv) **co-occurring neurodevelopmental or medical conditions**.

- Can autistic children who have very low **intellectual abilities** or severe **autistic features** develop strong language skills?
- What kinds of **language trajectories** can be observed in autistic children? Will a child without language at age 6 ever develop (strong) language skills? Do **minimally speaking** autistic children understand language? Do such children also have limited intellectual abilities?
- Do **autistic girls** develop language differently from autistic boys?
- What effect do co-occurring neurodevelopmental or medical conditions, such as ADHD or epilepsy, have on language development in autistic children?

Anchoring

Autism Spectrum Disorder (ASD) is a complex neurodevelopmental condition, whose phenotypical realizations have been reported to differ from person to person in severity, range, and combination of symptoms. As we saw in Chapter 1, when a child is diagnosed on the autism spectrum, clinicians are required to indicate whether (s)he presents one or more **co-occurring conditions** that may develop during different phases of the lifespan, the so-called **descriptive specifiers** of the DSM-5-TR. These include LI and DID, which are given a primary position in both the DSM-5 and the ICD-11 (see Chapter 1), and a number of other conditions, medical, neurodevelopmental, and genetic.

The diagnostic criteria in the DSM-5 attempted to maximize clinical consensus under the label "spectrum." However, diagnostic manuals do not clearly tease apart possible interpretations of this term, apart from noting

---

[1] We remind readers that this book uses the term Disorder of Intellectual Development (DID) to refer to what was previously labeled Intellectual Disability (ID) (see Chapter 1). DID is the term used in the ICD-11; it corresponds to the term Intellectual Developmental Disorder used in the DSM-5.

that the "full range" of intellectual and language abilities can be observed (ICD-11). Several meanings of "spectrum" can be retrieved in relation to autism (see Figure 10.1). Besides the reference to (i) the dimensional nature of the diagnostic criteria for ASD, which are categorized into a First Dimension covering an array of social communication difficulties and a Second Dimension covering restricted and repetitive behaviors, both of which may be instantiated somewhat differently; (ii) the continuity between the general population and the autistic population; and (iii) the categorical division of autism into subgroups or profiles of abilities (see Lai et al. 2013), "across the spectrum" may also refer to (iv) the variability (in number and severity) of diagnostic criteria features and associated factors within each individual at a given moment in his/her developmental trajectory. Finally, "across the spectrum" can also evoke (v) a longitudinal interpretation since individuals on the autism spectrum can present consistent differences in developmental changes: progress, plateauing, and regression are all observed in language trajectories, also when language is put into relation with most (if not all) core (diagnostic criteria features) and associated factors. In other words, autism is a spectrum in many different ways that reflect the wide variation in the type(s) and degree(s) of strengths and difficulties people experience: autism is different for every autistic person.

> **Acronym and Terminology Reminder**
> **ADHD:** Attention Deficit and Hyperactivity Disorder.
> **ALI:** Autism Spectrum Disorder with Language Impairment.
> **ALN:** Autism Spectrum Disorder, Language is Normal.
> **Co-occurring Condition:** Multiple diagnoses ("comorbidity").
> **DID:** Disorder of Intellectual Disability. ICD-11 category for intellectual disability.
> **Expressive Language:** Using language to label objects and actions, to put words together in sentences to express thoughts and desires (requests, answers, and descriptions).
> **First Dimension (Diagnostic Criteria):** Autistic diagnostic symptoms related to "deficits in social communication and social interaction" (DSM-5).
> **LI:** Language Impairment.
> **Language Regression:** Loss of language skills acquired early in childhood.
> **NVIQ:** Nonverbal intelligence quotient.
> **Receptive Language:** Ability to understand language.
> **Second Dimension (Diagnostic Criteria):** Autistic diagnostic symptoms related to "restricted, repetitive patterns of behavior, interests, or activities" (DSM-5).
> **Structural Language:** Formal aspects of language related to phonology, morphology, semantics, and syntax.
> **TD:** Typically developing.

Studies on language development in ASD have so far overwhelmingly focused on intellectually able autistic children who are also able to express themselves verbally (Silleresi, 2023). This focus excludes both the many individuals with DID and the many individuals who have limited/no speech. In addition, very few studies on language in autism have looked at longitudinal changes in autistic children,

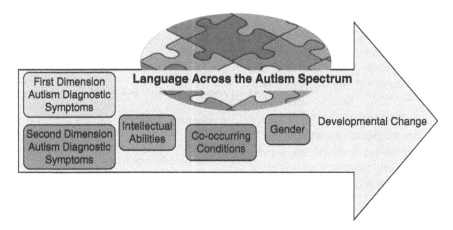

Figure 10.1 Language development across the spectrum. *Source:* Silvia Silleresi and Laurice Tuller.

even though it is well-known that unusual developmental trajectories are much more common in these children than in children without autism. Another notable lacuna concerns girls: girls are under-represented in all studies on ASD, including those focused on language. Finally, even very frequent co-occurring conditions (e.g. ADHD and epilepsy) are less investigated and often not controlled for in population samples in language studies. Since several co-occurring conditions are known to lead to language difficulties, independently of autism, it is likely that an autistic child who has one or more additional conditions could develop a specific language developmental profile. The scarcity of studies on these children does not represent a trivial obstacle to our understanding language in autism given the fact that these understudied children are so numerous and that these "special" cases raise "special" parental concerns, often centered on language development.

Language Development in Children Across the Autism Spectrum

Can Autistic Children Who Have Very Low Intellectual Abilities and/or Severe Autistic Features Develop Strong Language Skills?

For many years, the assumption that low intellectual abilities entail low language abilities has been taken for granted. However, this A PRIORI has been challenged both by clinical practice and research. From a clinical perspective, the ICD-11 identifies and describes five different profiles in ASD (Table 10.1).

Table 10.1 Diagnostic categories for Autism Spectrum Disorder.

	With mild or no impairment of functional language	With impaired functional language	With complete, or almost complete, absence of functional language
Without DID	Designated diagnostic category	Designated diagnostic category	No diagnostic category proposed
With DID	Designated diagnostic category	Designated diagnostic category	Designated diagnostic category

Source: World Health Organization (WHO) 2022.

Four of these profiles belong to the speaking (or verbal) part of the spectrum. They derive from all logically possible combinations of either spared or impaired functional language and intellectual abilities. Taking "functional language" to refer to structural aspects of language (see Chapter 1), this classification entails two homogeneous profiles, **ALN** (mild or no LI) without DID and **ALI** (with LI) with DID, and two discrepant profiles, ALI without DID and ALN with DID (see Chapter 1 for the distinction between ALI and ALN). A fifth profile concerns absence of functional language, which is found in minimally speaking children with ASD, combined with DID. In addition to what is reported in the ICD-11, a few studies have evoked a sixth profile, not mentioned in the ICD-11, characterizing minimally speaking children without DID (Munson et al. 2008; Bal et al. 2016). Although few studies have explicitly discussed the existence of this profile, if we take a careful look at the literature on minimally speaking children, we can see that many (if not all) studies included in their minimally speaking sample at least some children without DID (see Koegel et al. 2020). Finally, we note the lack of specific mention of children showing very high language and cognitive abilities, for whom there is no systematic empirical research in the literature. The possible existence of these profiles, and in particular those showing a discrepancy between linguistic and intellectual abilities, raises several theoretical considerations in the domain of research on language abilities in autism. First, it undermines the traditional assumption that spared (nonverbal) intellectual abilities necessarily lead to spared language abilities, and that impaired (nonverbal) intellectual abilities entail *ipso facto* impaired (or even absent) **structural language** skills. Moreover, the existence of these varied profiles provides a classical example of a **double dissociation** (Smith and Tsimpli 1995): language can be impaired or even absent in some children on the autism spectrum with otherwise intact intellectual abilities, and – more surprisingly – some children on the autism spectrum with DID may nonetheless have intact, or even enhanced, linguistic abilities. In the literature regarding structural language abilities in children with autism, there are very few studies that have reported all four profiles in the verbal portion of the autism spectrum, especially the ALN with DID profile (see Joseph, Tager-Flusberg, and Lord 2002; Silleresi et al. 2020), and even fewer that have found both intellectual ability profiles in the minimally speaking portion of the autism spectrum (Munson et al. 2008; Bal et al. 2016).

Why have these particular profiles been found so rarely and why do we know relatively little about them? One reason that may be behind both of these questions has to do with population sampling. The vast majority of studies investigating language abilities have concentrated exclusively on verbal children and on children without DID, which has led, in turn, to a lack of knowledge about language abilities in minimally speaking children (see Tager-Flusberg and Kasar 2013) and in children with DID (see Silleresi 2023). These gaps in the literature are troubling for many reasons: research has found that approximately 30% of children diagnosed with autism remain minimally speaking past age 5 (Tager-Flusberg and Kasari 2013), and current large-scale epidemiological studies have reported around 31% of children with ASD that were classified in the range of cognitive impairment (Wolff et al. 2022). Not including minimally speaking children and/or children with DID in research practice means lacking knowledge on language abilities of the corresponding 1/3 of the autism spectrum.

Besides intellectual abilities and language abilities, the core properties of autism concern the expression of autistic symptoms, which can be defined as features related to the two ASD symptom dimensions, social communication, the First Dimension, and restricted and repetitive behaviors, the Second Dimension. The term **severity** is generally used in relation to these features. However, it is not clear whether severity refers to the intensity of symptoms, the number of specific symptoms related to each of the two diagnostic dimensions (see Chapter 1), the ability to function with them, or if some symptoms should carry more weight in determining severity. The DSM-5 diagnosis for autism has clinicians assign a category to the two core diagnostic dimensions with reference to descriptions provided for three levels designed to reflect how much support a person is likely to need in their daily life: level 1 (requiring support), level 2 (requiring substantial support), and level 3 (requiring very substantial support). Research on autism makes use of measures of autism severity in terms of both the number of challenging behaviors/symptoms and their frequency. Commonly used measures are derived from the ADOS (based on direct clinical observation), notably the Calibrated Severity Score, and the ADI-R, a parental interview, notably the Reciprocal Social Interaction (for First Dimension features) and Restricted and Repetitive Behaviors (for Second Dimension features) measures.

In studies examining language development and autistic symptomatology, which are very few in the literature on language in ASD (see Silleresi 2023), the focus has mainly been on the First Dimension, and results have been mixed. Some studies have found significant correlations between the severity of autism and structural language abilities (e.g. Charman et al. 2005), while others have found no such link (e.g. Kjellmer et al. 2012). These contrasting findings are interesting since verbal language deficits are sometimes spoken about as being directly associated with or even explained by the autism itself and particularly by the severity of autistic symptomatology. The fact that studies have not found such correlations, especially in school-aged children, suggests that the idea that greater autism severity means that LI is more likely and more severe could be a myth. Some researchers have directly challenged the prevailing assumption on the basis of strengths among Second Dimension features (restricted and repetitive behaviors), notably reactivity to sensory input. They have suggested that sensory hypersensitivity could lead to unusually strong systemizing skills (hyper-systemizing), which in turn could be the base for strong statistical learning supporting the very strong structural language skills, which characterize some autistic individuals, including the autistic savant Christopher (Smith and Tsimpli 1995; Baron-Cohen 2009). In general, the link between sensory profiles and language (dis)abilities should be targeted in future research.

What Kinds of Language Trajectories Can Be Observed in Autistic Children? Will a Child Without Language at Age 6 Ever Develop (Strong) Language Skills? Do Minimally Speaking Autistic Children Understand Language? Do Such Children Also Have Limited Intellectual Abilities?

Most of the studies in the literature on language abilities in autism report on profiles of children on the autism spectrum at a given moment in their developmental trajectories. It is worth pointing out that changes take place in individuals with ASD, especially from a developmental perspective. In this sense, the term "spectrum" in ASD may have a further meaning, referring to variation within the developmental profile of each individual with ASD, through time. Linguistic abilities are certainly subject to developmental changes, due to aging, treatment and evolution of the wider clinical context. The picture becomes even more complex when we consider that other features (such as severity of symptoms, intelligence, and co-occurring conditions) are subject to developmental changes as well (Gotham, Pickles, and Lord 2012) and these other changes interact with language development trajectories.

Unusual childhood language trajectories are very frequent in autism, and they can include late language emergence, language regression, language "catch-up," and language plateauing. In general, much more is known about the development of spoken language abilities, as opposed to comprehension patterns, and this is true especially for minimally speaking or nonspeaking children (Slušná et al. 2021). In 2009, Tager-Flusberg and colleagues were the first ones to outline (spoken) language development benchmarks for autistic children, a framework that has been frequently adopted in more recent studies targeting expressive language trajectories (Kover, Edmunds, and Ellis Weismer 2016; Haebig et al. 2021). Based on current best evidence, they defined criteria to assign autistic children to four stages: (i) preverbal, (ii) first words, (iii) word combinations, and (iv) sentences. These benchmarks outline the minimum criteria for each stage across the domains of phonology, vocabulary, morphosyntax, and pragmatics. Verbal children are typically collocated at stage (iii) or (iv), while minimally speaking children at stage (i) or (ii).

Late language emergence is quite frequent in ASD; it is one of the most common reasons for initial consultation. While in neurotypical development first words and first word combinations (phrases or sentences) are found at around 12 and 24 months, respectively, in autism these milestones can be significantly delayed. For example, in a retrospective study of early development in 162 autistic children, 70% did not have phrases at age 33 months (Grandgeorge et al. 2009). **Language regression** (which is very often a component of general developmental regression) usually occurs within the first three years of life (ICD-11) and may be reported to be acute or gradual, with changes generally noted to occur over a few weeks to a few months. Published prevalence estimates of language regression in ASD range from about 25 to 40% (see Barger, Campbell, and McDonough 2013 for different types/rates of regression) and vary depending on the definition of regression, participant characteristics, sample size, and sampling methods. There is no clear rule specifying that a verbal child cannot regress to a minimally speaking stage, or a minimally verbal child cannot later catch up in language development. In fact, there is some evidence that many (perhaps most cognitively able) children who undergo early language regression may in fact have earlier language emergence than autistic children who did not experience language regression. They then go through a plateau during which language progresses very little, followed by slow improvement, and ultimately by attainment of at least some degree of fluent language (see Gagnon et al. 2021; Pickles et al. 2022). These conclusions are hampered by the way in which language skills were tested in these retrospective studies: global expressive communication and receptive communication scores from the VABS-II parental questionnaire or clinician appraisal of whether the child has "fluent speech," as defined by the ADOS ("spontaneous, flexible use of sentences with multiple clauses that describe logical connections within a sentence"). In other words, children with early language regression may later develop fluent language, but this language, though fluent, may display language impairment. No specific associations have been identified between language regression and genetic factors, but it may be that episodes of regression are associated with the manifestation and/or evolution of other co-occurring conditions (which, in turn, can change in severity during development), such as epilepsy and sleep disorders, though clarity on this question is so far lacking (see Giannotti et al. 2008; Barger, Campbell, and McDonough 2013; Backes, Zanon, and Bosa 2017).

Minimally speaking children are frequently affected by regression of speech. This phenomenon typically occurs in children with already limited or single-word vocabularies and appears in many cases to be accompanied by a loss of language comprehension. Besides regression, minimally speaking children can also show late language emergence, plateauing, or improvement/catch-up of language skills (Boterberg et al. 2019). Regarding receptive abilities, the picture is much more blurred. A more precise interpretation of language comprehension patterns in minimally speaking and nonspeaking children is currently still confounded by varying recruitment criteria. First, research has almost exclusively focused on minimally speaking school-aged children and adolescents. According to Pickles et al. (2022) beyond age 6, the rate of language development in ASD in general, enters a steady stage (plateauing), exhibiting little variation across the years and within different language outcome groups. So, the question that arises is what happens to minimally speaking children before age 6. Do they show different developmental trajectories from their older peers? Second, due to the long-held belief that children with DID are also children with impaired language abilities, researchers have often selected their samplings from a broader "low-functioning ASD population" without distinguishing either between speaking and nonspeaking children or between expressive/receptive language levels. This last point is very troubling, since lack of clarity remains over the relation between expressive and receptive capacities in children with ASD, especially since there is limited evidence pointing to a correlation (see, for mixed evidence, Kwok et al. 2015; Chenausky et al. 2018).

Systematic, separate investigation of expressive and receptive language trajectories would inform theories of language development in autism. In this vein, Kover, Edmunds, and Ellis Weismer (2016) suggested that it is possible, by age two and a half, to predict language growth for children with ASD across the preschool years and identify factors that discriminate between children who remain minimally speaking at age five and a half from those with high language proficiency. Namely, ages of expressive language milestones (i.e. first words, first phrases) could serve as predictors of developmental trajectories in very young children, though this picture could be muddled by the situation of language regression, which may be associated with early language milestones, as we saw above.

A critical additional question concerns the role of co-occurring primary and associated factors in this picture. Regarding intelligence, the picture varies according to chronological age: it seems, in fact, that in preschool children (especially those with minimal language), nonverbal intelligence at age 2 or 3 is one of the major predictors of later language gains for those children that acquire some language before age 5 (Thurm et al. 2015). Minimally speaking children who have a normal nonverbal IQ (NVIQ) seem to be likely to produce more words in their first years of life than their minimally speaking peers with DID (Bal et al. 2016), although there is no obvious correlation between enhanced nonverbal abilities and positive language development (as we saw before). In general, it has been noticed that, in contrast to the earlier life period when about one-third of the children can make dramatic gains, cognitive skills tend to remain stable or decline over this time span, especially after age 5. In parallel, it is worth noting that some researchers have evoked the possibility that discrepant profiles, such as ALN with DID, become statistically more frequent in ASD with age (in Joseph, Tager-Flusberg, and Lord 2002, they represented 8% of the population sample with a mean age of 5;5 and 28% of the population sample with a mean age of 8;11). This suggests that integrating a longitudinal/developmental perspective is fundamental when talking about profiles of language and intellectual abilities in children with ASD.

Concerning severity of autism symptoms, it appears that 5–6 years of age may also mark a milestone for language outcomes. Thurm et al. (2015) noted that, at age 3, scores on neither diagnostic dimension correlated with later phrasal language development in children who were minimally speaking or dichotomized children between minimally speaking and speaking. However, at age 5, scores in the First (social) Dimension constituted a valuable milestone in relation to language outcome in both minimally speaking and speaking children. This is consistent with previous findings from a retrospective study that reported lower social impairment on the ADI-R was related to positive development of verbal skills at least from age 4 (Wodka, Mathy, and Kalb 2013) and with recent studies (Georgiades et al. 2022) that have shown that autistic symptomatology, in relation to language and cognitive abilities, seems to either plateau (73% of the sample) or steadily improve (27% of the sample), after a turning point marking the period of transition to school (around age 6). It seems, nonetheless, that the relation between language abilities and severity of autism features goes in both directions: well-known studies such as Charman et al. (2005) found that low receptive and expressive language at young ages was related to increased autism symptom severity in the early school years.

Examining language abilities from a developmental perspective is particularly challenging since outcomes in expressive and receptive language skills seem to be somehow linked, on the one hand, to a sort of "sensitive" period (before age 6) and, on the other hand, to the severity of co-occurring factors. A possible strategy to cope with this *mare magnum* of difficulties could be to introduce into research (when possible) what Georgiades et al. (2022, and previous work) identified as **chronogeneity**, which can be defined as the heterogeneity of ability profiles in relation to the dimension of time, heterogeneity that affects not only language but all features of ASD. In other words, when looking into abilities in ASD, we should always consider that individuals on the autism spectrum are subject to (frequent) changes in a temporal dimension.

Do Autistic Girls Develop Language Differently from Autistic Boys?

Studies on ASD typically include many fewer females than males. Currently, females are diagnosed in lower numbers than males. 1:4 is the often-cited female-to-male ratio (DSM-5), but Loomes, Hull, and Mandy (2017) arrived at a ratio closer to 1:3. Small numbers of females in group studies have probably contributed to a lack of knowledge about the phenotypical realization of autism in females, which in turn could be a factor in missing or delayed diagnosis in girls (Lockwood Estrin et al. 2021). Among children without DID, the ratio of females to males appears to be even lower (perhaps as low as 1:8); in other words, there is a much higher proportion of girls in children with DID than in children without DID. Although this issue is currently the subject of controversy, the lower proportion of girls in children without DID might indicate that females with higher intellectual abilities have symptoms that are either different or more subtle than males and consequently more difficult to detect with current diagnostic criteria. Recent studies of social and behavioral variations have evoked the existence of a particular, so-called female phenotype (Hull, Petrides, and Mandy 2020), different from both that displayed by male children with ASD and male/female typically developing (TD) children. Females typically need to have more additional difficulties than males in order to receive an autism diagnosis, despite having equivalent levels of autistic characteristics (Dworzynski et al. 2012) and this could be due to their ability to "camouflage" their symptomatology more easily than males do. Under this view, it is therefore not surprising that females who do receive an autism diagnosis do so at a later age than males on average (Lockwood Estrin et al. 2021). Moreover, if they also exhibit other comorbidities (e.g. DID, behavioral difficulties) they tend to be diagnosed earlier than their female peers who do not display such co-morbid factors (Dworzynski et al. 2012). The detrimental implications of such potential gender bias have been highlighted as an area that needs urgent research attention.

Systematic investigation of language abilities in females, to see whether a "female language profile" exists in ASD, has just begun (Sturrock, Adams, and Freed 2021). Overall, these studies suggest that a specific profile of language and communication strengths and weaknesses for autistic females may exist. Generally, females with ASD have performed better than males on semantics, figurative language, language of emotions, and pragmatics, but no differences have emerged with respect to receptive and expressive vocabulary and syntax. In narrative abilities, Kauschke, van der Beek, and Kamp-Becker (2016) showed that girls with ASD verbalized internal processes more often than boys with ASD, showing a slightly different profile of narrative abilities. Although these results seem to suggest the existence of an "advantage" in females with ASD, practitioners report (informally) that as females with ASD grow up, pragmatic difficulties prove challenging within social interactions for them as well, though concrete evidence for this is so far meager. Future studies should include a comparison with both female and male TD children to see whether the so-called advantage of female participants is really due to a specificity of the ASD condition or to a general advantage of females over males in language development (see Adani and Cepanec 2019). Considering current knowledge on this topic, we cannot exclude the possibility that females on the autism spectrum may constitute a separate clinical group and might have some phenotypic language differences from male participants, though it should be emphasized that available evidence is so far quite limited.

What Effect Will Co-occurring Neurodevelopmental or Medical Conditions Have on Language Development in Autistic Children?

The DSM-5 reports that autism occurs along with an additional condition or diagnosis about 70% of the time and with two or more additional conditions or diagnoses about 40% of the time. There are likewise a number of neurodevelopmental, neurological, medical, genetic, and psychiatric conditions that are known to occur at higher rates in individuals with autism compared to individuals without autism. Beyond DID and LI itself, common co-occurring diagnoses are Attention Deficit and Hyperactivity Disorder (ADHD), epilepsy, sleep disorders, gastrointestinal disorders, Eating and Feeding disorders, Fragile-X Syndrome (see Chapter 11), anxiety, depression, Sensory Processing Disorder, and motor dysfunction. Some of these co-occurring conditions are known to be associated with high rates of LI, independently of autism, raising questions about their intersection with ASD and probable consequences. Two striking examples are ADHD, a Neurodevelopmental Disorder, and epilepsy, a neurological disorder.

ADHD is the most frequent joint diagnosis with ASD (40–70%), and its prevalence appears to be equivalent in autistic children whether they have DID or not (May et al. 2018). Autism appears likewise to be common among children with ADHD: these children frequently display ASD-like social difficulties and clinically identified ASD symptoms are also not unusual. Many children with ADHD experience language difficulties, at similar rates in those with or without comorbid autism (38% and 40% in Sciberras et al. 2014, a community-based study, though rates vary considerably from study to study – see May et al. 2018). These children's language skills have been found to be significantly weaker than those of TD peers in different linguistic areas, including formal aspects of language (Korrel et al. 2017). They also appear to experience greater pragmatic difficulties than their TD peers, even after controlling for structural LI, though their pragmatic difficulties may be less severe than those observed in autistic children (Carruthers et al. 2022). In a model study for language in autistic children with comorbid conditions, Boo et al. (2022) compared four groups of children: verbally fluent autistic children, nonautistic children with ADHD, children having diagnoses for both ASD and ADHD, and TD children. An analysis of narrative productions in different conditions revealed interesting differences and similarities in these children's language abilities: structural aspects were less complex in all three diagnostic groups compared to TD peers, but the comorbid ASD-ADHD group did not appear to perform less well than the ASD only or the ADHD only groups. This suggests that co-occurring conditions (or not all of them) may not necessarily entail greater language difficulties.

Epilepsy is another very frequent comorbidity in ASD. Its frequency in autism, which varies considerably from study to study, depending on population sampling, is much higher than that found in the general population (at least 10%, compared to 1%); likewise, the frequency of ASD among all children who have epilepsy far exceeds the general incidence of ASD (roughly one third). Epilepsy is diagnosed when a person experiences seizures, bursts of uncontrolled electrical activity between neurons, which are not related to an identified medical condition (e.g. brain trauma). The incidence of epilepsy is much higher in older compared to younger autistic children, reaching, in some studies, 25–30% of teenagers, and autistic individuals with DID compared to those with normal intellectual abilities. Even more frequent than clinical epilepsy in autism are EEG epileptiform abnormalities (sub-clinical epilepsy, in which there are no visible symptoms); these are found in significant proportions of even nonpileptic autistic children, including in younger children who may later develop epilepsy.

Developmental epilepsy is frequently associated with LI in children, and impaired language is a major characteristic of some epilepsy syndromes (e.g. Childhood Epilepsy with Rolandic Spikes, Epilepsy with Continuous Spike and Wave during Sleep, Landau-Kleffner Syndrome). Moreover, children with Developmental Language Disorder (DLD) present higher incidences of both epilepsy and epileptiform EEG abnormalities. It is therefore not surprising that associations with poorer language skills have frequently been found in studies of autistic children with epilepsy, clinical and subclinical.

Understanding the links between LI and epileptopathy in autism, however, is not an easy task, for several reasons. As noted above, epilepsy is associated with DID, independently of autism, but also in autism; DID is probably the major risk factor for associated epilepsy in autism. Some studies have reported language to be an independent risk factor for epilepsy in autism; others have not. Ewen et al. (2019), for example, found a relative independence for language level in the autism-epilepsy association. Viscidi et al. (2013) on the other hand, found that the association with language level disappeared when IQ was taken into account. While both of these studies can boast very large population samples (over 5000 participants), they both also illustrate how difficult it is to interpret language results from such studies, due notably to how language is measured. The Ewen et al. study uses the binary categories "late first word – yes/no," "abnormal spoken language – yes/no"; and Viscidi et al. report only a receptive vocabulary score, "current overall use of language" and "loss of language" based on parents' answers to two questions on the ADI-R. Of the ten studies on epilepsy in autism that report on language published starting in 2000, only four included direct measures of language, and these were either exclusively global language measures (e.g. a score for comprehension and a score for expression) or global derived categories (LI/no language) or exclusively a measure of receptive vocabulary (based on PPVT; see chapter 1). The other studies relied solely on parental reports (generally the ADI-R) or global clinical conclusions, resulting in very general categories such as "language absent/delayed/normal." More sophisticated and direct language measures will surely yield extremely interesting results; as Ewen et al. (2019) underline, "the ASD-epilepsy association needs detailed parsing of both ASD clinical phenotype and the epilepsy phenotype."

Summarizing, it is very likely that various comorbid conditions, notably ADHD and epilepsy, give rise to particular linguistic profiles in autistic children. The intersection with DID is just one of the challenges involved in the identification of such profiles. Widening the circle of complexity, not only are there probable links between language and ADHD and between language and epilepsy, but all of these appear to have associations with each other and with sleep disorders, another condition that has been shown to have links with LI, in both autistic and nonautistic children (Giannotti et al. 2008; Botting and Baraka 2018). Questions abound of course, whether comorbid conditions are more likely to result in language difficulties, but also whether the nature of observed difficulties is qualitatively or quantitatively distinct.

Focus on a Specific Study

We focus on Georgiades et al. 2022 for the following reasons: it is a very recent study, it is a very large study, and it is a longitudinal study that examined the trajectories of autism symptom severity in relation to language and cognitive abilities. A successive referral sample approach was used to enlist participants within four months after diagnosis in five hospital centers in Canada. A cohort of 187 children with ASD was assessed across four time points, from diagnosis at age 3, up to age 10. This study illustrates a possible methodological solution that takes into account how profiles of abilities develop from preschool years to early adolescence in relation to language, cognition, and severity of autism symptoms. Furthermore, the study employs well-known diagnostic tools (ADOS-CSS for severity of autism; Merrill-Palmer scales of Development for Cognitive Abilities), including direct language measures (PLS-4 for structural language – syntactic and semantic skills; see Chapter 1). It moreover uses innovative statistical analysis (unsupervised clustering methods) to (i) characterize the trajectory groups (clusters); (ii) identify possible trajectory turning points (changes in the slope for autism symptom severity); and (iii) explore individual child trajectory variability.

Results showed that children belonged to two different groups (clusters): Continuously Improving (27% of the population sample) and Improving then Plateauing (73% of the population sample). Findings also showed that children who followed continuously improving trajectories had lower ASD symptom severity and better cognitive, language, and adaptive functioning skills at diagnosis at age 3. A turning point was individuated within the period of transition into the school system. In line with previous investigations, group trajectories of symptom severity seem to, on average, diverge around age 6. Exploratory analysis of individual child trajectories within the two groups showed substantial variation in rates of change in symptom severity and in eventual age and number of turning points. This variation was more notable within the Continuously Improving trajectory.

The identification of language, cognitive, and adaptive functioning skills as trajectory correlates supports the utility of these constructs as clinical specifiers in the DSM-5 approach to describing ASD heterogeneity. Nonetheless, although this study is a good starting point for investigating how profiles in ASD unfold over time, several things could be added. First, to gain a better understanding of developmental trajectories we need to start thinking about informative trajectory specifiers: level and rate of change in primary factors (language, intelligence, autism severity) and co-occurring conditions (co-morbid neurodevelopmental or medical conditions), as we explained before, as well as turning points in child trajectories in relation to trajectory correlates. Furthermore, two aspects that were not explored in this study could profitably be included in future research: (i) the possible existence of a phenotypical female profile in ASD, which could present specific developmental patterns, and (ii) the role of co-occurring conditions in relation to language abilities. Finally, and importantly, such a study employing linguistic domain-specific language measures (rather than global language scores) would allow for a much more refined view of potential language changes over time, as changes could differ (considerably) from one linguistic component to another and interact differently with extralinguistic factors in autism.

Conclusion

This chapter set out to address the following questions:

- Can autistic children who have very low intellectual abilities or severe autistic features develop strong language skills?
- What kinds of language trajectories can be observed in autistic children? Will a child without language at age 6 ever develop (strong) language skills? Do minimally speaking autistic children understand language? Do such children also have limited intellectual abilities?
- Do autistic girls develop language differently from autistic boys?
- What effect do co-occurring neurodevelopmental or medical conditions, such as ADHD or epilepsy, have on language development in autistic children?

In order to arrive at a comprehensive view of language development across the autism spectrum, we considered the many ways in which autistic children differ from each other: their specific autistic diagnostic features, in both the First and Second Dimensions, the degree to which these affect children's daily life and distinguish them from their peers without autism, their intellectual ability, their gender, the presence and number of associated conditions and their severity, and the trajectories they are following in all areas of development. All of these contribute to the wide heterogeneity observed in autism and many of them appear likely to influence language development. Although knowledge about the intersection of many of these aspects with language is currently sketchy, what we do know presents a kaleidoscope view of how heterogeneous language in autism may be. There is clear evidence for homogenous profiles: autistic children with significant language difficulties who also have other significant cognitive difficulties and autistic children who have strong language skills who also have stronger nonlinguistic profiles. However, we have also observed a variety of discrepant profiles, such as intellectually able children with severe structural LI, children with DID and strong language skills, minimally speaking children with ordinary intellectual ability, minimally speaking children with DID with language comprehension, children with strong language skills, and very severe autistic symptomatology, etc. These latter types of profiles, whose relative frequency is currently not understood, fly in the face of many commonly held beliefs about autism and about language development.

Most autistic children, moreover, are not simply autistic, but have at the same time a diagnosis for another condition. Many of these other conditions, such as ADHD and epilepsy, are associated with language difficulties, in nonautistic children. Unsurprisingly, this appears to be the case for autistic children as well, though, again, LI with these and other co-occurring conditions is not an automatic consequence; it is merely more likely than not. We know very little about the effects on language development of the accumulation of more than one co-occurring condition, something that is relatively frequent in autism. It may be that LI in such cases is not necessarily more severe (see also Chapter 13).

Future studies on language development in autism should include serious consideration of children across the spectrum, in all their diversity. Knowing about language in verbally able children without DID and with no co-occurring conditions provides only a glimpse of a much richer picture. Exploration of the richer picture would undoubtedly advance our knowledge of both autism and of human language and its development. Better understanding of all the factors that determine how language progresses in children with autism will help clinical diagnosis and prognosis and also pave the way for development of specific, tailored strategies for parents, caregivers, therapists, teachers, and other actors that will help ameliorate quality of life for these children, wherever they fall on the spectrum.

> **What Do You Know Now?**
> Language development in autism is very heterogeneous and may be linked to the presence of associated factors; however, these associated factors do not necessarily entail single possible language outcomes.
> - While Christopher, a language savant, is clearly exceptional, having spared language skills along with (very) low intellectual ability is a possible ASD profile, as is the opposite profile (impaired language with normal intellectual ability). Different combinations of spared/impaired language and cognitive abilities are found in autistic children, though their relative frequency appears not to be equivalent, for reasons not yet understood.
>
>   It is not at all clear that the severity of core autism symptoms necessarily implies impaired language and vice-versa. The contradictory findings on the relationship between language and autism severity may largely stem from differing methodologies.
> - While more studies are sorely needed, there is some evidence that females on the autism spectrum may show different language profiles from males.
> - Generally, children who are already speaking at a young age do not regress into minimally speaking or nonspeaking. On the other hand, minimally speaking and nonspeaking children can either plateau, regress (from minimally to nonspeaking), or catch up with their peers. More generally there seems to be a period where changes are more frequent (before age 6) and more dramatic (gain or loss), after which developmental language outcomes seem to be more stable and subject only to plateauing or slow regression.
> - At least some co-occurring conditions, notably ADHD and epilepsy, appear to increase the likelihood of language difficulties in autistic children compared to autistic children who do not have this additional condition, though language difficulties may not be greater.

Suggestions for Further Reading

If you would like to learn more about language in children across the autism spectrum, we suggest the following readings: Silleresi et al. 2020 and Silleresi 2023, on language and intellectual ability profiles, Kjellmer et al. 2012, on language and autism severity, Hull, Petrides, and Mandy 2020, on language and gender, Slušná et al. 2021, on minimally speaking children, Pickles et al. 2022, on language trajectories, and Fernell and Gillberg 2023, on co-occurring conditions.

References

Adani, S. and Cepanec, M. (2019). Sex differences in early communication development: behavioral and neurobiological indicators of more vulnerable communication system development in boys. *Croatian Medical Journal* 60 (2): 141–149.

Backes, B., Zanon, R.B., and Bosa, C.A. (2017). Language regression in Autism Spectrum Disorder: a systematic review. *Psicologia: Teoria e Prática* 19 (2): 242–268.

Bal, V.H., Katz, T., Bishop, S.L. et al. (2016). Understanding definitions of minimally verbal across instruments: evidence for subgroups within minimally verbal children and adolescents with Autism Spectrum Disorder. *Journal of Child Psychology and Psychiatry* 57 (12): 1424–1433.

Barger, B.D., Campbell, J.M., and McDonough, J.D. (2013). Prevalence and onset of regression within Autism Spectrum Disorders: a meta-analytic review. *Journal of Autism and Developmental Disorders* 43 (4): 817–828.

Baron-Cohen, S. (2009). Autism: the empathizing-systemizing (E-S) theory. *Annals of New York Academy Science Journal* 1156 (1): 68–80.

Boo, C., Alpers-Leon, N., McIntyre, N.S. et al. (2022). Conversation during a virtual reality task reveals new structural language profiles of children with ASD, ADHD, and comorbid symptoms or both. *Journal of Autism and Developmental Disorders* 52 (7): 2970–2983.

Boterberg, S., Charman, T., Marschik, P.B. et al. (2019). Regression in Autism Spectrum Disorder: a critical overview of retrospective findings and recommendations for future research. *Neuroscience and Biobehavioral Reviews* 102: 24–55.

Botting, N. and Baraka, N. (2018). Sleep behaviour relates to language skills in children with and without communication disorders. *International Journal of Developmental Disabilities* 64 (4–5): 238–243.

Carruthers, S., Taylor, L., Sadiq, S. et al. (2022). The profile of pragmatic language impairments in children with ADHD: a systematic review. *Development and Psychopathology* 34 (5): 1938–1960.

Charman, T., Taylor, E., Drew, A. et al. (2005). Outcome at 7 years of children diagnosed with autism at age 2: predictive validity of assessments conducted at 2 and 3 years of age and pattern of symptom change over time. *Journal of Child Psychology and Psychiatry* 46 (5): 500–513.

Chenausky, K., Norton, A., Tager-Flusberg, H. et al. (2018). Behavioral predictors of improved speech output in minimally verbal children with autism. *Autism Research* 11 (10): 1356–1365.

Dworzynski, K., Ronald, A., Bolton, P. et al. (2012). How different are girls and boys above and below the diagnostic threshold for Autism Spectrum Disorders? *Journal of the American Academy of Child and Adolescent Psychiatry* 51 (8): 788–797.

Ewen, J.B., Marvin, A.R., Law, K. et al. (2019). Epilepsy and autism severity: a study of 6,975 children. *Autism Research* 12 (8): 1251–1259.

Fernell, E. and Gillberg, C. (2023). Autism under the umbrella of essence. *Frontiers in Psychiatry* 14: 1–7.

Gagnon, D., Zeribi, A., Douard, E. et al. (2021). Bayonet-shaped language development in autism with regression: a retrospective study. *Molecular Autism* 12 (1): 35.

Georgiades, S., Tait, P.A., McNicholas, P.D. et al. (2022). Trajectories of symptom severity in children with autism: variability and turning points through the transition to school. *Journal of Autism and Developmental Disorders* 52 (1): 392–401.

Giannotti, F., Cortesi, F., Cerquiglini, A. et al. (2008). An investigation of sleep characteristics, EEG abnormalities and epilepsy in developmentally regressed and nonregressed children with autism. *Journal of Autism and Developmental Disorders* 38 (10): 1888–1897.

Gotham, K., Pickles, A., and Lord, C. (2012). Trajectories of autism severity in children using standardized ADOS scores. *Pediatrics* 130 (5): 1278–1284.

Grandgeorge, M., Hausberger, M., Tordjman, S. et al. (2009). Environmental factors influence language development in children with Autism Spectrum Disorders. *PLoS One* 4: e4683.

Haebig, E., Jiménez, E., Cox, C.R. et al. (2021). Characterizing the early vocabulary profiles of preverbal and minimally verbal children with Autism Spectrum Disorder. *Autism* 25 (4): 958–970.

Hull, L., Petrides, K.V., and Mandy, W. (2020). The female autism phenotype and camouflaging: a narrative review. *Review Journal of Autism and Developmental Disorders* 7 (4): 306–317.

Joseph, R.M., Tager-Flusberg, H., and Lord, C. (2002). Cognitive profiles and social-communicative functioning in children with Autism Spectrum Disorder. *Journal of Child Psychology and Psychiatry* 43 (6): 807–821.

Kauschke, C., van der Beek, B., and Kamp-Becker, I. (2016). Narratives of girls and boys with Autism Spectrum Disorders: gender differences in narrative competence and internal state language. *Journal of Autism and Developmental Disorders* 46 (3): 840–852.

Kjellmer, L., Hedvall, Å., Fernell, E. et al. (2012). Language and communication skills in preschool children with Autism Spectrum Disorders: contribution of cognition, severity of autism symptoms, and adaptive functioning to the variability. *Research in Developmental Disabilities* 33 (1): 172–180.

Koegel, L.K., Bryan, K.M., Su, P.L. et al. (2020). Definitions of nonverbal and minimally verbal in research for autism: a systematic review of the literature. *Journal of Autism and Developmental Disorder* 50 (8): 2957–2972.

Korrel, H., Mueller, K.L., Silk, T. et al. (2017). Research Review: language problems in children with attention-deficit hyperactivity disorder – a systematic meta-analytic review. *Journal of Child Psychology and Psychiatry* 58 (6): 640–654.

Kover, S.T., Edmunds, S.R., and Ellis Weismer, S. (2016). Brief report: ages of language milestones as predictors of developmental trajectories in young children with Autism Spectrum Disorder. *Journal of Autism and Developmental Disorders* 46 (7): 2501–2507.

Kwok, E.Y., Brown, H., Smyth, R.E. et al. (2015). Meta-analysis of receptive and expressive language skills in Autism Spectrum Disorder. *Research in Autism Spectrum Disorders* 9: 202–222.

Lai, M.C., Lombardo, M.V., Chakrabarti, B. et al. (2013). Subgrouping the autism "spectrum": reflections on DSM-5. *PLoS Biology* 11 (4): 1–7.

Lockwood Estrin, G., Milner, V., Spain, D. et al. (2021). Barriers to Autism Spectrum Disorder diagnosis for young women and girls: a systematic review. *Review Journal of Autism and Developmental Disorders* 8 (4): 454–470.

Loomes, R., Hull, L., and Mandy, W.P.L. (2017). What is the male-to-female ratio in Autism Spectrum Disorder? A systematic review and meta-analysis. *Journal of the American Academy of Child & Adolescent Psychiatry* 56 (6): 466–474.

May, T., Brignell, A., Hawi, Z. et al. (2018). Trends in the overlap of Autism Spectrum Disorder and attention deficit hyperactivity disorder: prevalence, clinical management, language and genetics. *Current Developmental Disorders Reports* 5 (1): 49–57.

Munson, J., Dawson, G., Sterling, L. et al. (2008). Evidence for latent classes of IQ in young children with Autism Spectrum Disorder. *American Journal on Mental Retardation* 113 (6): 439–452.

Pickles, A., Wright, N., Bedford, R. et al. (2022). Predictors of language regression and its association with subsequent communication development in children with autism. *Journal of Child Psychology and Psychiatry* 63 (11): 1243–1251.

Sciberras, E., Mueller, K.L., Efron, D. et al. (2014). Language problems in children with ADHD: a community-based study. *Pediatrics* 133 (5): 793–800.

Silleresi, S. (2023). *Developmental Profiles in Autism Spectrum Disorder: Theoretical and Methodological Implications*. Amsterdam: John Benjamins.

Silleresi, S., Prévost, P., Zebib, R. et al. (2020). Identifying language and cognitive profiles in children with ASD via a cluster analysis exploration: implications for the new ICD-11. *Autism Research* 13 (7): 1155–1167.

Slušná, D., Rodríguez, A., Salvadó, B. et al. (2021). Relations between language, nonverbal cognition, and conceptualization in non or minimally verbal individuals with ASD across the lifespan. *Autism and Developmental Language Impairments* 6: 1–12.

Smith, N.V. and Tsimpli, I.M. (1995). *The Mind of a Savant: Language Learning and Modularity*. Hoboken, NJ: Blackwell Publishing.

Sturrock, A., Adams, C., and Freed, J. (2021). A subtle profile with a significant impact: language and communication difficulties for autistic females without intellectual disability. *Frontiers in Psychology* 12: 1–9.

Tager-Flusberg, H. and Kasari, C. (2013). Minimally verbal school-aged children with Autism Spectrum Disorder: the neglected end of the spectrum. *Autism Research* 6 (6): 468–478.

Tager-Flusberg, H., Rogers, S., Cooper, J. et al. (2009). Defining spoken language benchmarks and selecting measures of expressive language development for young children with Autism Spectrum Disorders. *Journal of Speech Language and Hearing Research* 52 (3): 643–652.

Thurm, A., Manwaring, S.S., Swineford, L. et al. (2015). Longitudinal study of symptom severity and language in minimally verbal children with autism. *Journal of Child Psychology and Psychiatry* 56 (1): 97–104.

Viscidi, E.W., Triche, E.W., Pescosolido, M.F. et al. (2013). Clinical characteristics of children with Autism Spectrum Disorder and co-occurring epilepsy. *PLoS One* 8 (7): 677–697.

Wodka, E.L., Mathy, P., and Kalb, L. (2013). Predictors of phrase and fluent speech in children with autism and severe language delay. *Pediatrics* 131 (4): 1128–1134.

Wolff, N., Stroth, S., Kamp-Becker, I. et al. (2022). Autism spectrum disorder and IQ – a complex interplay. *Frontiers in Psychiatry* 13: 856–884.

World Health Organization (WHO) (2022). *ICD-11: International Classification of Diseases* (11th revision). Available at https://icd.who.int/en/ (accessed 15 November 2023).

11

Language in Autism Compared to Language in Other NDDs

Alexandra Perovic and Kenneth Wexler

> **What Do You Think?**
> Sam, an 8-year-old boy with the diagnosis of autism, has joined a new school. Sam's teachers expected him to have difficulties in pragmatic language use; however, they were surprised to hear grammatical errors in his utterances, such as *Mary tickling me*; *Me go*. The special education teachers believed such errors are only heard in children with Developmental Language Disorder, or with Down Syndrome. Do you agree with them? What does this tell us about the nature of grammatical difficulties in autism compared to other Neurodevelopmental Disorders?

Introduction

A major question of interest is whether language difficulties experienced by many autistic individuals are unique, and characteristic of this condition only, or whether they are similar to those observed in other Neurodevelopmental Disorders (NDDs). The answer to this question is relevant for the provision of tailored support to people on the autism spectrum, but also for the development of all-encompassing models of human grammar (the term is used here in the broad sense to mean the human language capacity). The challenge lies in the heterogeneity of both linguistic and cognitive abilities in Autism Spectrum Disorder (ASD). Some individuals with ASD have intellectual disability, while some are highly educated. Some are minimally verbal, while others may have only subtle difficulties in the domain of pragmatics (see Chapters 6–8 and 10). Yet others may have grammatical difficulties reminiscent of those observed in other NDDs, which may manifest differently in different languages. To determine parallels and differences in the linguistic profile of autism condition, compared to other NDDs, it is necessary to go beyond the general descriptions of language

Language in Autism, First Edition. Edited by Jeannette Schaeffer et al.
© 2025 John Wiley & Sons Ltd. Published 2025 by John Wiley & Sons Ltd.

difficulties derived from assessments commonly used by clinicians. While useful, such assessments rarely provide information sophisticated enough to aid our quest for the linguistic ASD phenotype. We will show that linguistic theory is crucial in guiding our interpretation of language difficulties in (a)typical development across different languages. This chapter focuses on **grammar** (the term we shall use interchangeably with **morphosyntax**), addressing the following questions:

- How do general language abilities compare between ASD and other NDDs?
- How do grammatical abilities compare between ASD and other NDDs for tense marking on verbs?
- How do grammatical abilities compare between ASD and other NDDs for reference of pronouns and reflexives?

Anchoring

The DSM-5 (see Chapter 1) defines Neurodevelopmental Disorders (NDDs) as "a group of conditions with onset in the developmental period. The disorders typically manifest early in development, often before the child enters grade school, and are characterized by developmental deficits that produce impairments of personal, social, academic, or occupational functioning" (see Chapter 1). This term covers a diverse group of childhood-onset conditions: autism spectrum, ADHD, intellectual disability, communication disorders, specific learning disorders, and motor disorders. Despite high levels of overlap, this group is highly heterogeneous, both in terms of causes and clinical characteristics and outcomes.

While there are valid reasons to compare autism to a wide range of conditions that may overlap with autism in some domains (see DSM-5), here we focus on comparisons with Down Syndrome (DS), Williams Syndrome (WS), Fragile X Syndrome (FXS), and Developmental Language Disorder (DLD; also known as Specific Language Impairment, or SLI). These conditions have been chosen because their linguistic phenotypes (observable linguistic characteristics) may be relatively familiar to clinicians, linguists, and psychologists, although, as it will become clear from our review, there is a paucity of research in different linguistic (and cognitive) domains for each. Furthermore, comparisons of language abilities in autism and DS, WS, and FXS may shed more light on the role of genetic factors involved in the process of language acquisition, since for these NDDs the genetic basis is much better understood. Note that, as in autism, language delays and/or intellectual disability are present in many other NDDs; however, a pattern of strengths and weaknesses in both language and cognitive abilities is a characteristic of all the NDDs examined here. In autism, studies commonly distinguish between minimally verbal autistic individuals (those with little functional communication), individuals with language impairment (autism + language impairment: ALI), and individuals with typical language (autism + "normal" language: ALN).

Down Syndrome (DS) is one of the most common causes of intellectual disability, affecting one in 1000 people (Wu and Morris 2013). It is caused by a partial or full duplication of chromosome 21. Language skills, especially grammar, seem to be more affected than general cognitive and social skills.

Williams Syndrome (WS) is caused by a deletion of about 26–28 genes on the long arm of chromosome 7, affecting around one in 7500 people (Strømme, Bjørnstad, and Ramstad 2002). People with WS show an unusual pattern of strengths and weaknesses: grammar and especially vocabulary appear to be stronger, despite delays in the emergence of first words and utterances, and the presence of an intellectual disability (Mervis et al. 2000).

Fragile X Syndrome (FXS) is an inherited form of intellectual disability caused by the mutation of a single gene, FMR1, on the long arm of chromosome X (Protic et al. 2022). It affects approximately one in 7000 males and one in 11 000 females (Hunter et al. 2014), with more pronounced intellectual and language difficulties reported in males. FXS has attracted little

---

Acronym and Terminology Reminder

ALI: Autism with language impairment.
ALN: Autism with normal language.
Binding Theory (Principles): A module of grammar that regulates the distribution and interpretation of reflexive and personal pronouns.
Command, Domination: Linguistic concepts that describe the hierarchical relationship between words or phrases within a sentence.
DS: Down Syndrome – a genetic condition caused by a partial or full duplication of chromosome 21.
DLD: Developmental Language Disorder – language abilities below age expectations not attributable to any other condition.
Finiteness: Tense and agreement marking on the verb.
FXS: Fragile X Syndrome – an inherited form of intellectual disability caused by the mutation of a single gene, FMR1.
NDD: Neurodevelopmental Disorder – a group of conditions with onset early in the development, characterized by developmental deficits that produce impairments of personal, social, academic, or occupational functioning.
NVIQ: Nonverbal intelligence quotient.
Personal Pronouns: Words such as *I, me, you, she, they*.
OI: Optional Infinitive – a developmental stage where young children use infinitival (untensed/nonfinite) verbs instead of finite/tensed verbs.
Reference: Relationship between linguistic expressions (e.g. noun phrases, pronouns) and entities in the world. For example, *the bottle* refers to some particular bottle in the context, and *her* refers to some particular female person in the context.
Reflexive Pronouns: Words such as *herself, himself*.
TD: Typically Developing.
WS: Williams Syndrome – a genetic condition caused by a deletion of about 26–28 genes on the long arm of chromosome 7.
NVIQ: Nonverbal intelligence quotient.

attention from developmental linguists, despite grammatical difficulties observed in spontaneous speech and on standardized, norm-referenced language assessments (Hilvert and Sterling 2019).

Like autism and FXS, Developmental Language Disorder (DLD) is more common in boys than girls, although its genetic basis is less well understood than in FXS. Despite its high prevalence (approximately 7.5%, Tomblin et al. 1997), this condition remains relatively unknown outside the fields of linguistics, special education, and speech and language therapy. Developmental linguists have long been interested in DLD because it is a disorder specific to language; thus, existing linguistic theories of language difficulties in DLD are probably the most sophisticated compared to other NDDs. This population is frequently compared to autism, due to early claims that grammatical impairments in DLD and autism may be on a continuum (Bishop 2003) (see Chapter 3 for comparisons of domains not reported here).

An increased prevalence of autism has been reported in FXS, DS, and WS, compared to its prevalence in the general population. Comorbidity of ASD diagnoses in individuals with FXS is the most common, reported in over 70% of individuals, although rates depend on the diagnostic instruments used (Fielding-Gebhardt et al. 2021). For WS, 48% of individuals meet diagnostic criteria for ASD, although this number drops to 30% when only individuals with better language skills are included (Klein-Tasman, van der Fluit, and Mervis 2018). For DS, Kirchner and Walton (2021) report 22.4% of individuals screening positive on a parent report of autistic symptoms. Interestingly, the presence of autism has been argued to make language skills more vulnerable in at least some NDDs with secondary ASD diagnosis. This is observed in FXS (Sterling 2018; see our discussion on finiteness), as well as in DS. Hamner et al. (2020) report that on norm-referenced language and cognitive measures, children with DS+ASD perform worse than children with only DS or only ASD. The paucity of research in this field makes it difficult to establish precise effects of secondary autism diagnosis in NDDs (see Chapter 10).

Yet, few pairwise comparisons across conditions exist in the literature, even though the 2005 review by Rice and colleagues recognized that "the field is in need of research that systematically compares these disorders" (p. 7). Studies of language in NDDs have traditionally focused on vocabulary, phonology, and phonetics (Crystal 2013). Even when morphosyntax is investigated, spontaneous speech samples and standardized, norm-referenced assessments commonly used by clinicians are the measures of choice. While omnibus standardized tests used in clinical settings provide useful scores for general receptive (comprehension) or expressive language (production), these are often inadequate. The description of linguistic knowledge by linguists involves a theoretical understanding of a wide range of sophisticated linguistic processes, over a wide range of languages, which makes important predictions about which aspects of grammar may be affected in different languages (see Guasti 2017).

The phenomenon of tense marking (**finiteness**) is a good example. Hearing that a child omits -s from a third-person singular verb in English (uttering *Mary run* instead of *Mary runs*), a clinician might suspect that the problem has to do with the child's sound production, a problem with pronouncing the sound /s/. However, decades of research have established that there is a little problem with plural -s that attaches to nouns only (singular *toy* becomes plural *toys*). Clinical assessments often include both tense marking and plural on nouns, without differentiating the two in the final score obtained (see Chapter 1 for discussion of various language assessment tools).

Another example concerns the use of reflexive pronouns, for example, *herself*, *himself* (subsumed under the linguistic module of **binding**, to be discussed in more detail below), also rarely included in clinical assessments. We will see that some children with autism have a particularly difficult time with these linguistic expressions. Reflexives illustrate several properties of the semantic concept of **reference** (relationship between linguistic expressions, e.g. noun phrases, pronouns, and entities or concepts they represent in the world), an essential element in interpreting language, that is, in understanding (parts of) the semantics of language. It may be that autistic children have difficulty in interpretation, either limited to referential processes or more generally. A general language score does not tell us enough about what is going on.

This chapter focuses on two specific grammatical phenomena: finiteness and binding. These phenomena and the methodology used to investigate them, in autism and other NDDs, will be used as a test case for comparing grammatical acquisition in ASD and other NDDs. The acquisition of these two phenomena will furthermore illustrate how linguistic theory guides our research in NDDs. We refer the reader to Chapter 3, which provides more details of autistic children's difficulties in morphosyntax and includes comparisons with DLD for some constructions.

Difficulties with finiteness are probably one of the best-known issues among clinicians in the English-speaking world: close collaboration between linguists and clinicians has led to greatly improved methodology for assessing this part of grammar and to a number of intervention studies targeting these difficulties in a range of NDDs. The earliest well-documented, detailed phenomena observed in early morphosyntax are those found in the Optional Infinitive (OI) stage (Wexler 1994) where a young typically developing (TD) child uses infinitival (untensed/nonfinite) verbs instead of finite/tensed[1] verbs. For example, young French children often say (1), while the adult form is (2).

---

[1] We use the terms "finite" and "tensed" interchangeably: while the term "finite" is more appropriate, since it includes both tense and agreement on verbs, the term "tensed" may be more familiar to nonlinguistic audiences.

(1) Jean pas parler.
    John not speak
    'John isn't speaking.'

(2) Jean (ne) parle pas.
    John speaks not
    'John isn't speaking.'

The infinitive *parler* ('to speak') is formed by adding the special infinitive suffix *-er* to the verb stem *parl*. The present tense verb for third-person singular subjects is *parle*, pronounced *parl*. The infinitival verb is more phonologically complex than the present tense verb, containing two syllables rather than one – thus, simplicity of verb form does not account for a child's overuse of infinitives.

Despite omitting tense from their sentences, children know the properties of grammar, including the language-specific properties. From the youngest age, young children are able to form constituents, **merge**[2] them into larger constituents, and interpret them according to their structure. The young child also knows language-specific properties: for example, in French, the tensed verb (2) occurs before the negation *pas*, but if the verb is an infinitive (1), then the verb occurs after *pas*. Children do the same in close to 100% of their utterances. In another OI language, English, children use the nonfinite/stem verb such as *push* ("Sue push the box") instead of the tense form for third-person singular, *pushes* ("Sue pushes the box"). Crosslinguistic studies have amply confirmed these basic properties of the OI stage (see Guasti 2017).

Crucially, children in this developmental stage do not simply omit any suffix, only certain suffixes. For example, they do not omit *-ing* on a participle; they do not say *Sue is go*. They also understand tense: when the past tense is elicited, they either use the past tense or the OI, never the present tense. For example, in a past context, children say *Sue pushed* or *Sue push*, never *Sue pushes*. In a present context, they never say *Sue pushed*.

We refer the reader to a detailed explanation of a computational model of finiteness (Wexler 1998, 2011).[3] This model explains a wide range of morphosyntactic processes and data across languages in this age range. One example (among several others) is the phenomenon of null subjects, the fact that young

---

2 **Merge** is the operation of joining two elements to create a larger element.
3 The model is called the **unique checking constraint (UCC)**. In simplistic terms, it says that the child has trouble including two features in a computation so omits one of them, for example, omitting tense or agreement from a sentence, thus making it nonfinite. The model also predicts vast differences across languages, (e.g. Spanish and Italian will not show an OI stage and children will omit weak object pronouns – clitics – in French, Italian, and Catalan but not in Spanish or Greek) and across populations (only in some languages will children with SLI omit clitics, e.g. Italian but not Greek). (See Wexler 2011, 2014 for more details and Chapter 3 for a discussion of object clitics in autism.)

children display considerable subject omission in languages such as English or French, where this is not grammatical in the adult language, e.g. *want cookie* versus *I want cookie*.

Importantly, there is evidence that the requirement that all verbs are marked for tense is not "learned" (Wexler 2003). Finite verbs are more frequent in the input than untensed verbs; nevertheless, the youngest children often overwhelmingly use the infinitive. Numerous studies have shown that environment (e.g. socioeconomic status, as measured by maternal education) has a strong influence on vocabulary development but no influence on finiteness development. Behavioral genetic studies have confirmed the biological explanation of finiteness. For example, finiteness was the most heritable of the abilities studied in Bishop, Adams, and Norbury (2006).

The other linguistic module we will use to illustrate the importance of cross-syndrome comparisons is that of binding. Binding refers to the relations of reference between different words in a sentence (see Chomsky 1981, for the original theoretical definition). For example, a speaker who says *the dog* refers to some particular dog, mentioned previously, or obvious from the context. In contrast, reflexive pronouns such as *herself* do not have inherent reference. A name like *Sue* will refer to a person named Sue who is in the discourse context. But *herself* will have to get its reference from another phrase in the sentence. Thus, we cannot say (3) even if there is a woman in the context.

(3) *John likes herself.

Reflexives have a special grammatical property: they must be **bound** by another noun phrase that precedes them (their **antecedent**) and "pick up" their reference from this noun phrase that is in the correct grammatical position. We can say (4):

(4) Mary likes herself.

But we cannot say (5a) or (5b), even though the sentence contains a potential antecedent for the reflexive pronoun *herself*, namely *Mary* (as *Mary* is a single, feminine individual):

(5) a. *The husband of Mary likes herself.
     b. *Mary's husband likes herself.

The problem with (5a, b) results from the position of the potential antecedent for the reflexive, which must be in a particular structural relationship with the reflexive: it has to **command**[4] the reflexive. The subject *Mary* in (4) is

---

[4] The linguistic concepts "command" and "dominate" describe the hierarchical relationship between different words or phrases within a sentence. These are typically represented as syntactic trees. For technical definitions, please consult (online) resources recommended in Chapter 1.

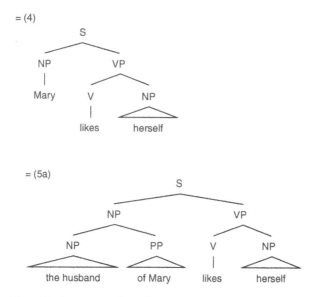

Figure 11.1 Hierarchical representations of sentences (4) and (5a). *Source:* Alexandra Perovic.

immediately dominated by the sentence since it constitutes the entire subject, and the sentence also dominates the reflexive (see Figure 11.1). This configuration gives rise to a grammatical sentence. In (5), in contrast, *Mary* is immediately dominated by another noun phrase (*the husband of Mary* in (5a), *Mary's husband* in (5b)). In other words, *Mary* does not constitute the entire subject; it is only part of the subject, and this subject does not dominate *herself*, rendering (5a, b) ungrammatical. The reflexive pronoun gets its reference from (is bound by) only the noun phrase that commands it.

Personal pronouns such as *her/him* are subject to a rather different principle: they must refer to (be bound to) the noun phrase in the pronoun's clause that commands the pronoun:

(6) **Mary** likes **her**.

The construction in (6) is fine if *her* refers to another person, mentioned previously, e.g. Sue. However, if *her* refers to Mary, the sentence is ungrammatical because *Mary* commands *her*.

We thus have two principles regulating the distribution of reflexive and personal pronouns that seem equally difficult and refer to the same concepts. However, in typical development, these principles seem to develop at different ages: children correctly interpret reflexives (such as *herself*) by age 4, possibly earlier, while their interpretation of personal pronouns (such as *her*) remains problematic even at the age of 6.

What causes this delay? Pronouns are heard in the input more frequently than reflexives and appear earlier in spontaneous speech, so this cannot be the reason for the delay. The most generally accepted answer (Wexler and Chien 1985; Chien and Wexler 1990 and much further literature) is that sentences like (6) use a **pragmatic** rule (a rule on the *use* of language) in addition to grammatical principles. This pragmatic rule prevents the pronoun from referring back to a specific noun phrase under certain conditions.

Binding is a topic that has been studied in great detail in theoretical linguistics, and some patterns of its acquisition are well-known in the field of typical language acquisition. However, the patterns of difficulties with binding in NDDs such as DS and, as we shall see, ALI, are less well known.

Language in Autism Compared to Language in Other NDDs

Comparison of language abilities in ASD versus DS, DLD, FXS, and WS may shed more light on the role of genetic factors in the process of the acquisition of grammar in idiopathic autism (autism not associated with a known genetic syndrome). Language delay is present in all NDDs discussed here; however, the end point achievement can be very different both between individuals with a given condition as well as between conditions (e.g. when comparing DS and WS, it is likely that individuals with WS will achieve a higher level of competence in grammar compared to DS). Furthermore, intellectual disability is present in all three NDDs with a clear genetic etiology (DS, FXS, and WS), but also in a significant proportion of autistic individuals (see Chapter 10 for discussion of cognitive and language profiles in autism).

Grammatical difficulties are present in DS, FXS, and WS, as well as in a large proportion of verbal people with autism, in ways that are not attributable to pragmatic factors. The clearest findings come from studies that specify the characteristics of their autistic participants in terms of the presence or absence of general language impairments: ALI and ALN (see Chapter 1).

However, the heterogeneity of linguistic and cognitive abilities in autism makes comparisons challenging, in addition to affecting the representativeness of samples. For example, it is difficult to find variables on which to match individuals with autism to individuals with DS: some autistic individuals have relatively intact grammar, while others experience grammatical difficulties comparable to those observed in DS. Likewise, some individuals will have a nonverbal IQ (NVIQ) in the average range, while others will fall within a severely impaired range (see Chapter 10). For this reason, studies comparing different NDDs may avoid matching altogether or include participants with too wide a range of abilities, which makes their results difficult to interpret.

This chapter focuses on studies that go beyond general language skills and omnibus scores, examining instead fine-grained patterns of linguistic functioning, illustrated here by the grammatical principles governing the distribution of reflexive and personal pronouns, or the omission of tense marking.

How Do Grammatical Abilities Compare Between ASD and Other NDDs for Production of Tense Marking on Verbs?

Based on the findings of a large body of literature on English, Dutch, French, and several other languages, it has been argued that omission of tense/finiteness is a clinical marker of language impairment. The OI stage (the period during which children regularly omit finiteness) in DLD is observed at a much older age compared to typical development: Rice and Wexler's spontaneous speech and elicited production studies showed that 5-year-old children with DLD had lower rates of finiteness marking than 3-year-old TD children. However, these same children also showed knowledge of the grammatical properties that TD children show; they did not omit the aspectual suffix -*ing* from a verb when it was required and rarely made agreement errors, e.g. using a third-person auxiliary instead of a first-person auxiliary (**I is laughing*). The DLD stage of OIs is referred to as the Extended Optional Infinitive Stage because finiteness rates are lower than in the OI stage in typical development, and it lasts longer (Rice and Wexler 1996).

Early studies typically examined verb inflection in children's spontaneous speech samples. While this is one of the most natural methods, it may not be the most efficient or accurate: a child may not produce a sufficient number of contexts of different types of verb inflections that would allow the researcher to determine with certainty whether finiteness has been successfully acquired. Moreover, contexts often are unclear about which verbal morpheme is required. Rice and Wexler used both methods.

The joint work of linguists and clinicians on finiteness in DLD led to the development of a now widely used diagnostic test in the English-speaking world, the Rice/Wexler Test of Early Grammatical Impairment (TEGI; see chapter 1; Rice and Wexler 2001). This test is an improvement on general, omnibus language tests of morphosyntax, as it focuses on relevant verb suffixes and distinguishes between regular (e.g. *play*, *watch*) and irregular (e.g. *write*, *see*) verbs, also allowing for an initial assessment of the child's ability to produce sounds required to mark finiteness in different phonological contexts.

Given the demonstrated grammatical difficulties in autism, the question arises as to whether there is a late OI stage in autism. Crucially, we should expect different patterns in ALI than in ALN: we should see an extended OI stage in ALI but not in ALN. We also expect ALN and ALI children to know the particular properties of their language's grammar that are relevant. Many predictions follow from this: ALI children should know the properties of word order associated with finiteness and nonfiniteness, as do TD and children with DLD.

Modyanova, Perovic, and Wexler (2017) is a large study with careful matching of ALI and ALN groups (ages 6–16) to TD control groups based on standardized tests. On the test of finiteness, TEGI, children in the ALI group (mean age: 10.6 years) scored significantly lower than all other groups tested, with only 57% correct. In contrast, the nonverbal mental age (MA)-matched TD group (mean age: 6) scored about 92%, which was similar to the result for the group with ALN (mean age: 9.5) and their own TD control group (mean age: 9.5) matched on nonverbal MA.

It is striking that in the ALI group, none of the eight measures of finiteness (e.g. past tense, simple present, the use of auxiliary verbs, and others) were significantly correlated with age, whereas in the ALN group, this was the case for all measures: this suggests that the ALI group has stalled in their finiteness performance. At the same time, the children in the ALI group knew other relevant properties of grammar that are consistent with the typical development: they did not omit the –*ing* from participial forms, they showed correct subject-verb agreement, they correctly used present tense in present-tense contexts and past tense in past-tense contexts, and they showed higher subject omission rates for untensed than tensed verbs, which is also predicted by the model of Wexler (1998). The most plausible explanation for these data is that ALI grammar is a genetically extremely delayed development of the OI stage, leaving open the question of whether older ALI children ever come close to adult performance.

While there are no studies directly comparing finiteness in autism and DLD, Roberts, Rice, and Tager-Flusberg (2004) and Modyanova, Perovic, and Wexler (2017) compared their participants' data on the TEGI task with those reported by Rice, Wexler, and Cleave (1995) for children with SLI/DLD. In Roberts, Rice, and Tager-Flusberg (2004), from 5- to 15-year-old autistic children were divided into three groups according to language skills: "normal," "borderline," and "impaired." Their "impaired" group, aged 8–9 years (which can be considered ALI), performed worse than children with DLD in the same age range for both third-person singular and regular past tense. The well-defined ALI group of Modyanova and colleagues (mean age: 10.6) showed a delay of about two years compared to Rice et al.'s DLD group.

This suggests that finiteness production is well mastered in DLD by age 8, whereas children with ALI show many errors even two years later. ALI is thus not simply autism + DLD; at the very least, the development is much slower in ALI than in DLD. In contrast, the children with ALN in Modyanova et al. (mean age: 9.5) performed similarly to both the younger 6-year-old TD controls and their 9-year-old age control group. This suggests that the ALN children are only slightly behind their TD peers.

In a study that directly compared finiteness in ASD and FXS, where participants with FXS had an additional ASD diagnosis (Sterling 2018), different patterns between the conditions were observed. Adolescents with FXS+ASD scored only 50% on the past tense probe, compared to 79% for ASD. Both groups found the present tense probe easier: FXS+ASD achieved 86% correct, and the ASD group 95% correct. While it appears that the FXS+ASD diagnosis has a more detrimental effect on grammar than the ASD diagnosis alone, the heterogeneity of ability between the two groups makes it difficult to draw definitive conclusions. The groups were matched on ASD symptom severity and were similar on a measure of expressive language, but significantly different in NVIQ, with the FXS+ASD group scoring almost at floor. No information is reported on the overall grammatical ability of the two groups, though the ASD group possibly contained a proportion of participants with ALN: this group had significantly higher scores on both vocabulary comprehension and production than the FXS+ASD group. The findings suggest that children with FSX+ASD appear linguistically similar to children with ALI, though further research is needed.

There are no direct comparisons of finiteness between autism and DS. However, finiteness seems to be particularly vulnerable in DS, probably even more so than in ALI. In a recent study with a larger than average number of participants, 52 children with DS aged 7-11 years scored at the minimum level on TEGI past tense and simple present probes (Baxter et al. 2022). Adolescents with DS aged 10-19 years (Laws and Bishop 2003) also showed low performance on the TEGI, not unlike the much younger children with DLD (from 4- to 7-year-olds).

There are likewise no studies comparing finiteness in autism and WS, though few finiteness difficulties have been reported in WS (Clahsen and Almazan 1998). We would therefore not expect a difference between ALN and WS, but children with WS may well do better than children with ALI (below we will discuss some revealing results from a comparison of WS with ALI and ALN on another part of grammar, pronoun reference).

The data presented above suggest considerable difficulty in mastering finiteness in ALI, DS, and possibly FXS+ASD, but not ALN. ALI shows lower scores and a longer developmental delay than DLD. It seems possible that mastering finiteness in DS is more problematic than ALI. There is a need for more comprehensive cross-syndrome and crosslinguistic research (including languages like Italian, predicted to not show finiteness effects) with carefully defined samples (especially ALN vs. ALI) before we conclude that our generalizations are correct and the search for detailed biological exploration can seriously proceed.[5]

---

[5] See Wexler (2003) for examples of how this was done in a comparison of children with DLD and with typical development.

However, it is equally important to establish what is not missing in these children's grammar. The most fundamental process of grammar, the joining of two elements to create a larger element (operation Merge), does not seem to be missing. In the studies reviewed in this chapter (and generally in the literature), all the children seem to have Merge. For example, a very young child's *Mommy go* is interpreted as something like *Mommy is going*, rather than just some string of words with no relation to one another. Just like young TD children, children with autism, DS, or FXS are able to form constituents, merge them into larger constituents, and interpret them according to their structure; there is no evidence that verbal children in the populations studied here are any different in this respect.

How Do Grammatical Abilities Compare Between ASD and Other NDDs for Understanding the Reference of Pronouns and Reflexives?

What should we expect about the knowledge of principles that guide the binding conditions, the conditions that regulate the reference of personal pronouns and reflexive pronouns, in autism? One of the most widely studied characteristics of autistic children is that they have more difficulties with the pragmatic use of language (see Chapter 6), how to use language in context, than TD children.

Given this view, we would expect that autistic children would have more difficulties in understanding personal pronouns, whose interpretation depends on particular pragmatic factors that take a longer time to resolve in TD children than in understanding reflexive pronouns, whose interpretations rely on pure grammatical principles. The reasonable expectation turns out to be wrong. In Perovic, Modyanova, and Wexler (2013a), English-speaking autistic children had considerable difficulties interpreting reflexives, but not so much pronouns, while Terzi et al. (2014) report little difficulty with reflexives in Greek-speaking autistic participants. The inconclusive pattern in the two studies could be explained by the lack of differentiation between participants with ALI and ALN in their samples. It seems that most participants in the study by Perovic and colleagues were children with ALI. In Terzi et al. (2014), most participants seemed to be ALN, though three participants who could be classified as ALI were excluded from the original counts. Intriguingly, the authors write that these three participants demonstrated poor knowledge of reflexives, just like the English-speaking children with ALI, suggesting an ALI/ALN reflexive grammar difference.

While there are no direct comparisons of binding in autism with DS, DLD, or FXS, there is one study that compared the knowledge of binding in children with ALI, ALN, and WS. This study improves on the studies of Perovic and colleagues and Terzi and colleagues as it distinguishes between ALI and ALN populations, crucial for delineating the precise linguistic phenotype in the autistic population, known for its heterogeneity of language and cognitive abilities.

Focus on a Specific Study

The study reported in Perovic, Modyanova, and Wexler (2013b) (PMW) provides an illustration of how a careful comparison of NDDs on a particular piece of grammar is carried out, though results need to be replicated. This study investigates both grammar and pragmatics: the interpretation of personal and reflexive pronouns. It controls for the heterogeneity of language abilities in autism, dividing participants into ALI and ALN, and includes a comparison to WS. While sharing atypicalities at genetic, neural, and behavioral levels (Vivanti, Hamner, and Lee 2018), autism and WS both present with socio-communicative difficulties, though these involve opposing social phenotypes: hyposociability in autism versus hypersociability in WS (Klein-Tasman, van der Fluit, and Mervis 2018).

PMW's participants included 26 ALI and 22 ALN children, selected based on scores on standardized tests of receptive and expressive language. The ALI group was matched to the WS group on nonverbal MA, while all three experimental groups, ALI, ALN, and WS, were matched on age (range: 6–16, mean around 11). Recall that six is the approximate age at which TD children have mastered both binding principles, the principle governing personal pronouns, and that governing reflexive pronouns. The WS group performed better on normed tests of vocabulary and grammar than the ALI group but not as well as the ALN group.[6]

Two control groups of TD children were included. The ALI-TD control group was selected by finding a TD match on gender and nonverbal MA for each of the children in the ALI group: the ALI group had a mean age of nearly 12 years, while their TD mental age matches had a mean age of 6. The same matching procedure was followed for the ALN-TD control group, but here the ALN group and their matched ALN-TD group were also similar in age. The experimental setup thus controlled for gender and general (nonverbal) reasoning and then measured behavior on one specific aspect of grammar, binding principles. If one group of autistic children and their matched TD controls showed poorer grammatical performance, this would suggest that the difference is due to a specific language delay rather than differences in general intelligence (or gender). The experiment used four types of stimuli (see Wexler and Chien 1985):

(7) Name-Reflexive: *Lisa's mom is pointing to herself.*

(8) Name-Pronoun: *Bart's dad is washing him.*

---

6 Note that groups were not matched on any language measure: while ALI and WS groups were matched on nonverbal MA, to control for the influence of general nonverbal skills, the lower scores of the ALI group on both vocabulary and grammar prevented their matching to the WS group in these domains. Since the focus of the study was grammar, rather than general cognitive skills, it would have been desirable to match participants on grammar too.

(9) Control-Name: *Lisa is touching Mom.*

(10) Control-Possessive: *Bart's dad is petting a dog.*

While the sentences in (7) and (8) involve the actual pronouns and reflexives, the sentences in (9) and (10) do not. The purpose of (9) is to establish whether the child understands the basic sentence pattern, with a proper name instead of a pronoun or a reflexive, and (10) tests the knowledge of the possessive noun phrase, again with no pronoun or reflexive.

In this two-choice picture task, children heard a sentence and saw two pictures, and were asked to select the picture that the sentence described. For (7) and (8), the child always had a choice of two noun phrases in the sentence for the coreferent. Here the incorrect picture always entailed an action performed on the wrong character. Understanding the picture would demand knowing the rules for the interpretation of reflexives, or pronouns, respectively. In (7), for example, the correct picture showed Lisa's mom pointing to herself, the mom. The incorrect picture shows Lisa's mom pointing to Lisa.

Table 11.1 presents data on the four participant groups. On the two control conditions, Control Name and Control Possessive, which did not involve either pronouns or reflexives, groups with no language impairment performed at ceiling: the two TD groups and ALN. Even the WS group, known to have some language difficulties, performed well. These children know the grammatical facts that are necessary to understand these sentences with ordinary noun phrases. The ALI children performed somewhat worse but still know a good deal of grammar.

A different situation was observed with the Name-Reflexive sentences. The ALN group and two control groups showed an almost ceiling performance.

Table 11.1 Estimated mean probabilities correct (standard error) per condition and participant group.

	ALI	TD controls for ALI	ALN	TD controls for ALN	WS
Control Name	0.79 (0.04)	0.98 (0.01)	0.98 (0.02)	0.98 (0.01)	0.94 (0.02)
Control Possessive	0.77 (0.04)	0.96 (0.02)	0.99 (0.01)	0.98 (0.01)	0.93 (0.02)
Name-Reflexive	0.49 (0.05)	0.93 (0.03)	0.96 (0.02)	0.97 (0.02)	0.88 (0.03)
Name-Pronoun	0.71 (0.05)	0.73 (0.05)	0.83 (0.04)	0.78 (0.05)	0.75 (0.05)

Source: Adapted from Perovic, Modyanova, and Wexler (2013b) (table 2).

The WS group performed slightly worse but not statistically significantly different from the TD controls and ALN. However, the estimated mean probability for the ALI group was only 0.49, indicating severe difficulties in understanding how the reflexive affects meaning. Since the ALI participants performed much better on the control condition that contains an ordinary noun phrase instead of a reflexive, the natural conclusion is that the grammatical constraint governing reflexives remains unknown to them. The ALI group exhibited a considerably greater lack of knowledge compared to ALN and WS.

On the Name-Pronoun condition, the estimated mean probabilities correct ranged from 0.71 to 0.83, with no statistically significant difference between the groups, including the autism groups, despite the fact that this condition has an essential pragmatic component. What is striking is how all these groups, with hugely different grammatical abilities (as in the Name-Reflexive results), were all distinctly less than perfect on the principle guiding the interpretation of pronouns and not much different from each other. This result mirrors in many ways the fact that the Name-Pronoun condition showed at best very little development in the age range of 2;6–6.0 in the original experiment with TD children.

We have seen that only the ALI children displayed an absence of knowledge of the piece of grammar that regulates the interpretation of the reflexive. In particular, the WS group patterned more closely to the TD group than to the ALI group. Despite the presence of intellectual disability in WS, as evidenced by their nonverbal reasoning test scores comparable to those of the ALI group, this result cannot be explained by nonverbal reasoning skills. The extreme lack of knowledge of the grammar of reflexives in ALI is in stark contrast to both TD children and those with WS or ALN, as this study demonstrated by using carefully matched groups. Consequently, neither intellectual functioning nor autism itself can account for this impairment. It appears to be a grammatical loss, likely attributable to genetic factors in ALI. However, given the current lack of understanding regarding the genetics of autism and the genetics of language, these factors remain poorly understood.

Two other groups that appear to be similar to ALI on their scores for comprehension of reflexives are very young TD children, aged about two-and-a-half (Wexler and Chien 1985), and individuals with DS (Perovic 2006, 2008). Perovic replicated the Wexler and Chien experiment with English-speaking and Serbo-Croatian-speaking adults with DS, revealing their lack of knowledge of the constraints governing the interpretation of reflexives. This finding was further confirmed for Greek-speaking adults with DS (Sanoudaki and Varlokosta 2014).

In sum, by age 11, grammatical knowledge of reflexives develops in TD, ALN, and WS but not in ALI. Whether it will develop later is unknown.

We have described a carefully designed study that highlights a significant, likely genetically determined, impairment of one part of grammar among ALI children.

Conclusion

This chapter attempted to answer the following questions:

- How do general language abilities compare between ASD and other NDDs?
- How do grammatical abilities compare between ASD and other NDDs for tense marking on verbs?
- How do grammatical abilities compare between ASD and other NDDs for reference of pronouns and reflexives?

We showed that to get a clearer picture of the parallels and differences in linguistic profiles in autism compared to other NDDs, it is crucial to control for heterogeneity in linguistic ability across research participants. The grammar of children with ALN seems close to typical development and better than that of various other NDDs. In contrast, aspects of grammar of children with ALI are severely impaired, in some cases, more so than in WS and DLD, and seem close to the language skills of children with DS (see Chapter 3 for discussion of various morphosyntactic constructions). As such, ALI does not seem to simply be a comorbidity of Autism + DLD.

Cross-syndrome comparisons help us understand how language development takes place, allowing us to unravel the role of different factors affecting language learning in a way that is not dissimilar to "natural experiments." However, our review revealed that there are very few experimental studies comparing grammar in autism and other NDDs, especially ones that take into account the heterogeneity of abilities in autistic children. We hope that this will be rectified in future research. Furthermore, we have shown that crosslinguistic research is essential because it is an important aid in testing theoretical models and necessary for clinical purposes.

What Do You Know Now?
The grammatical abilities of autistic children with language impairment (ALI) often resemble those found in Down Syndrome, in some cases more so than those found in Williams Syndrome or even DLD.
- Going back to our example in the "What Do You Think?" section at the beginning of this chapter, *Mary tickle me*, we now know that omission of tense (*tickle* here, instead of *tickled*) is common in some children with autism as well as children with DLD and DS, and even WS. However, within the autism spectrum, only children with grammatical impairment, the ALI group, will show difficulties with tense, but not those without grammatical impairment, ALN.

(Continued)

(Continued)

> - Our discussion of binding in autism and WS confirms that grammar in some children with autism (ALI) can be compromised independently of pragmatic impairments commonly associated with autism. It can be impaired independently of language delays and intellectual disability, both common to many NDDs.

Suggestions for Further Reading

For an introductory textbook on language acquisition guided by linguistic theory, we recommend Guasti 2017. For a general comparison of language in some NDDs please see Hilvert and Sterling 2019 and Rice, Warren, and Betz 2005. For an introduction to the Optional Infinitive stage, see Wexler 2003, 2011.

References

Baxter, R., Rees, R., Perovic, A. et al. (2022). The nature and causes of children's grammatical difficulties: evidence from an intervention to improve past tense marking in children with Down Syndrome. *Developmental Science* 25 (4): e13220.

Bishop, D.V.M. (2003). Autism and Specific Language Impairment: categorical distinction or continuum? In: *Autism: Neural Basis and Treatment Possibilities* (eds. G. Bock and J. Goode), 213–234. Novartis Foundation Symposium 251. Chichester, UK: Wiley.

Bishop, D.V.M., Adams, C.V., and Norbury, C.F. (2006). Distinct genetic influences on grammar and phonological Short-Term Memory deficits: evidence from 6-year-old twins. *Genes, Brain and Behaviour* 5: 158–169.

Chien, Y.C. and Wexler, K. (1990). Children's knowledge of locality conditions in binding as evidence for the modularity of syntax and pragmatics. *Language Acquisition* 1: 225–295.

Chomsky, N. (1981). *Lectures on Government and Binding*. Dordrecht: Foris.

Clahsen, H. and Almazan, M. (1998). Syntax and morphology in Williams Syndrome. *Cognition* 68 (3): 167–198.

Crystal, D. (2013). Clinical linguistics: conversational reflections. *Clinical Linguistics & Phonetics* 27 (4): 236–243.

Fielding-Gebhardt, H., Bredin-Oja, S.L., Warren, S.F. et al. (2021). Rethinking measurement standards of autism symptomology in adolescents with Fragile X Syndrome. *Journal of Autism and Developmental Disorders* 51: 4520–4533.

Guasti, M.T. (2017). *Language Acquisition, Second Edition: The Growth of Grammar*. Cambridge, MA: MIT Press.

Hamner, T., Hepburn, S., Zhang, F. et al. (2020). Cognitive profiles and autism symptoms in comorbid Down Syndrome and Autism Spectrum Disorder. *Journal of Developmental and Behavioral Pediatrics* 41 (3): 172–179.

Hilvert, E. and Sterling, A. (2019). Vocabulary and grammar development in children with Autism Spectrum Disorder, Fragile X Syndrome, and Down Syndrome. In: *International Review of Research in Developmental Disabilities* (eds. R.M. Hodapp and D.J. Fidler), 57: 119–169. Cambridge, MA: Academic Press.

Hunter J., Rivero-Arias O., Angelov A. et al. (2014). Epidemiology of Fragile X Syndrome: a systematic review and meta-analysis. *American Journal of Medical Genetics Part A* 164A (7): 1648–1658.

Kirchner, R.M. and Walton, K.M. (2021). Symptoms of Autism Spectrum Disorder in children with Down Syndrome and Williams Syndrome. *American Journal on Intellectual and Developmental Disabilities* 126 (1): 58–74.

Klein-Tasman, B.P., van der Fluit, F., and Mervis, C.B. (2018). Autism spectrum symptomatology in children with Williams Syndrome who have phrase speech or fluent language. *Journal of Autism and Developmental Disorders* 48 (9): 3037–3050.

Laws, G. and Bishop, D.V.M. (2003). A comparison of language abilities in adolescents with Down Syndrome and children with Specific Language Impairment. *Journal of Speech, Language and Hearing Research* 46: 1324–1339.

Mervis, C.B., Robinson, B.F., Bertrand, J. et al. (2000). The Williams Syndrome cognitive profile. *Brain and Cognition* 44 (3): 604–628.

Modyanova, N., Perovic, A., and Wexler, K. (2017). Grammar is differentially impaired in subgroups of Autism Spectrum Disorders: evidence from an investigation of tense marking and morphosyntax. *Frontiers in Psychology* 8: 320.

Perovic, A. (2006). Syntactic deficit in Down Syndrome: more evidence for the modular organization of language. *Lingua* 116 (10): 1616–1630.

Perovic, A. (2008). A crosslinguistic analysis of binding in Down Syndrome. In: *First Language Acquisition of Morphology and Syntax: Perspectives Across Languages and Learners* (eds. P. Guijarro Fuentes, M.P. Larrañaga, and J. Clibbens), 235–267. Amsterdam: John Benjamins.

Perovic, A., Modyanova, N., and Wexler, K. (2013a). Comprehension of reflexive and personal pronouns in children with autism: a syntactic or pragmatic deficit? *Applied Psycholinguistics* 34 (4): 813–835.

Perovic, A., Modyanova, N., and Wexler, K. (2013b). Comparison of grammar in Neurodevelopmental Disorders: the case of Binding in Williams Syndrome and autism with and without language impairment. *Language Acquisition* 20 (2): 133–154.

Protic, D.D., Aishworiya, R., Salcedo-Arellano, M.J. et al. (2022). Fragile X Syndrome: from molecular aspect to clinical treatment. *International Journal of Molecular Sciences* 23 (4): 1935.

Rice, M.L. and Wexler, K. (1996). Toward tense as a clinical marker of Specific Language Impairment in English-speaking children. *Journal of Speech and Hearing Research* 39 (6): 1239–1257.

Rice, M.L. and Wexler, K. (2001). *Rice/Wexler Test of Early Grammatical Impairment*. San Antonio: The Psychological Corporation.

Rice, M.L., Warren, S.F., and Betz, S.K. (2005). Language symptoms of Developmental Language Disorders: an overview of autism, Down Syndrome, Fragile X, Specific Language Impairment, and Williams Syndrome. *Applied Psycholinguistics* 26 (1): 7–27.

Rice, M.L., Wexler, K., and Cleave, P.L. (1995). Specific Language Impairment as a period of extended optional infinitive. *Journal of Speech and Hearing Research* 38: 850–863.

Roberts, J.A., Rice, M., and Tager-Flusberg, H. (2004). Tense marking in children with autism. *Applied Psycholinguistics* 25 (3): 429–448.

Sanoudaki, E. and Varlokosta, S. (2014). Pronoun comprehension in individuals with Down Syndrome: deviance or delay? *Journal of Speech, Language, and Hearing Research* 57 (4): 1442–1452.

Sterling, A. (2018). Grammar in boys with idiopathic Autism Spectrum Disorder and boys with Fragile X Syndrome plus Autism Spectrum Disorder. *Journal of Speech, Language, and Hearing Research* 61 (4): 1–13.

Strømme, P., Bjørnstad, P.G., and Ramstad, K. (2002). Prevalence estimation of Williams Syndrome. *Journal of Child Neurology* 17 (4): 269–271.

Terzi, A., Marinis, T., Kotsopoulou, A. et al. (2014). Grammatical abilities of Greek-speaking children with autism. *Language Acquisition* 21 (1): 4–44.

Tomblin, J.B., Records, N.L., Buckwalter, P. et al. (1997). Prevalence of Specific Language Impairment in kindergarten children. *Journal of Speech, Language, and Hearing Research* 40 (6): 1245–1260.

Vivanti, G., Hamner, T., and Lee, N.R. (2018). Neurodevelopmental Disorders affecting sociability: recent research advances and future directions in Autism Spectrum Disorder and Williams Syndrome. *Current Neurology and Neuroscience Reports* 18 (12): 94.

Wexler, K. (1994). Optional infinitives, head movement and the economy of derivations. In: *Verb Movement* (eds. D. Lightfoot and N. Hornstein), 305–350. Cambridge, UK: Cambridge University Press.

Wexler, K. (1998). Very early parameter setting and the unique checking constraint: a new explanation of the optional infinitive stage. *Lingua* 106 (1–4): 23–79.

Wexler, K. (2003). Lenneberg's dream: learning, normal language development and Specific Language Impairment. In: *Language Competence Across Populations: Toward a Definition of Specific Language Impairment* (eds. Y. Levy and J. Schaeffer), 11–62. Mahwah, NJ: Erlbaum.

Wexler, K. (2011). Grammatical computation in the optional infinitive stage. In: *Handbook of Generative Approaches to Language Acquisition* (eds. J. de Villiers and T. Roeper), 53–118. New York: Springer.

Wexler, K. (2014). The unique checking constraint as the explanation of clitic omission in normal and SLI development. In: *Developments in the Acquisition of Clitics* (eds. T. Neokleous and K. Grohmann), 288–344. Cambridge Scholars Publishing.

Wexler, K. and Chien, Y. (1985). The development of lexical anaphors and pronouns. In: *Papers and Reports on Child Language Development (PRCLD)*, 138–149. Stanford University.

Wu, J. and Morris, J. (2013). The population prevalence of Down's syndrome in England and Wales in 2011. *European Journal of Human Genetics* 21: 1016–1019.

12

Language in Autistic Adults

Marta Manenti and Philippe Prévost

> **What Do You Think?**
> You are invited with your cousin to a lecture entitled "Do language skills improve in autism from childhood to adulthood?" Your cousin thinks it is obvious that linguistic abilities improve over time. Do you agree with him?
> A friend of yours told you about her internship experience at an education center for autistic children. She noticed that some of them produce and understand language better than others and wonders whether this may portend what their life will be when they grow up. What do you think?
> In a health science class, the professor is explaining how **cognitive decline** affects language in typical and atypical aging. Among the conditions involving the atypical influence of aging on language, the professor mentions autism. One of your colleagues is very surprised and asks why. What would you answer?

Introduction

The understanding of autism has undergone significant change over time. One of the major changes concerns the acknowledgment of the lifelong persistence of this disorder. Due to historical and epidemiological reasons, autism research and clinical practice have long been oriented toward children, but interest in autistic adults has been increasing over time. Studies on language abilities in autism over the lifespan have sought to determine whether the language difficulties that have been identified in children, in particular language impairment, persist into adulthood. Given that autistic children are very diverse in terms of their (linguistic and nonlinguistic) cognitive profiles, studies have also tried to map their different developmental pathways across the life course. Further important questions concern the role of autism severity on the development of language abilities and the pattern of cognitive aging in autism. According to some scholars, the latter

---

Language in Autism, First Edition. Edited by Jeannette Schaeffer et al.
© 2025 John Wiley & Sons Ltd. Published 2025 by John Wiley & Sons Ltd.

could diverge from the pattern observed in the general population. Although current evidence on adult and older age outcomes in autism, including language skills, remains limited, this chapter aims to discuss what is known to date about language development in adulthood and aging adults by providing answers to the following questions:

- What is the pattern of change in the language of autistic individuals from childhood to adulthood?
- What are the language abilities of autistic adults across the spectrum?
- What are the predictive factors of adult outcomes in autism?
- How does aging impact on language functioning in autism?

Anchoring

Autism is a lifelong disorder, and, although a minority of individuals move off the spectrum, continuity in autism diagnosis from childhood to adulthood has been consistently reported. In parallel, despite many autistic individuals (especially those with lower intellectual abilities) remaining significantly impaired and dependent on the assistance of others for daily living, the severity of autistic symptoms appears to decrease with time. However, research on how autistic characteristics are perceived by autistic individuals has highlighted a peak in self-reported autism characteristics among middle-aged adults (39–59 years), suggesting that some of these characteristics may be more heavily experienced during middle adulthood rather than younger adulthood (19–39 years).

There is evidence for an increasing number of individuals (sometimes referred to as "the lost generation") seeking and receiving a diagnosis of autism later in life (Lai and Baron-Cohen 2015). If autism (as well as all other Neurodevelopmental Disorders) can be diagnosed only in individuals who presented symptoms in the early developmental

> **Acronym and Terminology Reminder**
> **Cognitive Decline:** Gradual loss of some skills, whether verbal or nonverbal (e.g. problem-solving, memory, perception...), due to advancing age.
> **Cross-sectional:** Study of a population sample at a single time-point.
> **DID:** Disorder of Intellectual Development.
> **Expressive Language:** Using language to label objects and actions, to put words together in sentences to express thoughts and desires (requests, answers, descriptions).
> **IQ:** Intelligence Quotient.
> **Lexicon:** Knowledge about words – their pronunciation, meaning, grammatical properties, and how they are connected to each other.
> **Morphosyntax:** Word and sentence structure, i.e. the way words and phrases combine.
> **Pragmatics:** Language use in context (including conversations).
> **Receptive Language:** Ability to understand language.
> **Verbal Fluency:** Ability to produce as many words as possible based on a specific rule in a limited timeframe.

period, why did these people not come to clinical attention sooner? The reasons may be manifold: a weak degree of impairment (e.g. in individuals with average/above-average cognitive abilities requiring medium to low levels of support) considered until a few decades ago as evidence that a diagnosis was not warranted (as explained below), the effects of perceived social stigma, which can lead parents to resist seeking a diagnosis for their children and autistic individuals to develop coping strategies, or autistic symptoms that only become manifest at a time when the individual's capacities are no longer sufficient to meet increasingly complex social demands, as explicitly stated in the last version of the DSM (i.e. DSM-5-TR). Regarding females specifically, there is flourishing evidence showing that autism is largely overlooked, misdiagnosed, or identified late (see Chapter 10).

In addition, the increased awareness of autism in adults among the general population and mental health professionals has largely contributed to the rise in the number of diagnoses. According to some scholars, broader societal factors might also be at play, such as pressure on clinicians for an autism diagnosis for reasons of access to services.

Gaining a better understanding of the linguistic abilities of this growing population has important clinical implications in terms of diagnosis, prognosis, and post-diagnostic support. This concerns, among other things, obtaining information on the nature of language impairment in autistic adults with respect, for instance, to the presence of potential discrepancies in receptive-**expressive language** and how language skills and nonlanguage cognitive abilities interact in this population. This is also relevant for the characterization of the subcategories proposed by the last version of the International Classification of Diseases (ICD-11) to account for the variability of cognitive profiles in autism (see Chapter 10). Research on language in autistic adults, including older individuals, might also inform on how atypical aging differs from typical aging in terms of cognitive decline.

Despite great heterogeneity across individuals, a general slowing/decline in a variety of cognitive functions, notably processing speed and Working Memory, and cognitive plasticity, accompanies healthy aging. With respect to language, different domains seem to be affected differently by aging. For instance, the size of the mental **lexicon** (our knowledge about words) remains preserved or keeps on growing. In contrast, older adults are slower than younger adults in recognizing and retrieving words from their lexicon, probably due to overall slowed processing and deficits in Executive Functions (e.g. inhibition, switching, and planning). Likewise, reduced comprehension of syntactically complex sentences (e.g. syntactic structures like relative clauses, see Chapter 3), has been reported, which is likely to stem from more general changes in cognitive abilities (e.g. Working Memory). Age effects have also been explored on tasks tapping **verbal fluency**, in which participants are asked to provide responses that either start with a specific letter (e.g. B, F, and L; phonemic/phonetic fluency) or fit into a specific semantic category (e.g. animal; semantic/category fluency) in a limited timeframe. Some studies found a negative effect of age on verbal fluency in general (Barnes et al. 2003).

This chapter discusses the literature on language in autistic adults in light of some methodological concerns (e.g. sample representativity, challenges of language evaluation) that need to be addressed in order to assess the knowledge that has been acquired so far on the linguistic abilities of these individuals.

Language in Autistic Adults

What Is the Pattern of Change in the Language of Autistic Individuals from Childhood to Adulthood?

The language abilities of autistic individuals have been investigated via **cross-sectional** (i.e. inter-group comparisons at a single time-point, including groups of different ages) and longitudinal (i.e. intra-group comparisons over time) studies. This section focuses on studies using a longitudinal approach, including studies that are retrospective (where information about the past of the individuals being sampled is collected and used). We summarize results from these studies, describing the language trajectories of autistic individuals, namely the progression of their linguistic skills over time.

In keeping with decreasing autistic symptoms (see the "Anchoring section"), overall improvement in linguistic skills from childhood to adulthood (i.e. catch-up) represents a robust finding within autism research, despite considerable interindividual variability (Magiati, Tay, and Howlin 2014). For instance, Pickles, Anderson, and Lord (2014) explored the development of expressive and **receptive language** in 192 children referred early for possible autism and assessed on six occasions between ages 2 and 19 via the Vineland Adaptive Behavior Scales (VABS; a standardized, semi-structured, parent interview designed to assess adaptive functioning). The authors observed that, despite overall improvement, trajectories were characterized by great variation. This is illustrated in Figure 12.1, showing that the linguistic development of individuals referred early for autism, while globally remaining under normative expectations, follows slightly different trajectories for individuals belonging to different subgroups.[1]

A qualitative difference in language development has been observed between early life (i.e. before age 6) and later stages of development (i.e. from middle

---

[1] Pickles and colleagues did not discuss whether the individuals displaying (varying degrees of) language delay could be considered to be linguistically impaired.

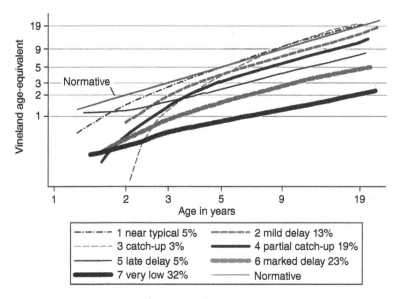

Figure 12.1 Change of overall language age-equivalents from childhood to young adulthood for autistic participants divided into seven subgroups based on developmental patterns. *Source:* Pickles et al. (2014). Reproduced with permission of Wiley Blackwell.

childhood to adolescence). Early life is characterized by greater variability, while later development presents much flatter curves. One possible explanation for this discrepancy in development is that language skills expected to develop during adolescence are particularly difficult for autistic individuals to acquire (Sigman and McGovern 2005). Adolescence is in fact a time of drastic changes at several levels (physical, cognitive, and emotional), with new challenges to be addressed (such as acquiring independence) and more complex social environments to navigate. Finally, evidence for stability or worsening in language abilities has also been provided, in particular for individuals with low Intelligence Quotient (**IQ**) levels (see Chapter 10).

What Are the Language Abilities of Autistic Adults Across the Spectrum?

Despite a growing body of research, language outcomes in autism remain to date poorly understood. It is consistently agreed upon that great heterogeneity exists in adulthood as well as in childhood, with language abilities ranging from very good to very poor (Baghdadli et al. 2018). A recent study on conversational language in autistic adults reported wide variation across participants on several measures, including the total number of utterances and of different words produced. Some adults produced fewer than 10 utterances, versus 50 or more for others, and the number of different words ranged from 1 to 306, illustrating interindividual differences in talkativeness (the total number of utterances produced in a given time period) and vocabulary skills (Friedman et al. 2019).

It should be pointed out that, in general, the older the studies, the poorer the reported outcomes. The cohorts, including participants diagnosed several decades ago, are in fact not representative of individuals diagnosed with autism today, in terms of profiles and access to intervention. In the 1980s, the concept of autism was narrower than it is today. Regarding language, the diagnostic criteria for what was named "infantile autism" included gross deficits in language development (DSM-III). Individuals who spoke well and did not have Disorder of Intellectual Development (**DID**) did not come to clinical attention at the time.[2] Therefore, they did not take part in research, which may explain the poor outcomes of those who did participate in research. The transition from the third to the fifth (latest) version of the DSM was accompanied by a widening of diagnostic criteria, which includes the elimination of language impairment from the core diagnostic dimensions of autism. This ensured that individuals with a different (somehow milder) presentation of the disorder participated in adult outcome studies, so much so that today verbal individuals with average/above-average IQ have become the main focus of autism studies. As for access to intervention, the prospects of autistic individuals have improved markedly over time, with many children diagnosed and provided with special educational programs early on, which raises hopes for better outcomes.

Finally, it has been held for a long time that the development of receptive language lagged behind that of expressive language in autism. Even though this production-comprehension discrepancy is mentioned in the DSM-5-TR, it has not been confirmed by empirical evidence in autistic children (Kwok et al. 2015). What about autistic adults? Some studies suggested that this discrepancy may be less marked than in childhood (Pickles, Anderson, and Lord 2014; Girolamo and Rice 2022), but too little attention has been paid to this issue from a developmental point of view to reach a firm conclusion. We turn now to specific language abilities of autistic adults.

---

2 Historically, different terms have been used to describe what is referred to as DID in the last version of the ICD-11, namely the conditions characterized by intellectual functioning that is approximately two or more standard deviations below the mean, which corresponds to a standard score <70 (World Health Organization [WHO] 2022). Since ICD-11 is the most recent nosological classification, the term DID will be used throughout this chapter, including to refer to conditions originally defined by a different terminology.

The term **morphosyntax** (also referred to as "grammar") encompasses both morphology and syntax and refers to the set of formal rules and principles that govern the internal structure of words (and their meaningful parts) and the structure of sentences. Based on these principles, the degree of complexity of different structures in a given language can be determined. Complexity has been proposed to depend on the nature and the number of syntactic operations needed for the construction of a syntactic structure. For example, passive sentences, in which the object of the verb becomes the subject (e.g. *the mouse was eaten by the cat*), have been claimed to be more complex than active sentences, which do not involve such an operation (e.g. *the cat ate the mouse*). Likewise, object relative clauses (e.g. *the man that my sister knows*) have been shown to be more complex than subject relatives (e.g. *the man that knows my sister*; see Chapter 3).

The few cross-sectional studies on autistic adults that included a measure of morphosyntax yielded different results, largely depending on the population sample. Individuals with average to high IQ seem to have age-appropriate morphosyntactic skills, showing low sensitivity to complexity. For example, the comprehension of passive (and active) sentences has been shown to be unimpaired, although adults with a diagnosis of autism have been found to display difficulties understanding relative clauses in contrast to nonautistic adults (Pijnacker et al. 2009), in particular object relative clauses (Durrleman et al. 2015). This latter result is in line with findings on children (see Chapter 3). When the language capacities of cohorts with low to average IQ were assessed, results differed across individuals to a larger extent. For example, the young autistic adults with and without DID tested by Girolamo and Rice (2022) via a grammaticality judgment task performed persistently (across three time-points between 18 and 20 years) either below age expectations, qualifying for language impairment, or at ceiling. Similarly, Manenti et al. (2023) showed that autistic adults with ranging intellectual abilities vary significantly in their performance on a sentence repetition task. Conducting (language) studies on heterogeneous samples is therefore important to obtain results that are as representative as possible of all individuals on the spectrum.

A handful of longitudinal studies that included measures of morphosyntax/grammar have been carried out on autistic adults, but they tend to report morphosyntactic scores at only one time-point (Szatmari et al. 2009; Whitehouse et al. 2009; LeGrand et al. 2021), leaving open the question of how these skills develop into adulthood.

Along with **pragmatics** (see below), lexicon, measured by vocabulary score, is the linguistic domain that has been targeted the most in studies on autistic adults, mirroring what has been reported in studies on autistic children (see Chapter 2). Note that, although present in many studies, lexical measures have sometimes been used as a variable of language development for matching groups of participants or as childhood predictors for adult outcomes, meaning that details on lexical competence are not always provided. Based on studies reporting participants' lexical knowledge, it appears clear that some autistic individuals continue to display difficulties in adulthood. There is evidence for a consistent number of autistic adults showing a wide gap between their chronological age and the age-equivalent obtained from expressive and receptive vocabulary tasks (picture naming and picture matching, respectively), suggesting the presence of language impairment (Howlin 2003). Differences between autistic (with or without speech onset delay) and nonautistic individuals have also been identified, as well as between autistic adults and adults with a receptive language disorder (Mawhood, Howlin, and Rutter 2000). Despite a large body of evidence pointing at a difference between autistic and nonautistic individuals with respect to lexical knowledge, some studies reported no differences. For example, Baxter et al. (2019) found that autistic and neurotypical adults performed alike (i.e. within norms) in terms of correctly defining words. However, it is not clear whether these conflicting results should be imputed to differences in methodological designs.

As one would expect given the first diagnostic dimension of autism, namely persistent deficits in social communication and interaction, pragmatic and communication skills have received much attention in autism research, including in adults (see Chapter 6). One of the earliest studies documenting the communicative abilities of autistic adults (mostly with DID) diagnosed with autism as children showed that 55% of those involved in institutional/home facilities and 25% of those living at home lacked speech in adulthood (Wolf and Goldberg 1986). Even for individuals with high IQ, Szatmari et al. (1989) report communication scores to be affected, as measured by a standardized parent interview, though a third of the individuals scored higher than the mean. Overall poor communicative skills were reported by subsequent studies, with autistic adults displaying higher production of pragmatically inappropriate utterances, emptier conversional turns, and lower conversation initiation ratios than adults with a developmental receptive language disorder. Autistic individuals have also been found to experience difficulties understanding inference, appreciating humor, and producing emphatic stress (i.e. the placing of emphasis on a particular word of a sentence) to convey meaning in speech.

Finally, communication (and socio-interaction) problems common in autism, such as limited reciprocity, atypical intonation, and prosody, seem to persist into adulthood to a higher extent than other typical childhood autistic symptoms (e.g. emotional problems and maladaptive behaviors), although improvement throughout the lifespan has been regularly reported.

The findings on language abilities in autistic adults should be interpreted in light of some limitations mainly concerning: (i) population sampling (in terms of heterogeneity of age and cognitive functioning), (ii) the design of longitudinal studies, and (iii) the measures used to assess language. Regarding sample composition, there are three stumbling blocks that are worth making explicit. First, the age range of "adult" cohorts can be quite wide in some studies, including both adolescents and adults (e.g. 13–41 years) or both young and old adults (e.g. 18–67 years).[3] This might not be optimal for exploring the development and the adult functioning of (linguistic and nonlinguistic) cognitive abilities in a population as inherently heterogeneous as the autistic population. When combining results from individuals at different developmental stages who may differ in terms of physiological and cognitive functioning, particular attention should be paid to the potential effect of age on performance. For one, adolescence might be an especially vulnerable period for the developmental trajectory and outcomes of autism (as seen above); moreover, the definition of "aging" within the domain of autism research is still a matter of debate (as explained below). For this reason, cognitive aspects of mental functions should also be controlled to ensure that (older) participants' performance is not affected by cognitive decline. The second reason why it is hard to draw general conclusions about language in autism in adulthood has to do with the level of intellectual functioning of the participants in existing studies. Individuals with DID are estimated to represent around 30% of the autistic population, including adults. Yet, individuals with low IQ are rarely integrated into experimental cohorts. Language-related studies on adults are no exception since most of them focus on individuals in the high range of intellectual functioning. Excluding people with DID from autism research stems partly from methodological concerns, as designing tasks accessible to these individuals is particularly challenging. Thirdly, individuals who are minimally verbal are seldom integrated into autism research. In addition to experimental cohorts that should be more representative of the heterogeneity characterizing the autism spectrum, future research would benefit from studies in which autistic adults are compared to nonautistic adults with DID as well as nonautistic adults with Developmental Language Disorder (DLD). The first comparison would make it possible to understand whether the language difficulties displayed by autistic individuals with DID are (exclusively) due to their intellectual disability, whereas the second comparison would help define whether language impairment in autism and DLD share the same etiology and characteristics (see Chapter 11).

Another limitation to our knowledge of language abilities in autistic adults concerns the way longitudinal studies are designed. Longitudinal studies dating back as far as 30 years reported results for only two to at most three

---

3 We acknowledge that defining adolescence is not an easy undertaking, since adolescence and adult age may overlap in more than one aspect.

observation time-points, separated by about a decade. Some of the most recent studies are designed to follow individuals more systematically, thus increasing the possibility of characterizing developmental tendencies and the timing of changes more precisely. Finally, many longitudinal studies on autistic adults that have included a language measure have not assessed the same abilities both in childhood and adulthood. Future studies should therefore evaluate language skills more thoroughly.

One final barrier to drawing meaningful conclusions about the linguistic abilities of autistic adults is the dearth of focused and appropriate measures of language. Given the lack of tests standardized on adults, many of the studies to date have made use of tasks normed on children (e.g. the BPVS-3; see Chapter 1), a vocabulary test normed up to 16 years of age. Moreover, in some studies, verbal IQ scores or parental/caregiver questionnaires for assessing autistic symptoms were used as proxies for language. While providing us with invaluable information on the overall linguistic and communication skills of the participants, these tools provide global and indirect measures, respectively. This limits the possibility of drawing accurate conclusions on the linguistic abilities of autistic individuals who are likely to be differently (and potentially selectively) impaired in different language domains (see Chapter 16).

In addition, standardized tests designed to assess a certain language skill have been used to measure a different type of ability. It is the case, for instance, of phonology, namely the ability to perceive and manipulate speech sounds (see Chapter 4). The phonological abilities of autistic adults have virtually never been assessed. Yet, when they were targeted, they were evaluated via tools meant to test other abilities, such as auditory discrimination and phonetics (e.g. Pijnacker et al. 2009).

Experimental tasks also present limitations. Many factors may specifically influence language performance in autistic individuals (see Chapter 16), which is why assessing linguistic abilities in this population, including adults, is far from being straightforward. Information on the test construction process, i.e. how factors that might affect language performance have been controlled for, is missing in many studies. Designing tasks for adults involves further challenges because, depending on their cognitive capacities and how their language skills have developed over time, they may present with a mental age that differs greatly from their chronological age. In this sense, the gap that may exist between adults at different levels of functioning can be much wider than the gap that may be found across children, especially concerning language abilities. This should be carefully considered when creating language tasks with the aim of making them accessible to the entire adult autistic spectrum. It has been shown that nonword and sentence repetition tasks (where participants are asked to repeat items that target particular sound and sentence structures), which involve limited pragmatic and memory demands, display a particularly high completion rate (>80%) when administered to autistic children and adults, including those with borderline to low IQ (Manenti et al. 2023; Tuller et al. in press).

What Are the Predictive Factors of Adult Outcomes in Autism?

Research has been increasingly attempting to identify predictive variables associated with adult functioning ever since the earliest follow-up report in the 1970s. In this section, the evidence on language is addressed from two different perspectives: considering language as a predictor variable (i.e. what are the outcomes that can be anticipated based on language functioning?) and as a variable to be predicted (i.e. what are the factors whose level of functioning can predict linguistic abilities?). Early language skills, often referred to as early "childhood functional/useful speech," are one of the most researched contributing factors of later outcomes in autism, together with childhood IQ. Speech and language acquisition before age 5 or 6, better childhood language/communication skills, and rate of language change from childhood to adulthood have consistently been found to be very strong predictors of adolescent and adult outcomes, in terms of general cognitive and linguistic abilities, employment, social relationships/participation, independent living, autistic symptoms, adaptive behaviors, social interaction, and daily functioning (Howlin and Moss 2012).

This picture mirrors findings from recent longitudinal studies. Baghdadli et al. (2018) showed that absence of functional speech, as well as more severe autistic symptoms and a low developmental quotient (an IQ-equivalent measure of the gap between developmental age and chronological age), predicted low developmental trajectories in the autistic population from childhood to adulthood. Early language (and cognitive) level appears to also be related to verbal functioning, educational level, and social and independent functioning (Sevaslidou, Chatzidimitriou, and Abatzoglou 2019). Simonoff et al. (2020) observed that language, together with schooling type (mainstream vs. specialized), predicted adult IQ.

One issue of particular interest concerns the potential interrelation between language skills and the severity of autism symptoms. In other words, do children with low language skills tend to develop more severe autistic symptoms with time, presumably because they cannot rely on their language capacities to improve their intersocial skills? The answer to this question is far from established yet. While autistic children with language impairment have been found to develop more severe autistic symptoms in late adolescence than autistic children with no language impairment (Szatmari et al. 2009), language was not found to be related to the developmental trajectory of autism symptoms in the longitudinal study by Simonoff et al. (2020). More research is clearly needed in this area.

Given that language is an established predictor of later outcomes in autism, including adult linguistic abilities, we might ask what specific features of childhood language skills best predict adult outcomes. By exploring the linguistic trajectories of 29 4-year-old autistic children over 20 years, LeGrand et al. (2021) found that verb diversity (i.e. number of different verbs produced) in childhood was the best predictor for the outcomes of young autistic adults, concerning verbal IQ, socio-communication, and receptive vocabulary. This may be due to the fact that verbs play both a syntactic and semantic role, which makes them ideal for shedding light on skills in multiple linguistic areas. Other studies showed that it was adult language abilities (proportion of elaborate utterances and number of different words) rather than childhood language abilities that best predicted functional outcomes (independence and friendships) five years later (Friedman et al. 2019). Further research is thus warranted on this issue as well.

Compared to language as a predictor of later outcomes, language as a predicted outcome has received far less attention. As mentioned above, linguistic skills in childhood, in particular verb diversity, seem to predict linguistic outcomes in adulthood. More generally, previous studies have identified childhood receptive vocabulary as a factor contributing a large part to language level in adulthood (Mawhood, Howlin, and Rutter 2000). In addition to linguistic skills, fine motor skills, functional play, responsiveness to joint attention, and initiation of requesting behaviors have been found to predict language outcomes in autism (Sigman and McGovern 2005; Bal et al. 2020). A significant and positive relationship has also been observed between cognitive level and adult communication (Ballaban-Gil et al. 1996). However, research on the predictors of linguistic outcomes, in addition to being characterized by the methodological shortcomings mentioned earlier, is still too limited for any meaningful conclusion to be drawn.

How Does Aging Impact on Language Functioning in Autism?

Older age research in autism is a rapidly growing field, but there is still a wide knowledge gap about what happens to the linguistic skills of autistic people as they approach older age. Why is it so? As mentioned above, how to define "aging" in autism is still a matter of debate. While in the general population, the threshold for examining the aging process is usually set at around 60 years, there are reasons to think that, for the autistic population, the threshold should be set at a younger age, around 50 years. First, there is evidence suggesting that the risk of premature death is two to three times higher for the autistic than for the neurotypical population. Moreover, co-occurring (physical and/or mental) health conditions (e.g. diseases of the digestive system, Obsessive-Compulsive Disorder), which are frequent in the autistic population, imply pharmacological treatments that might adversely affect cognitive functioning, including by favoring neurodegenerative symptoms (Roestorf et al. 2019).

Concerning language, a retrospective study on the adult outcomes of 74 participants aged 30–70 years that have been part of the same community program for 20–35 years found that more than three-quarters of them presented with some degree of atypical linguistic behaviors or language impairment (determined by the psychologist's clinical experience and knowledge of each individual), from abnormal prosody, perseveration, or echolalia to minimal verbal skills (one/two-word phrases, or no speech; Wise, Smith, and Rabins 2017). It should be noted that many among them also had mild to severe DID. Over 90% of the autistic adults aged 50 and over had some degree of language impairment, even though no global difference was detected when compared with younger adults (<50 years). A significant difference between younger and older adults was observed in a subsequent study by Fombonne et al. (2020), who reported on language impairment (measured via a questionnaire on current everyday language level) being strongly associated with age. The prevalence of nonfluent language was about one-third among the youngest participants (18–19 years) versus about 50% in the older ones (over 40 years). However, this trend (parallel to that of DID, diagnosed in nearly half of the total sample) could be due to improved access to autism-specific intervention in younger participants or to the widening of autism diagnostic criteria resulting in younger generations with milder phenotypes (i.e. a set of observable symptoms characterizing an individual).

To date, no studies have been conducted to investigate whether and how specific language abilities change in autism during older age, except for (phonemic and semantic) verbal fluency. One of the reasons why verbal fluency has received such an interest is that it requires Executive Function capacities, such as flexible processing and inhibition, known to be affected by both aging and autism. Studies of verbal fluency in older autistic adults, which focused exclusively on individuals with average to high intellectual abilities, have come to different conclusions, even when similar tasks were used. Looking at phonemic fluency, Geurts and Vissers (2012) found that with increasing age, autistic individuals gave less correct responses than age-matched neurotypicals (51–83 years). Importantly, only in the control group did fluency show a strong negative relationship with age, suggesting that aging might affect autistic and neurotypical adults differently, at least in certain cognitive domains. However, evidence for older autistic adults being less prone to age-related effects than older neurotypicals has not been replicated. Davids et al. (2016) found a significant negative correlation between age and semantic fluency for both autistic adults (age 50–84 years) and age-matched controls (age 50–79 years), which can be interpreted as a finding in favor of parallel decline. Baxter et al. (2019) reported no effect of age on semantic and phonemic fluency in either the control group (14 young adults, M = 21 years; 20 middle-aged adults, M = 50 years) or the autism group (18 young adults aged, M = 21 years; 24 middle-aged adults, M = 53 years). However, they reported on a group effect for semantic (but not phonemic) fluency, with participants in the control group generating significantly more answers than those in the autism group. Similarly, recent cross-sectional studies found that, although verbal fluency was one of the cognitive domains in which autistic adults showed most difficulties, performance was not linked with age (Torenvliet et al. 2022; age 31–85 years). In a subsequent study, Torenvliet et al. (2023) found that verbal fluency was affected by longitudinal change in older autistic adults, but no difference was observed in the pattern of change between autistic (age 24–79 years) and nonautistic adults (age 30–85 years). In addition to verbal fluency, the effect of aging was explored on encoding and recalling speech. Mayer and Heaton (2014) assessed the ability of autistic (age 23–59 years) and typically developed (age 25–52) individuals to perform a verbatim recalling of 15-word sentences recorded and manipulated to generate three different speed conditions (normal, moderate, and fast). In contrast to what was found for controls, increased perceptual disturbance from fast speech was significantly and positively related to increasing age in autistic participants.

To sum up, evidence has been provided for both decreased and increased age-related effects, although most studies seem to agree on the existence of similar age-related effects in autistic and nonautistic adults. These lines of evidence echo the aging patterns that have been proposed for cognitive decline in autism, namely protective, accelerated, or parallel (with respect to typical aging). While some authors have speculated that older autistic adults might be at increased risk of cognitive decline or dementia, others have hypothesized that a hyperplasticity state associated with autism could act as a protector against age-induced cognitive decline or the development of dementia (Roestorf et al. 2019). To date, the cognitive functions of older autistic adults need to be investigated further, and language abilities are yet to be explored.

Note that, along with the population sampling issues pointed out earlier, most studies on cognitive functions in autistic aging have recruited individuals who received an autism diagnosis late in life. Therefore, the findings mentioned above, in addition to being in need of replication, are not generalizable to all people on the autism spectrum. Finally, the number of participants aged over 50 included in these studies was not always made explicit, limiting the interpretation and replicability of the results.

Focus on a Specific Study

To illustrate some of the points discussed throughout this chapter, we briefly report on the method and the results presented by Howlin et al. (2014). We chose this seminal study because, in addition to presenting several methodological strengths (e.g. design, sample size, age range) and providing largely replicated evidence, it exemplifies many of the challenges faced when exploring language abilities in autistic adults (e.g. recruiting a representative cohort, identifying autism-friendly tests that ensure controlled evaluation and comparable results).

In view of providing a picture of cognitive abilities after early adulthood in autism, Howlin and colleagues explored the developmental trajectories and the predictive factors of change in a sample of 60 autistic individuals first diagnosed as children (mean age = 6 years 9 months; range 2–13) and followed up to mid-later adulthood (mean age = 44 years 2 months; range 29–64). Some of the participants (44/60) also took part in an experimental protocol during what the authors defined as early adulthood (mean age = 26 years 1 month; range 16–46). The two cognitive measures included in the study were IQ and language. For IQ, assessment measures varied over time. Therefore, a "Best Estimate" IQ was derived for each participant. For language, a parental/caregiver questionnaire was used to obtain an "Overall language level" expressed on a three-level scale, from functional use of spontaneous/echoed phrases to no speech. In addition, lexical tasks (picture naming and picture matching) were used to obtain a measure of expressive and receptive language at follow-up.

The authors reported general IQ stability (despite considerable variability in individual patterns of change) and language improvement by adulthood (see Figure 12.2), with only 5% of the cohort (three participants) remaining without

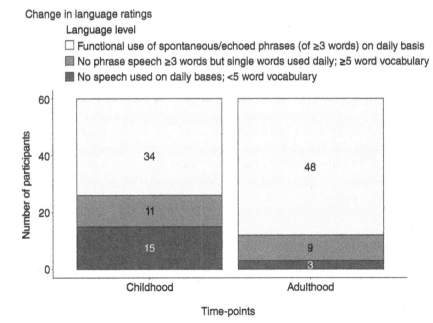

Figure 12.2 Change in language ratings from childhood to adulthood. *Source:* Adapted from Howlin et al. (2014) (table 3). Reproduced with permission of Wiley Blackwell.

useful speech. Only four participants showed deterioration in language abilities over time, three of whom had also shown clinically meaningful decline in IQ. Interestingly, no significant discrepancy was reported for expressive and receptive language. This is in line with the hypothesis that differences between production and comprehension, if any in autism (as has often been argued despite lack of clear empirical evidence), decrease with age. Finally, poor language (both in childhood and at follow-up) was one of the variables most significantly associated with the inability to complete formal intelligence tests in adulthood.

In addition to being longitudinal, this study has the great merit of including adults older than 40 in a larger-than-average sample. However, only some of the participants were assessed at three time-points, limiting, as explained above, the scope and generalizability of the conclusions about developmental patterns. Moreover, only individuals with a nonverbal childhood IQ ≥70 (i.e. without DID) were included, mirroring much of the existing literature on the topic (see Chapter 10). Finally, given the wide age range, including participants aged over 60 years, it would have been interesting to explore potential differences between the performances of younger and older adults. The study of Howlin and colleagues, similarly to many studies on adulthood, did not include discrete age groups and did not use age as a predictor of relevant characteristics.

As for cognitive evaluation, due to the heterogeneity of participants' abilities (some of whom, for instance, had difficulties with long assessments), no single task could be employed to assess intellectual functioning, exemplifying the challenges that must be faced when evaluating the cognitive abilities of autistic adults. Concerning language assessment, different measures were used at Time 1 and Time 2. This raises issues concerning both interindividual comparability and the comparability of different developmental stages. Moreover, vocabulary was used as a proxy for expressive and receptive language. Since the participants' ages were above ceiling in expressive vocabulary, it was not possible to calculate standard scores. Similarly, the receptive vocabulary task has normative data available only up to age 16. This illustrates how the lack of appropriate language measures for adults often leads to the use of tasks that might be too easy for (some) participants, thus obscuring potential areas of difficulty.

Conclusion

This chapter attempted to answer the following questions:
- What is the pattern of change in the language of autistic individuals from childhood to adulthood?
- What are the language abilities of autistic adults across the spectrum?

- What are the predictive factors of adult outcomes in autism?
- How does aging impact on language functioning in autism?

Results from longitudinal studies indicate that language difficulties decrease over time, showing a trend toward improvement. However, both developmental trajectories and adult outcomes are characterized by great interindividual variability, since mixed trajectories have been observed and both very poor and very good linguistic skills have been reported.

Studies focusing on language domains such as morphosyntax and vocabulary pointed to the existence of two different profiles in the adult autistic population: some individuals seem to display severe language impairment while others present with age-appropriate linguistic skills. In line with evidence on children, pragmatics has been argued to be the area that best differentiates autistic from nonautistic adults. Also worth noting is that information on the phonological abilities of autistic adults is altogether missing (while impairment in this domain has been reported for autistic children).

Good linguistic skills have been consistently reported to play an important role in the prediction of better social and adaptive functioning and independent living. In contrast, the factors contributing to good linguistic skills in adulthood are yet to be determined.

Similarly, how cognition is affected by aging in autism remains unclear, as evidence has been provided for all logical patterns (protective, accelerated, or parallel pattern with respect to typical aging), although parallel aging appears to be, to date, the most consistent result. Moreover, no purely linguistic domain has been investigated in older adults.

Findings on language in autistic adults need to be replicated by further studies, which should ideally be designed in such a way as to avoid several pitfalls. For instance, the results from different developmental stages should not be combined without controlling for the potential effects of age on performance, and, when older participants are involved, cognitive decline should be measured. In addition, language abilities should be assessed across the whole spectrum of intellectual functioning so that findings are generalizable to the full range of autistic individuals. It would be interesting to compare the profiles of those diagnosed as children and the profiles of those diagnosed as adults (based on the same diagnostic criteria). It is also important to consider language in autism developmentally, following individuals at several time-points not too far apart from each other. Finally, future research should benefit from the use of tasks designed to ensure a controlled assessment of linguistic abilities while minimizing the influence of external factors on performance (e.g. attention deficits and/or difficulties in integrating stimuli coming from different sources).

Even though many important questions on linguistic abilities in autism at adult age remain, research has made considerable progress since the first report on autistic adults, allowing us to gain a better understanding of the language developmental trajectories across the lifespan and the language profiles that can be found in adulthood, but also of how the tools commonly used to obtain this information can be refined in order to be more accurate and suitable for a larger range of individuals on the autism spectrum.

> **What Do You Know Now?**
> The developmental trajectories and adult outcomes of autistic individuals are characterized by great interindividual variability.
> - Language skills display mixed patterns of development from childhood to adulthood (improvement, stability, decline) in autism.
> - The language of individuals with low intelligence levels seems to improve less with time. Typical language acquisition during early development and better childhood language abilities strongly predict later outcomes in several domains, including linguistic and nonlinguistic cognition but also social relationships, daily living skills, and professional achievements. To date, no conclusions can be drawn about the relationship between language ability and autism severity.
> - On the one hand, older autistic adults have been claimed to be partially protected against an age-related decrease in cognitive functioning. On the other hand, aging in autism has been claimed to disproportionately affect specific cognitive processes (e.g. cognitive flexibility). Research on this topic, however, is still too limited for any firm conclusions to be drawn.

Suggestions for Further Reading

If you want to know more about outcomes in adulthood for autistic individuals, we recommend reading the study by Magiati, Tay, and Howlin 2014. The authors conducted a systematic review of existing literature on cognitive, language, social, and behavioral outcomes in autistic adults. If you are interested in learning more about how the linguistic skills of autistic individuals develop over time, we recommend that you read Brignell et al. 2018. It is a recent systematic review and meta-analysis that provides a narrative description of language outcomes in autism and has the merit of discussing current evidence in light of the type of language tools that have been used to obtain this evidence and overall methodological shortcomings.

References

Baghdadli, A., Michelon, C., Pernon, E. et al. (2018). Adaptive trajectories and early risk factors in the autism spectrum: a 15-year prospective study. *Autism Research* 11 (11): 1455–1467.

Bal, V.H., Fok, M., Lord, C. et al. (2020). Predictors of longer-term development of expressive language in two independent longitudinal cohorts of language-delayed preschoolers with Autism Spectrum Disorder. *Journal of Child Psychology and Psychiatry* 61 (7): 826–835.

Ballaban-Gil, K., Rapin, I., Tuchman, R. et al. (1996). Longitudinal examination of the behavioral, language, and social changes in a population of adolescents and young adults with autistic disorder. *Pediatric Neurology* 15 (3): 217–223.

Barnes, L.L., Wilson, R.S., Schneider, J.A. et al. (2003). Gender, cognitive decline, and risk of AD in older persons. *Neurology* 60 (11): 1777–1781.

Baxter, L.C., Nespodzany, A., Walsh, M.J.M. et al. (2019). The influence of age and ASD on verbal fluency networks. *Research in Autism Spectrum Disorders* 63: 52–62.

Brignell, A., Morgan, A.T., Woolfenden, S. et al. (2018). A systematic review and meta-analysis of the prognosis of language outcomes for individuals with Autism Spectrum Disorder. *Autism and Developmental Language Impairments* 3.

Davids, R.C., Groen, Y., Berg, I.J. et al. (2016). Executive Functions in older adults with Autism Spectrum Disorder: objective performance and subjective complaints. *Journal of Autism and Developmental Disorders* 46: 2859–2873.

Durrleman, S., Hippolyte, L., Zufferey, S. et al. (2015). Complex syntax in Autism Spectrum Disorders: a study of relative clauses. *International Journal of Language and Communication Disorders* 50 (2): 260–267.

Fombonne, E., Green Snyder, L., Daniels, A. et al. (2020). Psychiatric and medical profiles of autistic adults in the SPARK cohort. *Journal of Autism and Developmental Disorders* 50: 3679–3698.

Friedman, L., Sterling, A., DaWalt, L.S. et al. (2019). Conversational language is a predictor of vocational independence and friendships in adults with ASD. *Journal of Autism and Developmental Disorders* 49: 4294–4305.

Geurts, H.M. and Vissers, M.E. (2012). Elderly with autism: Executive Functions and memory. *Journal of Autism and Developmental Disorders* 42: 665–675.

Girolamo, T. and Rice, M.L. (2022). Language impairment in autistic adolescents and young adults. *Journal of Speech, Language, and Hearing Research* 65 (9): 3518–3530.

Howlin, P. (2003). Outcome in high-functioning adults with autism with and without early language delays: implications for the differentiation between autism and Asperger Syndrome. *Journal of Autism and Developmental Disorders* 33: 3–13.

Howlin, P. and Moss, P. (2012). Adults with Autism Spectrum Disorders. *The Canadian Journal of Psychiatry* 57 (5): 275–283.

Howlin, P., Savage, S., Moss, P. et al. (2014). Cognitive and language skills in adults with autism: a 40-year follow-up. *Journal of Child Psychology and Psychiatry* 55 (1): 49–58.

Kwok, E.Y., Brown, H.M., Smyth, R.E. et al. (2015). Meta-analysis of receptive and expressive language skills in Autism Spectrum Disorder. *Research in Autism Spectrum Disorders* 9: 202–222.

Lai, M.C. and Baron-Cohen, S. (2015). Identifying the lost generation of adults with autism spectrum conditions. *The Lancet Psychiatry* 2 (11): 1013–1027.

LeGrand, K.J., Weil, L.W., Lord, C. et al. (2021). Identifying childhood expressive language features that best predict adult language and communication outcome in individuals with Autism Spectrum Disorder. *Journal of Speech, Language, and Hearing Research* 64 (6): 1977–1991.

Magiati, I., Tay, X.W., and Howlin, P. (2014). Cognitive, language, social and behavioural outcomes in adults with Autism Spectrum Disorders: a systematic review of longitudinal follow-up studies in adulthood. *Clinical Psychology Review* 34 (1): 73–86.

Manenti, M., Tuller, L., Houy-Durand, E. et al. (2023). Assessing structural language skills of autistic adults: focus on sentence repetition. *Lingua* 294: 103598.

Mawhood, L., Howlin, P., and Rutter, M. (2000). Autism and developmental receptive language disorder – a comparative follow-up in early adult life. I: cognitive and language outcomes. *The Journal of Child Psychology and Psychiatry and Allied Disciplines* 41 (5): 547–559.

Mayer, J.L. and Heaton, P.F. (2014). Age and sensory processing abnormalities predict declines in encoding and recall of temporally manipulated speech in high-functioning adults with ASD. *Autism Research* 7 (1): 40–49.

Pickles, A., Anderson, D.K., and Lord, C. (2014). Heterogeneity and plasticity in the development of language: a 17-year follow-up of children referred early for possible autism. *Journal of Child Psychology and Psychiatry* 55 (12): 1354–1362.

Pijnacker, J., Hagoort, P., Buitelaar, J. et al. (2009). Pragmatic inferences in high-functioning adults with autism and Asperger Syndrome. *Journal of Autism and Developmental Disorders* 39: 607–618.

Roestorf, A., Bowler, D.M., Deserno, M.K. et al. (2019). "Older adults with ASD: the consequences of aging." Insights from a series of special interest group meetings held at the International Society for Autism Research 2016–2017. *Research in Autism Spectrum Disorders* 63: 3–12.

Sevaslidou, I., Chatzidimitriou, C., and Abatzoglou, G. (2019). The long-term outcomes of a cohort of adolescents and adults from Greece with Autism Spectrum Disorder. *Annals of General Psychiatry* 18 (1): 1–6.

Sigman, M. and McGovern, C.W. (2005). Improvement in cognitive and language skills from preschool to adolescence in autism. *Journal of Autism and Developmental Disorders* 35 (1): 15–23.

Simonoff, E., Kent, R., Stringer, D. et al. (2020). Trajectories in symptoms of autism and cognitive ability in autism from childhood to adult life: findings from a longitudinal epidemiological cohort. *Journal of the American Academy of Child and Adolescent Psychiatry* 59 (12): 1342–1352.

Szatmari, P., Bartolucci, G., Bremner, R. et al. (1989). A follow-up study of high-functioning autistic children. *Journal of Autism and Developmental Disorders* 19 (2): 213–225.

Szatmari, P., Bryson, S., Duku, E. et al. (2009). Similar developmental trajectories in autism and Asperger Syndrome: from early childhood to adolescence. *Journal of Child Psychology and Psychiatry* 50 (12): 1459–1467.

Torenvliet, C., Groenman, A.P., Radhoe, T.A. et al. (2022). Parallel age-related cognitive effects in autism: a cross-sectional replication study. *Autism Research* 15 (3): 507–518.

Torenvliet, C., Groenman, A.P., Radhoe, T.A. et al. (2023). A longitudinal study on cognitive aging in autism. *Psychiatry Research* 321: 115063.

Tuller, L., Silleresi, S., and Prévost, P. (in press). Autism and language modularity. In: *Footprints of Phrase Structure: Studies in Syntax in Honor of Tim Stowell* (eds. M. Arche, J.-W. Zwart, H. Demirdache, and N. Hyams). Amsterdam: John Benjamins.

Whitehouse, A.J., Line, E.A., Watt, H.J. et al. (2009). Qualitative aspects of developmental language impairment relate to language and literacy outcome in adulthood. *International Journal of Language and Communication Disorders* 44 (4): 489–510.

Wise, E.A., Smith, M.D., and Rabins, P.V. (2017). Aging and Autism Spectrum Disorder: a naturalistic, longitudinal study of the comorbidities and behavioral and neuropsychiatric symptoms in adults with ASD. *Journal of Autism and Developmental Disorders* 47: 1708–1715.

Wolf, L. and Goldberg, B. (1986). Autistic children grow up: an eight to twenty-four year follow-up study. *The Canadian Journal of Psychiatry* 31 (6): 550–556.

13

Multilingualism in Autism

Natalia Meir and Rama Novogrodsky

> **What Do You Think?**
> A 4-year-old bilingual boy has recently been diagnosed with autism. The parents contemplate abandoning Italian, the family language, which is not the dominant language in their community. Do you think autistic children can acquire more than one language? Does acquiring two languages aggravate the severity of autistic symptoms, or the presence of cognitive and language difficulties?
>
> An 8-year-old girl with ASD exposed to Russian at home and Hebrew for five years at school speaks only Russian. Do you think she has received enough exposure to Hebrew to support its acquisition? Are language skills affected by the quantity of language exposure? Are a child's skills in both languages affected by the quantity of exposure to both languages?
>
> A 7-year-old French-speaking boy with autism taught himself English through computer games and television programs. Despite attending a French-speaking school and only French at home, English has become his preferred language. The school teacher suggests focusing on French in all contexts, including digital media. What do you think about such advice?

Introduction

Today, **multilingualism** is part of the life experience of many children, both autistic and nonautistic. The term multilingualism is used to refer to children who grow up with two or more languages.[1] More than half of the world's children are raised in communities where multilingualism is the norm (De Houwer 2007; Grosjean 2010). It is therefore important to understand how exposure to multiple languages may affect language and cognitive development in autism.

---

1 Please note that the terms "bilingual" and "multilingual" are used interchangeably to refer to people who use more than one language.

This chapter addresses three questions, focusing on the effect of multilingualism on language difficulties in autism and the assumption of a **double delay**, the idea that multiple languages aggravate the symptoms of the disorder.

- Does multilingualism exacerbate language difficulties in children with autism?
- Do multilingual children with autism show a (double) delay in their cognitive abilities?
- How does language input affect development in multilingual autistic children?

Anchoring

There are different kinds of multilingual acquisition. We present the three common ones. **Simultaneous multilingualism** is when children acquire multiple languages simultaneously from birth. In **sequential multilingualism** (e.g. in contexts of migration, but not only), a child first acquires a Heritage Language (also known as a *home language, minority language*) until the onset of schooling and then is exposed to a Societal Language (the majority language) at school and through other daily interactions. Lastly, **diglossia**, where two varieties of a language are used by the same community, also presents a multilingual condition. For example, many children acquiring Arabic acquire the spoken dialect through interactive and spontaneous exposure and the standard variety, which is common to all Arabic speakers, through schooling and exposure to media and literacy (Saiegh-Haddad 2003). Multilingual acquisition can also be a mix of these three types. Each child represents a unique multilingual profile, as will be discussed in this chapter.

Although multilingualism is the norm for many communities, there is a common assumption, even among some professionals, that exposure to multiple languages might pose additional challenges to autistic children (Yu 2013; Hampton et al. 2017). One reason for this assumption might be the relative scarcity of research in this area. Additionally, current language assessment procedures are not always optimal, meaning that not all the languages that the child speaks can be assessed, making it challenging to get the full picture of the child's ability to acquire language. However, it is important to note that multilingualism itself does not cause language disorders (e.g. Kohnert 2010; Uljarević et al. 2016).

Before discussing the potential effects of multilingualism on language development in autism, we present an overview of typical multilingual language development. A multilingual child or adult, in broad terms, refers to someone who can use more than one language in comprehension, production, and both spoken and written modalities at any level.

Multilingual development follows the same milestones observed in monolingual language development. For example, multilingual children produce their first words and phrases at the same time as their monolingual peers (Tuller 2015). However, it is crucial to understand that children raised as multilinguals, including those with autism, are not simply the combination of two complete or incomplete monolinguals. They have unique and specific linguistic characteristics (Grosjean 2010). Multilingual individuals may differ from monolinguals as their language performance can be influenced by their knowledge of multiple languages across different domains.

Typically, multilingual children are **unbalanced multilinguals**, meaning they have one language that is dominant or preferred compared to their other language(s) (Grosjean 2010). Additionally, language skills in multilingual children may be distributed unevenly across and within the languages they speak (Kohnert 2010). For instance, a multilingual child might have greater knowledge of school-related words in their Societal Language, while having more familiarity with home-related words in their Heritage Language.

> **Acronym and Terminology Reminder**
>
> **Code-Switching (Language-Mixing, Code-Mixing, or Borrowing):** Alternating between two languages or inserting linguistic units from one language into another.
>
> **Crosslinguistic Influence:** Effects, positive or negative, on language acquisition and maintenance related to the similarities and differences between the languages.
>
> **Definiteness Marking:** How a noun phrase indicates that its referent is identifiable, e.g. the article "the" in English.
>
> **Diglossic Language:** Two varieties of a language are used by the same community.
>
> **Double Delay:** A common myth that exposure to multiple languages aggravates the symptoms of the disorder.
>
> **Multilingualism (/Bilingualism):** A term used to describe children who grow up with two or more languages.
>
> **Referential Expression:** An expression referring to an entity in the world or in discourse, e.g. *a dog, the dog, Spot, it/he/she, my old dog,* or *this one.*
>
> **Structural Language:** Formal aspects of language related to phonology, morphology, semantics, and syntax.
>
> **Unbalanced Multilingualism:** One language is dominant or preferred compared to other language(s).

When assessing the linguistic development of multilingual children, it is important to consider language skills in all languages spoken by the child. However, this is not always possible: multilingual children are often assessed in only one of their languages and compared to language test norms designed for monolingual children. This practice leads to a fragmented picture of the child's linguistic abilities. For example, when assessed in only one language, multilingual children often score lower than their monolingual peers on vocabulary measures. This is because multilingual individuals use their languages in specific contexts and may encounter certain words in only one of their languages. It is crucial to consider all languages spoken by multilingual children, whether they are autistic or nonautistic, during language assessment and therapy. When this is not possible, due to the multiplicity of home languages in many contexts, or the unavailability of language-specific assessment tools and clinicians who can administer them, indirect measures such as questionnaires can offer a partial solution. These questionnaires provide information about language history milestones in the language(s) spoken by the child (both Home Languages and Societal Languages), including those that are not spoken by the clinician, such as speech and language therapist, special education teacher, psychologist, and clinical linguist (Tuller 2015; Novogrodsky and Meir 2020).

Several factors contribute to individual differences in the language skills of multilingual children (for an overview, see Paradis 2023). These factors include child-internal factors, such as the age of onset of bilingualism, cognitive abilities, and socio-emotional well-being. Additionally, child-external factors, such as the quantity and quality of language exposure, parental language proficiency, and family identity, influence language skills of a child. As mentioned earlier, children can acquire their languages simultaneously from birth or sequentially, where one language is acquired first, followed by additional languages later in life. The age of onset of bilingualism also plays a role in the trajectory of language acquisition. For example, a 6-year-old child exposed to a language from the age of 2 will likely demonstrate higher proficiency in that language compared to a child exposed to the same language from the age of 5, assuming they have the same amount of weekly exposure to the languages. Moreover, the quantity and quality of language exposure (language input) can vary among children. For instance, one child may have exposure divided between two languages as 20–80%, while another child may have a 50–50% distribution. Children tend to demonstrate dominance in the language with greater exposure (e.g. Armon-Lotem and Meir 2019). Finally, socio-emotional and motivational aspects also play a role in determining language proficiency. For example, family identity and positive attitudes toward a language have been found to be associated with higher proficiency in that language (Mak et al. 2023).

Children raised in multilingual environments exhibit various language contact phenomena, such as code-switching and crosslinguistic influence, mirroring the behavior of multilingual members in their communities. **Code-switching**, also known as **language-mixing, code-mixing**, or **borrowing**, refers to the insertion of linguistic units from one language into another. Inter-sentential code-switching involves producing one sentence in one language and the following sentence in another language (e.g. in English and Spanish: *I like the red house! A ti cuál te gusta?*, meaning 'which one do you like?'), while intra-sentential code-switching involves inserting one or more words from one language into a sentence produced in another language (e.g. inserting the Spanish word *casa*, meaning house, into an English sentence: *The red casa is the one I like*). Code-switching is not a sign of confusion; rather, it is a common practice in bilingual communities. Code-switching is affected by internal and external variables, including who the participants in the conversation are, what the topic of the conversation is, and the relative status of both languages. For example, in everyday conversations, bilinguals code-switch more from their Heritage Language to the Societal Language. There is no evidence suggesting that code-switched utterances in a child's language input hinder children's language acquisition.

Another well-documented language contact phenomenon is **crosslinguistic influence**, which occurs across various language domains, including phonology (a foreign accent in one of the languages under the influence of the other language), lexicon (e.g. code-switching and literal word-for-word translation), and morphosyntax (see examples of plural marking and word order below). When there are similarities between the two languages, there can be a positive effect on language acquisition and maintenance. This means that multilingual individuals may have an advantage in acquiring a particular linguistic phenomenon (e.g. number marking like *dog* vs. *dogs*) due to exposure to that phenomenon in both languages. For example, bilingual children exposed to both Dutch and Greek, which both mark grammatical gender, might grasp the concept of gender faster than their monolingual peers (e.g. Egger, Hulk, and Tsimpli 2018). On the other hand, there can be a negative effect, also known as interference, when the two languages do not overlap in a specific linguistic phenomenon or morphosyntactic rule. In phonology, this can manifest as a nonnative accent. In terms of lexical abilities, it may be evident through literal translations and borrowed words. For example, an English–French multilingual child might say *I have hungry* instead of *I am hungry* in English, influenced by the French equivalent *J'ai faim* (literally: I have hungry) (Nicoladis 2019). In morphosyntax, crosslinguistic influence can be observed when the morphosyntactic properties of one language diverge under the influence of the other language. For instance, a multilingual child speaking both French and English might reverse the placement of adjectives in either language, producing *a monkey purple* in English, following the noun-adjective order of French. Crosslinguistic influence is a part of multilingual development. Among children, crosslinguistic influence during language development is bidirectional. This means that there are influences from the Heritage Language onto the Societal Language, as well as from the Societal Language onto the Heritage Language.

In summary, crosslinguistic influence can affect acquisition in different language domains, both positively and negatively. These effects can be observed in the rate and ease of acquisition, as well as the overall language skills of the child, and they are specific to the languages in contact.

Multilingualism in Autism

Does Multilingualism Exacerbate Language Difficulties in Children With Autism?

Overall, no detrimental effects of multilingualism have so far been reported in autistic children (Prévost and Tuller 2022). Nevertheless, despite available evidence, clinicians, and parents of multilingual autistic children often express concerns that exposure to multiple languages may burden these children and impede their language development (Yu 2013).

Although there is little research on the use of code-switching in autistic individuals, existing preliminary results suggest that autistic children resort to code-switching in a similar manner as their nonautistic peers. Meir et al. (2024) showed that autistic ($n = 10$) and nonautistic ($n = 10$) children engaged in code-switching more when communicating with a bilingual experimenter than with a monolingual experimenter during ADOS sessions, confirming that autistic bilingual children are sensitive to the linguistic context. Furthermore, when communicating with a bilingual experimenter, the autistic children code-switched more than their nonautistic peers. Specifically, they used more Russian words and phrases when communicating in Hebrew with a bilingual Russian–Hebrew experimenter. The link between increased frequency of code-switching with a bilingual adult and an autistic child points to the sensitivity of children with autism to the flow of the conversation and how the two languages are used in monolingual and bilingual settings.

Crosslinguistic influence is observed in both autistic and nonautistic children across different language domains. For instance, monolingual children with autism often face challenges in using pronouns. Novogrodsky (2013) found that monolingual English-speaking autistic children produce ambiguous pronouns. For example, one autistic child began his rendition of a wordless storybook with the following sentence, "Once upon a time there was a frog, and he said, 'Frog, where are you?'" – where *he* was meant to refer to the boy seen in the picture. However, no prior reference introduced the pronoun *he*, thus making the use of *he* in this context ambiguous. These ambiguous pronouns hinder the identification of the referent to which the child is referring. In multilingual children, crosslinguistic influence in pronominal use may arise when there is a divergence in pronominal systems between the languages spoken by the child. If the two languages have similar pronominal systems, wherein subject pronouns can be omitted (e.g. Spanish and Italian), there may be no divergence. However, in the case of different systems (e.g. English and Italian), multilingual children with typical language development, as well as their autistic peers, may exhibit divergence from their monolingual counterparts. For example, in a study that explored pronominals in a sentence elicitation task, children with ASD (monolingual and bilingual) were less accurate than their nonautistic peers (monolingual and bilingual) (Meir and Novogrodsky 2019). Bilingual children in this study were speakers of Russian and Hebrew, two languages that have similar pronominal systems, i.e. both languages allow pronoun omission, a fact that certainly contributed to the finding that the multilingual children did not perform differently from their monolingual peers in pronoun production.

In a study that examined Greek-speaking monolinguals and multilinguals with and without autism, the correct use of pronouns (e.g. *he, it*) in narratives produced by the children was compared (Peristeri et al. 2020). Importantly, the multilingual children in this study spoke a variety of languages, including Albanian, Russian, Swedish, and German, in addition to Greek. The multilingual children with autism scored higher than their monolingual peers, suggesting that pronoun use can be enhanced in multilingual autistic children. This finding suggests that social pragmatics (see Chapter 6), often reported to present difficulty to children with autism, is not necessarily negatively impacted by knowledge of multiple languages.

The assumption that multilingualism aggravates the symptoms of the disorder is unsupported. A recent systematic review by Gilhuber, Raulston, and Galley (2023, p. 1516) concluded that "available research provides no indication that being exposed to more than one language has adverse effects on the communication skills of autistic children." However, most of the studies reviewed, 12 out of 19, assessed multilingual children in only one of their languages, disregarding the language and communication abilities of these children in their other language. Furthermore, the comparison between nonautistic multilingual controls and their monolingual peers was not consistently present, and not all language domains were examined. When interpreting the results comparing multilingual and monolingual children with autism, it is important to consider whether the multilingual children were assessed in both languages and whether they were compared to their monolingual peers without autism.

Data reported by Meir and Novogrodsky (2020) provide evidence against the assumption of a double delay in multilingualism in autism. The authors compared morphosyntactic abilities in four groups of children. The study utilized sentence repetition tasks to evaluate the morphosyntactic skills of monolingual Hebrew-speaking and multilingual Hebrew–Russian-speaking children with or without autism. Importantly, the multilingual children were tested in both of their languages to obtain a comprehensive understanding of their language competence. Sentence repetition tasks are effective in identifying language impairment in monolingual and multilingual children. The children repeated sentences of varying morphosyntactic complexity, such as simple sentences with Subject–Verb–Object word order (e.g. *A cat pushed a ball*) and sentences with coordination and subordination. Meir and Novogrodsky (2020) demonstrated that Russian–Hebrew-speaking autistic children exhibited two profiles: one subgroup of multilingual children showed intact morphosyntactic skills, while the second subgroup demonstrated impaired morphosyntactic skills in both languages spoken by the child. These two profiles were previously documented in monolingual autistic children (for more details, see Chapter 3). Furthermore, the study by Meir and Novogrodsky (2020) revealed that the error patterns observed in multilingual autistic children were similar to those observed in monolingual and multilingual children with structural language impairment in the absence of autism, such as Developmental Language Disorder (DLD), where language abilities are below age expectations and not attributable to any other condition. Recall that some multilingual children may be unbalanced multilingual, showing good morphosyntactic performance in one language and poorer performance in the other language(s). However, such poor performance is not indicative of language impairment. Only children who experience difficulties in both/all of their languages, including children with autism, can be diagnosed with language impairment. Regarding the influence of multilingualism, there is no evidence that multilingualism poses an extra burden for multilingual children with autism. This is the case also for multilingual children with other developmental disorders, not just autism (Uljarević et al. 2016; Novogrodsky and Meir 2020).

Do Children with Autism Show a Double Delay in Their Cognitive Abilities?

Turning to the cognitive skills of multilingual children with autism, no evidence for a double delay has been reported here either. Several studies have reported that, compared to monolingual autistic peers, multilingual children with autism show similar or even greater advantages in nonverbal cognition (e.g. inhibition, sorting, shifting, Working Memory) and social cognition (e.g. Theory of Mind abilities; see Chapter 1) (Gonzalez-Barrero and Nadig 2019; Peristeri, Vogelzang, and Tsimpli 2021; for an overview see Prévost and Tuller 2022). Note that children with autism show difficulties in various cognitive functions compared with neurotypical children (e.g. Schaeffer et al. 2023). Here, we focus on the comparison between bilingual and monolingual autistic children. For example, Gonzalez-Barrero and Nadig (2019) demonstrated that Working Memory abilities were similar in monolingual and bilingual individuals with autism, while a bilingual advantage was observed in a task involving set-shifting. Set-shifting tasks assess the ability to unconsciously shift attention between different tasks, representing cognitive flexibility. Similarly, Peristeri, Vogelzang, and Tsimpli (2021) tested monolingual and bilingual autistic children on cognitive tasks, including attention switching (an Executive Function involving the ability to subconsciously shift attention between one task and another), Working Memory (the ability to hold information for a short time while performing a cognitive task), and Theory of Mind. They reported that multilingual autistic children outperformed their monolingual peers on Theory of Mind tasks. In the same vein, Montgomery et al. (2022) found that multilingual children with autism performed better than monolingual children with autism in an inhibitory control task. In contrast, some studies report no differences between monolingual and bilingual children with ASD. For example, Meir and Novogrodsky (2020) found that bilingual children with ASD were on par with their monolingual peers in verbal Short-Term Memory and Working Memory, as measured by forward and backward digit span. It is important to note that no negative effects of bilingualism have been reported on the cognitive abilities of children with ASD.

How Does Language Input Affect Development in Multilingual Autistic Children?

Both the quantity and quality of linguistic input play important roles in child language development, for monolingual as well as multilingual children (for an overview, see Armon-Lotem and Meir 2019). Among nonautistic children, language input variables are directly related to language outcomes: more exposure to a language leads to better performance. Gonzalez-Barrero and Nadig (2018) reported that for children with autism, similarly to nonautistic children, the child's current amount of exposure to each language was the strongest predictor of both vocabulary and morphological skills measured in the corresponding language.

However, despite the links observed between exposure and language outcomes, Gonzalez-Barrero and Nadig (2018) reported that not all autistic children who were exposed to multiple languages at a young age grew up to be proficient in them. Despite ample exposure, around 40% of the time, to another language, some children were not able to communicate in that language. Conversely, others who had little exposure to the other language, around 20%, were proficient in both languages. The discrepancy between linguistic exposure and language outcomes was also noted by Armon-Lotem and Meir (2022). Their study compared multilingual children with typical language development, with DLD, or with autism. In each of the three groups, an exposure-outcome gap was observed. Whereas increased language input was found to be associated with better language outcomes in children with typical language development and in children with DLD, this link was not straightforward for children with autism. For multilingual children with autism, increased exposure to a language was not linked to better outcomes. The finding highlights that while some children with autism benefit from increased language exposure, for others, increased exposure does not necessarily lead to better outcomes. The results of the study also underscore the diversity of language abilities among multilingual children with autism, revealing an exposure-outcome gap that parallels the observed heterogeneity in monolingual children with autism.

The complex relationship between exposure to a language and language outcomes in autism is further supported by individuals who demonstrate unexpected multilingualism. Several cases of independent and spontaneous acquisition of languages in unique conditions among autistic individuals have been reported. Language learning through noninteractional input has been described in several case studies. For instance, Vulchanova et al. (2012) reported on a 10-year-old girl with autism from Bulgaria who independently acquired German by watching television programs. This girl demonstrated high proficiency in both Bulgarian and German oral skills, vocabulary, and grammar. Zhukova et al. (2023) presented a case study of an 11-year-old boy with autism born into a Russian-speaking family who unexpectedly acquired English. Interestingly, his first words were in English rather than Russian, despite Russian being the ambient language in his communicative environment. The authors noted that the boy learned English by watching cartoons in English rather than through direct interaction with his family. Unexpectedly, his English skills developed while his Russian skills lagged behind. In another study, Hindi and Meir (2023) shared data from 46 English–Hebrew speaking children with and without ASD aged 4–12, divided into three groups. Two groups included bilingual children (i.e. with and without ASD) who acquired both languages in a naturalistic setting, as they were raised in an English-speaking environment and acquired English as a Heritage Language and Hebrew as the (dominant) Societal Language in educational settings. Another group with autism consisted of children who learned English unexpectedly via noninteractive sources such as YouTube, the Internet, and TV. Results showed that children in all three groups demonstrated comparable morphosyntactic skills, yet significant variability was noted across their languages. The findings demonstrate that paths to language acquisition in autism can be different. While many of these children acquire their two languages through interactive input at home and in educational settings (as in the case of natural bilinguals with and without ASD), at least some of them do so through noninteractive settings (the case for autistic children who acquired English via the internet).

Kissine et al. (2019) documented similar, unique patterns of language acquisition in a diglossic context, where two varieties of the same language exist side by side: a spoken dialect and a standard dialect. In their study, five Tunisian boys with autism exhibited an unusual preference for Modern Standard Arabic, which is not commonly used in everyday communication by Arabic speakers. Instead, it is primarily used in very formal, mostly written settings, as well as in television programs and cartoons broadcast across the Arabic-speaking world. They showed that these five children had a strong inclination toward noninteractional language learning.

In the same vein, Abd El-Raziq, Meir, and Saiegh-Haddad (2023) investigated the choice between Modern Standard Arabic and Palestinian Arabic in 57 children aged 4–11, split into three groups: autistic children with intact structural language skills, autistic children with impaired structural language skills, and nonautistic controls. Children in all three groups presented the same pattern of favoring the spoken variety over Modern Standard Arabic. However, when individual profiles were scrutinized, it emerged that a few children in each group exhibited extensive use of Modern Standard Arabic: lexical items and structures. These cases of unexpected language learning and language choice raise fundamental questions about the extent to which interactive input is essential for successful language acquisition among autistic children.

Focus on a Specific Study

To exemplify the complexity of interpreting findings aimed at evaluating multilingual language development, we discuss the methodology and results presented in Meir and Novogrodsky (2023). We chose this study because it highlights the importance of design in multilingual research: it involves a large sample of participants, who are matched on relevant variables, and crucially, assesses their competence in BOTH the Home Language and Societal Language.

The study compared four groups of children: monolingual children with or without autism, and bilingual children with or without autism. The four groups were matched in terms of chronological age and nonverbal IQ. Importantly, the two autistic groups did not differ in terms of autism severity, indicating that multilingualism does not exacerbate autistic symptoms, at least not in autistic children with normal nonverbal IQ, as discussed in the previous section. Parental questionnaires were utilized to collect detailed background information, including exposure variables. The bilingual children with or without autism in the study were assessed on vocabulary and morphosyntactic tasks in both of their languages, allowing for a comprehensive understanding of the child's linguistic repertoire. We emphasize the advantages of employing a four-group design in research to enhance the understanding of the separate and combined effects of bilingualism, autism, and language impairment on language abilities.

The study focused on **referential expressions**, which are ubiquitous in human language and require social pragmatic judgments in specific contexts (Ariel 2001), as well as grammatical competence. For instance, when referring to a dog, there are multiple options for referential expressions, such as *a dog, the dog, Spotty, it/he/she, my old dog,* or *this one*. Children with autism often struggle to select the appropriate linguistic expression based on its pragmatic relevance to a given context (e.g. Marinis et al. 2013; Novogrodsky and Edelson

2016). In narrative tasks (see Chapter 7), autistic children may employ under-informative referential expressions, such as *the dog* or *he*, without prior mention of the dog, or fail to provide explicit information about a specific dog when multiple dogs are present in the context, resulting in the interlocutor not knowing which dog is being referred to. These under-informative expressions disrupt the listener's ability to follow the discourse. The property of informativeness in referential expressions is a language-universal aspect of social pragmatics and is not influenced by multilingualism. Here, LANGUAGE-UNIVERSAL means that informativeness is required across different languages such that, in all languages, speakers need to make sure that the expressions they use successfully identify the entities they refer to. This is a universal requirement that holds therefore in every language because speakers wish to be understood. In contrast, grammaticalized **definiteness marking** is language-specific, with some languages using a definiteness marker (e.g. *the* in English; *la, le, les* in French), while others lack such markers (e.g. Russian). In languages without definiteness markers, alternative linguistic means, such as demonstratives (*this, that*) and different word orders, are available to express definiteness.

Meir and Novogrodsky (2023) investigated the use of referential expressions, specifically focusing on the informativeness principle, our universal capacity to be informative, and the language-specific ability to mark definiteness in bilingual Hebrew–Russian-speaking children with autism. Informativeness of referential expressions was evaluated in contexts that required contrastive use of referents (e.g. *a sad clown* vs. *a happy clown*). No effect of multilingualism was expected for informativeness, as it is considered a language-universal ability. In contrast, difficulties in acquiring the Hebrew definiteness marker *ha-* (as seen in example 1b) were expected to be observed in bilingual children due to the influence of their Russian, which lacks definite and indefinite morphological markers. The four-group design allowed for comparisons between bilingual and monolingual children in each group (typically developing children and children with autism), as well as within each language condition (monolingual and bilingual) between children with autism and those with typical development.

The elicitation task was conducted in Hebrew and included different types of contrasting conditions in order to evaluate the informativeness of referential expressions and conditions that required the use of the definiteness marker. Children were presented with two pictures and asked questions about these pictures (see Figure 13.1). In Figure 13.1a, the child needs to introduce the referents for the first time; therefore, no contrastive referential expressions and no definiteness marking are required. In this case, both *A sad clown and a happy clown* and *Two clowns* were correct responses (1a). However, in (1b), the two clowns must be contrasted with each other; therefore, the use of definiteness marking is required (e.g. *the sad clown and the happy clown*).

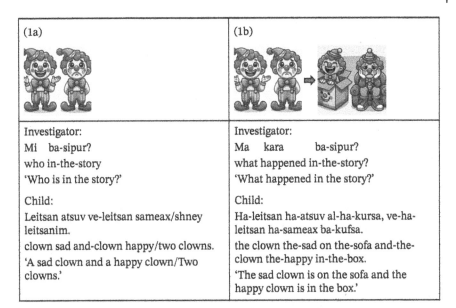

Figure 13.1 An item from the experiment used in Meir and Novogrodsky 2023, with an example question and the expected response – in Hebrew, with the accompanying word-by-word glosses, and the English translation. *Source:* Courtesy of Natalia Meir and Rama Novogrodsky.

The results revealed no differences between monolingual and multilingual children in terms of the informativeness of referential expressions. This means that multilingual children performed similarly to their monolingual counterparts, with and without autism, when using contrastive referential expressions. However, children with autism, regardless of their exposure to multiple languages, were less informative compared to their nonautistic peers. For example, when asked about what happened in the story, children with autism provided answers that did not distinguish between the two clowns, such as the responses in (2). These responses did not exhibit morphosyntactic errors, indicating that morphosyntax was not a major difficulty for these children. However, pragmatically, these noncontrastive examples lacked sufficient informativeness for the listener to understand which clown did what. It is noteworthy that most typically developing children, both monolinguals and bilinguals, did include information that differentiated between the two clowns. These findings align with the prediction that if the properties of the two languages overlap (as is the case for informativeness), multilingual children do not show divergence from their monolingual peers.

(2) a. Leitsan exad ba-kufsa ve-leitsan sheni al ha-sapa
   clown one in-the-box and-clown second on the-sofa
   'One clown is in the box and a second clown is on the sofa.'
   b. Hu ba-kufsa ve-hu al ha-sapa
   he in-the-box and-he on the-sofa
   'He is in the box, and he is on the sofa.'

However, different results were found for definiteness marking. Recall that the two languages spoken by the multilingual participants do not encode definiteness in the same way, with Hebrew using a definite marker and Russian not having a definite marker. The results revealed that multilingual children, both with and without autism, were more prone to omitting the definiteness marker in Hebrew, compared to the monolingual Hebrew-speaking children. The omission of definiteness marking in Hebrew was attributed to crosslinguistic influence from Russian, which lacks definiteness. Thus, as anticipated, multilingual children deviated from their monolingual peers under the influence of their knowledge of an additional language. In the case of children with autism, both monolingual and bilingual children omitted the definiteness marker, and this omission was linked to their difficulties with morphosyntax.

Importantly, no interaction between multilingualism and autism was detected for contrastive referential expressions and the use of definite markers. Let us refer to some statistical terms when explaining interactions in four-group design studies. If an interaction in such studies is detected, there are two possible scenarios for the source of the interaction: (i) an advantage for multilingual autistic children over their monolingual autistic peers, or (ii) a disadvantage for multilinguals compared to monolinguals. Meir and Novogrodsky (2023) demonstrated that there was no interaction between multilingualism and autism in their study. This absence of interactions between language condition (multilingual vs. monolingual) and clinical status (autistic vs. nonautistic) was found for both referential expressions and definiteness marking. This provides support for the notion that there is no multilingual disadvantage and there is no double delay or additional burden for multilingualism. In contrast to some of the aforementioned studies (e.g. Peristeri et al. 2020), no advantage was observed for multilingual children with autism. This study suggests therefore that, concerning the use of referential expressions, we can conclude that autism affects monolingual and multilingual children similarly.

The authors suggested that there are language-universal principles governing referential expression choice, such as contrasting referents for informativeness, as well as language-specific principles, such as definiteness marking (Ariel 2001). The study demonstrated that both language-universal and language-specific principles of referential choice are impacted by autism. These results suggest that clinicians should opt for testing universal pragmatic properties (using both linguistic and social pragmatic tasks), specifically when testing multilingual children. These properties might help identify the child's true pragmatic weaknesses, which are not affected by the knowledge of additional languages and language exposure.

Conclusion

This chapter aimed to address the following questions:

- Does multilingualism exacerbate language difficulties in children with autism?
- Do multilingual children with autism show a (double) delay in their cognitive abilities?
- How does language input affect development in multilingual autistic children?

The evidence provided in this chapter suggests that multilingualism is not detrimental for the development of language and cognitive skills in children with autism. In fact, some reports indicate that multilingualism may even enhance executive functioning and Theory of Mind skills in some children, both those with and without autism. Autistic children without intellectual disability are clearly capable of learning multiple languages. However, we note that there is a lack of studies on bilingualism in autistic children with intellectual disability or other co-occurring conditions (see Chapter 10), and thus the influence of multilingualism across the autism spectrum awaits future studies.

Multilingual autistic children, as well as their nonautistic peers, may exhibit different patterns of language dominance, influenced by the characteristics of the input they receive in each language within their communicative environment. Like their nonautistic multilingual peers, multilingual autistic children rely on all their languages to various degrees to function in their daily lives. However, the relationship between language exposure and language outcomes is more complex in autistic children compared to nonautistic children, as language exposure does not always directly translate into language production in autistic individuals. One apparently unique characteristic of multilingual autistic children is the varied paths to language acquisition that some of them demonstrate. Multilingualism can occur naturally, similar to what happens in children with typical development, where the quality and quantity of interactive input in multiple languages influences language skills. However, in autism, multilingualism can also involve unexpected paths, such as learning through noninteractive sources like television and computer games.

The presence of multilingualism complicates the language assessment of autistic children, often requiring the use of indirect language tools, such as questionnaires. Questionnaires can help bridge gaps in evaluating language skills when direct assessment is only possible in one language. Furthermore, language-universal pragmatic properties pose challenges for language acquisition in autistic children regardless of which languages they speak, unlike divergence in language-specific properties that may be attributed to the child's knowledge of another language and be prone to crosslinguistic influence as discussed above. Therefore, language-universal properties can be sensitive indicators for language assessment in multilingual autistic people. It is, however, also crucial not to overlook language-specific properties in diagnosis and intervention, as it is important to understand the difficulties that children face in each of the languages they speak and provide support for their communication needs in both languages.

> **What Do You Know Now?**
> Many autistic children become multilingual. However, the characteristics of their multilingualism may differ from those of nonautistic peers.
> - The relationship between language exposure and language outcomes is more complex in autistic children compared to nonautistic children, as language exposure does not always directly translate into language production in autistic individuals. Many children with autism learn multiple languages. This does not seem to worsen their language or cognitive skills, nor does it increase the severity of autism symptoms.
> - Like their nonautistic counterparts, children with autism raised in multilingual environments may display various patterns of language dominance, influenced by the quality and quantity of input that they receive in each language within their communicative environment. However, some autistic children show unique language patterns that are not directly related to input and may show spontaneous language acquisition of a language that is not the ambient language of their environment. Multilingual autistic and nonautistic children may mix their languages, similar to other individuals in multilingual communities where they are raised. They might show divergence from monolingual peers, as their communicative and language competence is affected by the knowledge of two languages.
> - While language exposure clearly affects language outcomes in nonautistic children, the situation is more complex with autistic children: language exposure is not always automatically transferred into the language output of autistic children, and autistic children might acquire language in a noninteractive manner.

Suggestions for Further Reading

If you want to learn more about bilingualism and cognition in children with autism, we recommend Gonzalez-Barrero and Nadig 2019, Peristeri, Vogelzang, and Tsimpli 2021, and Prévost and Tuller 2022. For an overview of multilingual language experience in ASD, see Hantman et al. 2023, and for an overview of factors that affect individual differences in language skills of multilingual children, see Paradis 2023. If you are interested in learning about the parental perception of bilingualism of children with autism, see Hampton et al. 2017.

References

Abd El-Raziq, M., Meir, N., and Saiegh-Haddad, E. (2023). Lexical skills in children with and without autism in the context of Arabic diglossia: evidence from vocabulary and narrative tasks. *Language Acquisition* 31 (3–4): 199–223.

Ariel, M. (2001). Accessibility theory: an overview. In: *Text Representation (Human Cognitive Processing Series)* (eds. T. Sanders, J. Schilperoord, and W. Spooren), 29–87. Amsterdam: John Benjamins.

Armon-Lotem, S. and Meir, N. (2019). The nature of exposure and input in early bilingualism. In: *The Cambridge Handbook of Bilingualism* (eds. A. De Houwer and L. Ortega), 193–212. Cambridge, UK: Cambridge University Press.

Armon-Lotem, S. and Meir, N. (2022). The differential impact of age of onset of bilingualism and language exposure for bilingual children with DLD and autism. *Linguistic Approaches to Bilingualism* 12 (1): 33–38.

De Houwer, A. (2007). Parental language input patterns and children's bilingual use. *Applied Psycholinguistics* 28 (3): 411–424.

Egger, E., Hulk, A., and Tsimpli, I.M. (2018). Crosslinguistic influence in the discovery of gender: the case of Greek–Dutch bilingual children. *Bilingualism: Language and Cognition* 21 (4): 694–709.

Gilhuber, C.S., Raulston, T.J., and Galley, K. (2023). Language and communication skills in multilingual children on the autism spectrum: a systematic review. *Autism* 27 (6): 1516–1531.

Gonzalez-Barrero, A.M. and Nadig, A.S. (2018). Bilingual children with Autism Spectrum Disorders: the impact of amount of language exposure on vocabulary and morphological skills at school age. *Autism Research* 11 (12): 1667–1678.

Gonzalez-Barrero, A.M. and Nadig, A.S. (2019). Can bilingualism mitigate set-shifting difficulties in children with Autism Spectrum Disorders? *Child Development* 90 (4): 1043–1060.

Grosjean, F. (2010). *Bilingual: Life and Reality*. Cambridge, MA: Harvard University Press.

Hampton, S., Rabagliati, H., Sorace, A. et al. (2017). Autism and bilingualism: a qualitative interview study of parents' perspectives and experiences. *Journal of Speech, Language, and Hearing Research* 60 (2): 435–446.

Hantman, R.M., Choi, B., Hartwick, K. et al. (2023). A systematic review of bilingual experiences, labels, and descriptions in Autism Spectrum Disorder research. *Frontiers in Psychology* 14: 1095164.

Hindi, I. and Meir, N. (2023). Different paths to bilingualism in Autism Spectrum Disorder (ASD): natural and unexpected. Talk presented at the International Symposium on Bilingualism (ISB14) at Macquarie University, Sydney, Australia (June, 2023).

Kissine, M., Luffin, X., Aiad, F. et al. (2019). Noncolloquial Arabic in Tunisian children with Autism Spectrum Disorder: a possible instance of language acquisition in a non-interactive context. *Language Learning* 69 (1): 44–70.

Kohnert, K. (2010). Bilingual children with primary language impairment: issues, evidence and implications for clinical actions. *Journal of Communication Disorders* 43 (6): 456–473.

Mak, E., Nichiporuk Vanni, N., Yang, X. et al. (2023). Parental perceptions of bilingualism and home language vocabulary: young bilingual children from low-income immigrant Mexican American and Chinese American families. *Frontiers in Psychology* 14: 1059298.

Marinis, T., Terzi, A., Kotsopoulou, A. et al. (2013). Pragmatic abilities of high-functioning Greek-speaking children with autism. *Psychology* 20 (3): 321–337.

Meir, N. and Novogrodsky, R. (2019). Prerequisites of third-person pronoun use in monolingual and bilingual children with autism and typical language development. *Frontiers in Psychology* 10: 2289.

Meir, N. and Novogrodsky, R. (2020). Syntactic abilities and verbal memory in monolingual and bilingual children with High Functioning Autism (HFA). *First Language* 40 (4): 341–366.

Meir, N. and Novogrodsky, R. (2023). Referential expressions in monolingual and bilingual children with and without Autism Spectrum Disorder: a study of informativeness and definiteness. *Journal of Child Language* 50 (2): 215–244.

Meir, N., Brants Yosefy, D., Rekun, O. et al. (2024). Code-switching in bilingual children with ASD: evidence from two studies. Talk presented at Language in Autism (MOLA) conference at Duke University, USA (March, 2024).

Montgomery, L., Chondrogianni, V., Fletcher-Watson, S. et al. (2022). Measuring the impact of bilingualism on executive functioning via inhibitory control abilities in autistic children. *Journal of Autism and Developmental Disorders* 52 (8): 3560–3573.

Nicoladis, E. (2019). "I have three years old": cross-linguistic Influence of fixed expressions in a bilingual child. *Journal of Monolingual and Bilingual Speech* 1 (1): 80–93.

Novogrodsky, R. (2013). Subject-pronoun use of children with Autism Spectrum Disorders (ASD). *Clinical Linguistics and Phonetics* 27 (2): 85–93.

Novogrodsky, R. and Edelson, L.R. (2016). Ambiguous pronoun use in narratives of children with Autism Spectrum Disorders. *Child Language Teaching and Therapy* 32 (2): 241–252.

Novogrodsky, R. and Meir, N. (2020). Multilingual children with special needs in early education: communication is the key. In: *The Handbook of Early Language Education* (eds. M. Schwartz and D. Prosic-Santovac), 1–29. Berlin: Springer.

Paradis, J. (2023). Sources of individual differences in the dual language development of heritage bilinguals. *Journal of Child Language* 50 (4): 793–817.

Peristeri, E., Baldimtsi, E., Andreou, M. et al. (2020). The impact of bilingualism on the narrative ability and the Executive Functions of children with Autism Spectrum Disorders. *Journal of Communication Disorders* 85: 105999.

Peristeri, E., Vogelzang, M., and Tsimpli, I.M. (2021). Bilingualism effects on the cognitive flexibility of autistic children: evidence from verbal dual-task paradigms. *Neurobiology of Language* 2 (4): 558–585.

Prévost, P. and Tuller, L. (2022). Bilingual language development in autism. *Linguistic Approaches to Bilingualism* 12 (1): 1–32.

Saiegh-Haddad, E. (2003). Linguistic distance and initial reading acquisition: the case of Arabic diglossia. *Applied Psycholinguistics* 24 (3): 431–451.

Schaeffer, J., Abd El-Raziq, M., Castroviejo, E. et al. (2023). Language in autism: domains, profiles and co-occurring conditions. *Journal of Neural Transmission* 130 (3): 433–457.

Tuller, L. (2015). Clinical use of parental questionnaires in multilingual contexts. In: *Assessing Multilingual Children: Disentangling Bilingualism from Language Impairment* (eds. S. Armon-Lotem, J. de Jong, and N. Meir), 301–330. Bristol: Multilingual Matters.

Uljarević, M., Katsos, N., Hudry, K. et al. (2016). Multilingualism and neurodevelopmental disorders – an overview of recent research and discussion of clinical implications. *Journal of Child Psychology and Psychiatry* 57 (11): 1205–1217.

Vulchanova, M., Talcott, J.B., Vulchanov, V. et al. (2012). Language against the odds, or rather not: the weak central coherence hypothesis and language. *Journal of Neurolinguistics* 25: 13–30.

Yu, B. (2013). Issues in bilingualism and heritage language maintenance: perspectives of minority-language mothers of children with Autism Spectrum Disorders. *American Journal of Speech-Language Pathology* 22 (1): 10–24.

Zhukova, M.A., Talantseva, O.I., An, I. et al. (2023). Brief report: unexpected bilingualism: a case of a Russian child with autism. *Journal of Autism and Developmental Disorders* 53 (5): 2153–2160.

14

Reading in Autism

Racha Zebib and Carole El Akiki

> **What Do You Think?**
> You meet a childhood friend, and the two of you give each other news about mutual old friends. Your friend tells you that one of these friends has a child with autism who apparently is going to attend a regular elementary school. Your friend seems skeptical and tells you that she thought that children with autism could not develop skills such as reading. What do you tell her?
>
> After his first day as an intern at a speech-language pathology practice, your roommate tells you that he has seen a child with autism who is able to read fluently an entire text. He comments that he knew that some individuals with autism could read really well, but that he had heard that these children never understand what they read. What do you think?

Introduction

Learning to read promotes academic and professional opportunities, independence into adulthood, as well as general quality of life. Reading in Autism Spectrum Disorder (ASD) remains a relatively understudied area, even though many individuals with autism learn how to read. Some individuals with autism have even become famous for their exceptional reading skills. One of the most striking examples is Christopher, a man with an autistic profile who is known for his ability to read (and speak) in more than 15 languages with various orthographic features (Smith and Tsimpli 1995). However, cases like Christopher's are not representative of all individuals with autism. Reading skills vary considerably from one autistic individual to another, and some have very weak or no reading skills. Findings reported in studies on reading in autism also vary considerably. Interstudy variability can be explained by methodological differences between studies, which sometimes reflect methodological limitations that impact study results and, more

Language in Autism, First Edition. Edited by Jeannette Schaeffer et al.
© 2025 John Wiley & Sons Ltd. Published 2025 by John Wiley & Sons Ltd.

globally, our knowledge of reading skills in children with ASD. Insight into the reading skills of individuals with ASD, including both strengths and weaknesses, and identification of the factors that predict them is needed to improve learning and make recommendations for more adequate intervention. This chapter presents what is currently known about reading skills in individuals with ASD by addressing the following questions:

- How well do autistic individuals read?
- Is there a specific reading profile associated with autism?
- What are the factors that predict reading skills in individuals with autism?

Anchoring

The main objective of reading is to access the meaning of what is read. One of the most influential frameworks defining reading ability is the **Simple View of Reading** (Gough and Tunmer 1986). We adopt this conception of reading due to its centrality in the field over the past decades and its use in studies on reading in autism. According to this view, Reading Comprehension is equal to the product of Word Recognition times Listening comprehension. We visualized this view in Figure 14.1. **Listening Comprehension** refers to receptive oral language skills – the ability to understand spoken words, sentences, and discourse. This section presents the processes involved in the two components that are specific to reading, i.e. written **Word Recognition** and **Reading Comprehension**, in other words, reading skills.

Word Recognition in reading is the ability to identify written words. It is usually measured by reading context-free words, words presented in isolation from other words, such as in a list. Although several models of Word Recognition have been proposed, two strategies remain central in many adult and acquisition models: (i) phonological decoding and (ii) lexical access.

Phonological decoding is based on grapheme-phoneme correspondences, the ability to convert letters or groups of letters into the corresponding sounds and then assemble these sounds in order to recognize a written word. For example, to recognize the word BEE via phonological decoding, the letter B is first converted into the sound /b/, then the letters EE are converted into the sound /iː/, and finally, the two sounds are assembled to form the word /biː/.

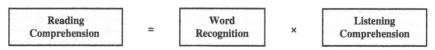

Figure 14.1 Visualization of the Simple View of Reading as proposed by Gough and Tunmer 1986.

Lexical access (sometimes called Sight Word Recognition) relies on mental representations of known words; these are stored in Long-Term Memory. Lexical access consists of direct recognition of these words without having to go through grapheme-phoneme correspondences. For instance, an English-speaking expert reader doesn't need to decipher the written word HOUSE as he/she has a mental (orthographic, phonological, and semantic) representation of the word stored in his/her Long-Term Memory, which allows him/her to identify it directly by associating the written word with this representation.

One of the most frequently cited models of Word Recognition in reading is Coltheart's **Dual Route Model** (Coltheart 2006). This model proposes that Word Recognition can be achieved through either of two routes that correspond to the two-Word Recognition strategies outlined above (Figure 14.2). The phonological decoding strategy corresponds to the right-hand route and the lexical access strategy to the left-hand route. Phonological decoding is an effortful strategy that is central to beginning readers. In more advanced readers, a switch in favor of lexical access is observed, although skilled readers continue to use both strategies. Lexical access is faster, more fluent, and less effortful, which allows more cognitive resources to be allocated to Reading Comprehension. Generally, in research and clinical settings, lexical access is evaluated via irregular Word Recognition (reading of words whose written form is irregular, such as *yacht*), as irregular words cannot be identified via the phonological strategy. Pseudoword/nonword decoding, on the other hand, is typically used to assess the phonological strategy, as it is impossible to have a stored mental representation of a pseudoword or nonword.

Acronym and Terminology Reminder

Cognitive Load: Number and complexity of items processed in Working Memory at the same time.

Grapheme: Smallest functional unit of a writing system (letters and letter combinations).

Inference Skills: Inferences made by the reader to complement explicitly provided information.

Letter Knowledge: Ability to recognize letter names and sounds.

Lexical Access/Sight Word Recognition: Direct recognition of a word without phonological decoding.

Listening Comprehension: Receptive oral language ability.

Long-Term Memory: System that stores information for an extended period of time.

Nonword/Pseudoword: Group of letters or speech sounds that may look or sound like a word but that is not a word.

Phonological Decoding: Ability to convert (groups of) letters into sounds and assemble sounds for Word Recognition.

RAN: Rapid automatized naming – ability to rapidly name familiar items (e.g. objects, letters, numbers).

TD: Typically Developing.

ToM: Theory of Mind – ability to infer and understand mental states (e.g. beliefs, true or false) in oneself and others.

Word Recognition: Ability to identify written words.

Working Memory: Ability to hold information for a short time while performing a cognitive task.

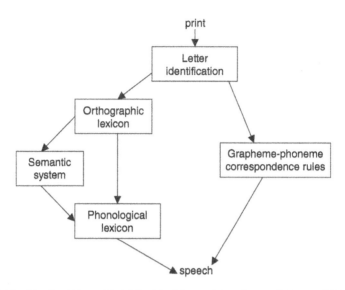

Figure 14.2 The Dual Route Model for Word Recognition. *Source:* Coltheart (2006). Reproduced with permission of Taylor & Francis.

Word Recognition is related to several cognitive abilities such as Working Memory (i.e. the ability to hold information in memory for a short time while performing a cognitive task), cognitive load (i.e. the number and complexity of items processed in Working Memory at a time), phonological awareness (i.e. the ability to identify and manipulate speech sounds, such as isolating or removing a syllable or phoneme in a word), letter knowledge (i.e. the ability to recognize letter names and letter sounds), and rapid automatized naming (i.e. the ability to rapidly name familiar items, such as familiar objects, letters, or numbers).

Reading Comprehension refers to the ability to access the meaning of what is read. As mentioned above, the Simple View of Reading describes Reading Comprehension as the product of Word Recognition skills times Listening Comprehension (see Figure 14.1). In other words, proficiency in Reading Comprehension depends on proficiency in Word Recognition (i.e. accuracy and fluency in Word Recognition) and on receptive oral language skills. The weight of Word Recognition and Listening Comprehension in Reading Comprehension varies during development: Word Recognition is the main predictor of Reading Comprehension performance in the early stages of reading acquisition, and Listening Comprehension becomes the main predictor later, in higher grades, after children have gained relative mastery of Word Recognition.

Reading Comprehension, similarly to Listening Comprehension, involves a number of factors and skills. For instance, as in Listening Comprehension, prior knowledge and inference skills are needed to ensure proper understanding of what is read. Prior knowledge consists of the reader's linguistic knowledge as well as prior knowledge of the subject being read about. It allows the reader to build a mental representation of what is read (Smith et al. 2021). For example, understanding a text that criticizes a new governmental decision or law requires the reader to have background knowledge about that decision or law. It also requires the reader to have prior knowledge of the vocabulary that is used and to be able to process linguistic information, such as the syntax of the sentences employed, based on his/her knowledge of the language. Prior knowledge furthermore includes interpersonal and social knowledge, which involves knowledge and understanding of emotions, behaviors, motivations, relationships, etc., skills that may be particularly challenging for individuals with ASD (Brown, Oram-Cardy, and Johnson 2013). Moreover, inference is necessary to ensure proper understanding of what is being read. Readers construct the meaning of a sentence or a text in light of the explicit information it contains, but also in light of inferences they make to complement the explicitly provided information with details or links that are not explicitly provided. For example, to understand why Little Red Riding Hood's mother warns her not to talk to strangers on the way to her grandmother's house, the reader must process the information that is explicitly provided in the text and rely on his/her prior knowledge concerning the potential risks of talking to strangers. When reading a text, comprehension is also modulated by the characteristics of the text, such as its linguistic complexity, its local coherence (i.e. the clarity of the links between consecutive sentences), and its global coherence (i.e. the clarity of the links at the text level). Interindividual variability in Reading Comprehension is furthermore predicted by several other cognitive processes, such as Working Memory and cognitive load (Smith et al. 2021). In sum, as laid out in Table 14.1, Reading Comprehension stems from the interaction between the reader's linguistic knowledge and cognitive skills and what is being read.

Table 14.1 Factors involved in Reading Comprehension.

Factors	Content, examples
Text characteristics	• Linguistic complexity • Local coherence • Global coherence
Reader's prior knowledge	• Linguistic knowledge • Knowledge of the topic being read about • Interpersonal and social knowledge
Reader's inference skills	• Ability to complement explicit information with information that is not explicitly stated
Other	• Working Memory • Cognitive load

Reading Skills in Autism

How Well Do Autistic Individuals Read?

Regarding **Word Recognition** skills, a number of early studies targeting reading skills in individuals with ASD reported that Word Recognition is generally preserved. However, more recent studies comparing word reading in ASD and in Typically Developing (TD) individuals have reported more mixed results, with a majority showing lower performance in individuals with ASD, but some showing similar performance or even better performance. In Vale, Fernandes, and Cardoso's (2022) literature review of 24 studies comparing word reading (which requires both lexical access and phonological decoding) and nonword reading (which relies solely on phonological decoding) performance in children with ASD and TD children, approximately 62% found no significant difference between the groups, 35% reported poorer performance for the ASD group, and only 4% found children with ASD to perform better than TD children. A closer scrutiny of the studies shows a considerable amount of heterogeneity among population samples. Although Word Recognition scores may be within norms at the group level, some autistic individuals score above average and others show below or substantially below-average performance (McIntyre et al. 2017; Solari et al. 2022). Additionally, the proportion of autistic individuals who have reading skills that are average for their age is considerably lower than that observed in the TD population. For example, in Solari et al. (2019), only 32.1% of the children with ASD achieved average reading scores, compared to the approximately 80% reported for samples of TD children with similar IQ levels. In summary, there is no clear evidence for a universal strength or weakness in Word Recognition in individuals with ASD: these individuals exhibit high interindividual variability in Word Recognition.

Little is known about how children with ASD process written words – whether they favor lexical access or phonological decoding, for instance. Vale, Fernandes, and Cardoso (2022) reported that only 54% of the studies in their review included measures of word and pseudoword reading, and only 1 out of the 13 studies compared the performance of children with ASD on tests assessing word versus nonword reading. An early study of just five participants, all having advanced reading skills (with respect to their age and their IQ), revealed superior decoding skills for pseudowords and regular words compared to irregular words (Welsh, Pennington, and Rogers 1987), indicating a dominant phonological strategy. However, more recent studies with larger population samples have found evidence for the predominance of a lexical access strategy over a phonological decoding strategy. For example, Henderson, Clarke, and Snowling (2014) reported that the children with ASD in their study exhibited strikingly low levels of nonword reading (phonological decoding), with 8/49 children unable to read any nonwords at all. However, all children obtained average scores on the word reading test (both lexical access and phonological decoding). These results suggest that the children with ASD relied on the lexical access strategy rather than the phonological decoding strategy. In addition, when matched with TD peers on word reading ability, they performed significantly worse on nonword reading tasks, indicating difficulty with the phonological decoding strategy. Similar results have been obtained in other studies (e.g. Nation, Clarke, and Wright 2006), suggesting that word reading and nonword reading abilities are not always the same in individuals with ASD and that some individuals with ASD may use nonphonological strategies for Word Recognition. According to some authors, this may be related to a strength in visual-spatial abilities in individuals with ASD, which is helpful for the recognition of orthographic patterns, facilitating lexical access, and, therefore, allowing for successful word reading. Relatively high lexical access abilities may lead to an overestimation of reading skills and thus mask phonological decoding difficulties in individuals with ASD.

The focus of studies on reading in individuals with ASD has been on **Reading Comprehension** skills. In general, these studies have shown discrepancies between Word Recognition skills and Reading Comprehension abilities in favor of Word Recognition. A meta-analysis reviewing 26 studies (Sorenson Duncan et al. 2021) reports that, at the group level, children with ASD have better word reading than Reading Comprehension. Reading Comprehension seems to be the main pitfall in these children's reading, affecting a large proportion of them (Solari et al. 2019). However, here too, interindividual variability has been observed, and having a diagnosis of ASD does not seem to predict Reading Comprehension skills as individual scores range from severe impairment to within-norm performance in this population (Brown, Oram-Cardy, and Johnson 2013). Moreover, besides interindividual variability, between-study variability has also been observed. While many studies have revealed Reading Comprehension impairment in individuals with ASD, others have not reached the same conclusion (e.g. Mayes and Calhoun 2006). Furthermore, when a difference is found in Reading Comprehension between individuals with and without ASD, the magnitude of this difference varies considerably from one study to another.

Although a discrepancy between Word Recognition and Reading Comprehension in individuals with ASD has been put forward at the group level,

Reading Comprehension does not seem to be independent of Word Recognition in this population. Reading Comprehension in ASD has been shown to be strongly correlated with both oral language abilities (in a variety of linguistic domains) and word reading skills, showing that both skills contribute to performance. In a meta-analysis covering 36 studies on Reading Comprehension skills in children with ASD, linguistic knowledge (in the review, focusing mainly on vocabulary) and Word Recognition came out as the strongest individual predictors of Reading Comprehension (Brown, Oram-Cardy, and Johnson 2013). As such, Reading Comprehension does not seem to be dissociable from Word Recognition in ASD (Sorenson Duncan et al. 2021). These findings support the Simple View of Reading (see Figure 14.1) for individuals with ASD as well.

In addition to Word Recognition and oral language skills, there are other factors influencing Reading Comprehension. Similar to what was presented in Table 14.1 for neurotypical people, Reading Comprehension in individuals with ASD has been shown to be related to inference skills and prior knowledge, although results are mixed. For example, some studies on ASD have reported that social knowledge strongly predicts Reading Comprehension. These studies found that the Reading Comprehension scores of individuals with ASD were lower for highly social texts (texts initially developed to test ToM) than for texts that can be interpreted with limited social knowledge, on which they had normal performance. According to these studies, individuals with ASD seem to have particular difficulties understanding a text that requires social knowledge. This is consistent with their known difficulties in social cognition (Brown, Oram-Cardy, and Johnson 2013). Regarding inference ability, some studies have shown that individuals with ASD have difficulties making inferences (see Chapter 6) and that these difficulties predict Reading Comprehension skills in children and adolescents with ASD (McIntyre et al. 2020). However, other studies have not reached the same conclusions. Saldaña and Frith (2007), for example, found no difference between adolescents with and without ASD in their ability to rely on background knowledge (either physical or social) and to draw inferences. The authors concluded that Reading Comprehension difficulties in individuals with ASD cannot be attributed to an impairment in reliance on background knowledge or in the ability to make implicit inferences. They argue that these difficulties may be related to other processes specific to text reading, as their experimental protocol involved isolated sentences, and not texts.

Other studies propose various other deficits that may explain Reading Comprehension impairment in individuals with ASD. For instance, it has been argued that these individuals have difficulties processing local coherence indices such as associating a pronoun with its referent (e.g. ***The boy*** *misses his father.* ***He*** *hasn't seen him since last year*) or processing the global coherence of a text, which was related to their reported weak central coherence (i.e. the ability to put together bits of information into a global and coherent pattern, see Chapters 6 and 8). However, here again, interindividual variability in the processes involved in Reading Comprehension in individuals with ASD has been found (Jolliffe and Baron-Cohen 2000).

In sum, individuals with ASD vary considerably in their Reading Comprehension skills. Reading Comprehension in this population does seem to be related to Word Recognition and oral language skills (which form the base for Listening Comprehension skills), as predicted by the Simple View of Reading (Figure 14.1). However, there is evident interindividual and inter-study variability in the processes involved in Reading Comprehension in individuals with ASD.

Is There a Specific Reading Profile Associated With Autism?

Reading profiles are based on reading skills, the ability to recognize words and the ability to understand written words, sentences, and texts. The most frequently reported reading profile for individuals with ASD is not in fact that frequent. **Hyperlexia**, Word Recognition skills that exceed Reading Comprehension abilities and verbal or intellectual functioning levels, is commonly believed to be associated with autism. Although frequently reported (Frith and Snowling 1983; O'Connor and Klein 2004; Newman et al. 2007), the normal/advanced Word Recognition with poor Reading Comprehension profile does not apply to all autistic readers. While autism is over-represented among reported cases of hyperlexia (84% in Ostrolenk et al.'s 2017 meta-analysis), as it is in other kinds of savant abilities, only a small proportion of autistic children have in fact been found to display this profile (4–21%, depending on the study, see Nally et al. 2018; Ostrolenk et al. 2017). Thus, the assumption according to which individuals with ASD have intact word reading with impaired Reading Comprehension cannot be applied to all. Indeed, as we have seen above, individuals with ASD vary considerably in both Reading Comprehension and word reading skills, which leads to a variety of reading profiles.

Recall from Figure 14.1 in the Anchoring section that the Simple View of Reading states that Reading Comprehension = Word Recognition × Listening Comprehension. Based on this view, three reading comprehension profiles are typically predicted and discussed in the general reading literature: (i) a profile with good Reading Comprehension, and thus good Word Recognition and good Listening Comprehension, (ii) a profile with poor Reading Comprehension associated with poor Word Recognition (with good or poor Listening Comprehension), and (iii) a profile with poor Reading Comprehension because of poor Listening Comprehension, despite good Word Recognition. This is schematized in Table 14.2, where the three reading profiles are in gray.

Table 14.2 Reading profiles (in gray) predicted by the Simple View of Reading in relation to Listening Comprehension.

Three reading profiles		Listening Comprehension
Reading Comprehension	Word Recognition	
Good	Good	Good
Poor	Poor	Poor/Good
Poor	Good	Poor

These three reading profiles have indeed been found in nonautistic individuals (Catts, Hogan, and Fey 2003). A few studies have explored reading profiles in individuals with ASD. McIntyre et al. (2017) found four reading profiles in children and adolescents with ASD, based on the first two columns in Table 14.2: a profile with average skills on both Word Recognition and Reading Comprehension (with intact cognitive and linguistic skills), a profile with average Word Recognition and impaired Reading Comprehension, (with impaired structural language and listening comprehension), and two profiles with impaired Word Recognition and impaired Reading Comprehension (with deficits in phonology, vocabulary, and Listening Comprehension), differing only in the severity of reading difficulties (a Global Disturbance profile and a Severe Global Disturbance profile).

Solari et al. (2019) conducted a longitudinal study over a 30-month period to verify whether reading profiles in children and adolescents with ASD are stable over time. At the first assessment time, they observed profiles roughly similar to the ones observed by McIntyre et al. (2017), with slight differences, notably concerning the profiles with global disturbance. They also found four profiles: a profile with average Word Recognition and Reading Comprehension, a profile with average Word Recognition and low Reading Comprehension as in McIntyre et al. (2017), as well as two profiles with below average Word Recognition and low Reading Comprehension (one with low linguistic skills, but intact receptive vocabulary, and the other one with generalized low linguistic skills). At the second assessment time (30 months later), they found the same profiles. However, they observed that a number of individuals with ASD transitioned from one profile to another, indicating that profile membership was not stable over time. Importantly, individuals with ASD who transitioned the most were the ones with average Word Recognition but low Reading Comprehension skills (the most documented profile in ASD), followed by the ones with below-average Word Recognition, Reading Comprehension, and linguistic skills (but intact vocabulary). Some individuals with these profiles improved with time to reach an average reading level. Thus, the prognosis of autistic children with Reading Comprehension deficits and average Word Recognition skills seems to be better than that of other profiles of autistic children with reading deficits, namely the profiles with impairment in both Reading Comprehension and Word Recognition. Interestingly, the average Word Recognition but low Reading Comprehension profile concerned only 28% of the sample at the first assessment time, but 47% of them transitioned to average reading skills in both Word Recognition and Reading Comprehension at the second assessment time. The percentage of individuals with this profile became then the lowest in the sample, which raises questions about its prominence in the scientific literature and in public imagination. It is noteworthy that, despite this developmental evolution, the prevalence of reading difficulties remained much higher in individuals with ASD than in the general population.

In sum, diverse reading profiles have been observed in individuals with ASD. These profiles include average global (Word Recognition and Reading Comprehension) reading skills, low global reading skills (Word Recognition and Reading Comprehension), and low Reading Comprehension with average Word Recognition skills.

What Are the Factors That Predict Reading Skills in Individuals with ASD?

Studies exploring predictors of reading skills in individuals with ASD are relatively scarce. Generally, these studies have explored the predictive value of factors such as age and gender, autism impact on daily life, oral language skills, ToM, as well as cognitive skills that are known to predict reading abilities in individuals without ASD, such as letter knowledge, phonological awareness, and rapid automatized naming.

Age and gender do not seem to predict reading profiles. Studies that have explored reading profiles in individuals with ASD have not found an effect of age or gender on identified profiles. Individuals of different ages are equally likely to fit any reading profile (McIntyre et al. 2017; Solari et al. 2019), and there is no reading profile that is associated with a certain age. However, age has been shown to be negatively associated with reading skills in children with ASD. When children get older and/or when reading tasks get more complex, the reading proficiency of individuals with ASD may fall behind (Nally et al. 2018).

Autism symptom severity, which refers to the impact of autism on how the individual is able to function and thus what kind of support is required in everyday life (see Section 2, Chapter 1), has been shown to negatively correlate with reading skills, notably Reading Comprehension skills. Higher autism symptom severity is associated with lower reading performance. Reading profiles characterized by more severe and generalized impairment (e.g. the *Severe Global Disturbance* profile proposed by McIntyre et al. 2017) have been found to be associated with higher autism severity. However, ASD symptom severity measured at a young age (around 3 years) does not seem to be a relevant predictor of later reading performance (Åsberg et al. 2019).

Intellectual ability, generally assessed via a measure of the Intellectual Quotient (IQ), has been claimed to be a poor predictor of reading performance. For instance, the meta-analysis by Brown, Oram-Cardy, and Johnson (2013) showed that nonverbal IQ explains merely 1.33% of the variance in Reading Comprehension performance. However, other studies have reached a different conclusion. For example, in a study by Westerveld et al. (2018), nonverbal cognition (a developmental quotient based on visual and fine motor skills) significantly predicted Word Recognition ability, explaining 17.9% of its variance. Åsberg et al. (2019) examined the role of nonverbal intellectual ability in different reading profiles of children with ASD. Their results showed distinct patterns of nonverbal cognitive skills as a function of profile type. While "Poor Readers" (poor Word Recognition and Reading Comprehension) had low nonverbal cognitive ability, "Skilled Readers" and "Poor Comprehenders" presented average nonverbal cognitive skills. It is noteworthy that most studies exploring reading skills in individuals with ASD have targeted individuals with normal IQs, thus excluding a significant proportion of the autism spectrum, which constitutes a pitfall in their sample representability.

Language skills, oral language abilities in production and reception in all linguistic domains, in individuals with ASD predict reading skills. As mentioned earlier, Reading Comprehension is associated with oral language skills, showing that the *Simple View of Reading* (Figure 14.1) is applicable in this population. In their meta-analysis, Brown, Oram-Cardy, and Johnson (2013) showed that lexical-semantic knowledge (receptive/expressive vocabulary and quality of lexical representations) is the strongest predictor of Reading Comprehension, independently explaining 57% of its variance. Davidson and Weisme (2014) examined predictors of reading in children with ASD in the early stages of reading acquisition. Their results showed that good oral language skills (as measured by omnibus comprehension and expressive scores), particularly at the expressive level, constitute a good predictor of good reading skills in these children. Moreover, children with ASD with language impairment perform significantly lower than children with ASD with normal language on a composite score of reading, including scores on decoding, Word Recognition, and Reading Comprehension (Lindgren et al. 2009, in which language impairment was determined by total language ability scores on the CELF [see Chapter 1] and/or on a test of nonword repetition), which suggests that language impairment may affect reading skills in individuals with ASD.

Theory of Mind (ToM), the ability to infer and understand mental states (e.g. beliefs, true and false) in oneself and others, has been shown to predict Reading Comprehension in individuals with ASD (McIntyre et al. 2018; Ricketts et al. 2013). This association seems, however, dependent on the type of text that is being read and on individual ToM ability. White et al. (2009) showed that text-Reading Comprehension is impaired only in children with ASD with impaired ToM who were reading texts involving biological agents (humans and animals). Conversely, Reading Comprehension was not impaired in this group when reading texts that did not involve agents (nature stories). Moreover, individuals with ASD with relatively preserved ToM did not significantly differ from individuals without ASD in Reading Comprehension, for all text types. The authors argue that a deficit in mental state processing may affect understanding of stories with biological agents.

Letter knowledge is considered one of the main predictors of reading ability in TD children and in children with learning difficulties and disorders. It has been argued that letter knowledge is not a good predictor of reading skills in individuals with ASD. According to some studies, individuals with ASD may perform very well on letter identification and letter naming tasks, but this performance does not necessarily correlate with their other reading-related skills. One possible explanation for this result is that individuals with ASD have strong visual processing abilities and/or may be particularly interested in letters and texts (an example of restricted interests in their Second Dimension autistic symptoms, see Chapter 1, and also the cover and accompanying text for this book), which may enhance their performance on these tasks (Solari et al. 2022).

Phonological awareness has been shown to be associated with Word Recognition in individuals with ASD, as in TD samples (Solari et al. 2022). In a longitudinal study conducted by Åsberg et al. (2022) with children with ASD without intellectual disabilities, phonological awareness predicted word reading accuracy and reading fluency. However, other studies report other results. For instance, Gabig (2010) examined the relationship between phonological awareness abilities and reading accuracy in TD children and children with ASD. The ASD group performed significantly worse on measures of phonological awareness (62% of children with ASD presented highly deficient phonological awareness skills), but there was no significant correlation with reading accuracy in this group. However, the small sample size in this study (only 14 participants with ASD) may bias this result. Other studies have observed different patterns of phonological abilities among reading profiles. McIntyre et al.'s (2017) "Average Readers" profile corresponded to average or above-average performance in phonological abilities (including expressive phonology/phonological memory, and phonological awareness); the "Poor Comprehenders" profile showed adequate phonological abilities;

and the "Global Disturbance" and "Severe Global Disturbance" profiles had lower phonological abilities. Thus, autistic individuals displaying Word Recognition difficulties seem to have lower phonological abilities.

Rapid Automatized Naming (RAN), which has been shown to be relatively low in individuals with ASD (White et al. 2006; Åsberg and Dahlgren Sandberg 2012; Vale, Fernandes, and Cardoso 2022), seems to predict reading performance. For instance, in a longitudinal study conducted by Åsberg et al. (2022), RAN contributed significantly to reading fluency. Similarly, in a longitudinal study by Westerveld et al. (2018), RAN measured in preschool predicted Word Recognition skills in grade 1.

In sum, studies exploring predictors of reading skills in individuals with ASD are not unanimous. Some studies have reported links between reading skills and autism severity, ToM, intellectual ability, language skills, phonological abilities, and Rapid Automatized Naming. However, contrary to what is found in nonautistic individuals, it has been argued that letter knowledge is not a good predictor of reading in individuals with ASD. Age and gender don't seem to be good predictors either.

Finally, a note on the recurrent inter-study inconsistencies is in order. As is true for work on language in autism more generally, there are a number of methodological limitations affecting results and thus our knowledge of reading in autism. Limitations include small sample size, lack of appropriate comparison groups, over-sampling of individuals without DID, and possibly of better oral language skills and of better Word Recognition skills. Moreover, factors such as age have autism-specific effects on differences between study results. Younger children are generally exposed to texts that require relatively limited inference skills, while the texts that are geared toward older children, adolescents, and adults require much more reliance on prior knowledge and inference skills, which would disadvantage older individuals with autism. Studies including samples of young children versus older participants may therefore reach different conclusions concerning the role of prior knowledge and inference skills in Reading Comprehension. Finally, tasks used to assess reading skills and other abilities, such as oral language skills, are not always appropriate for use with individuals with ASD. For instance, most Reading Comprehension tasks generally require an oral response, which can be detrimental to children with ASD who may be disadvantaged by their expressive communication and language difficulties.

Focus on a Specific Study

We have chosen to focus on the study by Åsberg et al. 2019 because it is one of the few studies exploring early predictors (at around age 3) of later reading profiles (at around age 8) in children with ASD. Besides its longitudinal nature, its methodological strength lies in the method used to recruit the participants.

Contrary to most other studies that include clinical samples, participants were identified via general population screening, which reduces sample-related bias. This screening concerned 97.5% of Swedish children, and the authors included in their study all children who screened positive for ASD for whom they had parental consent and who were in first or second grade at the second assessment time, at around age 8 ($n = 53$). Their sample was therefore more representative than those in other studies, which have generally been based on clinical samples and which often apply restrictive inclusionary criteria. Moreover, the authors compared the cohort intake scores of these 53 children with those of all the other children who screened positive for ASD in the general population screening but who did not participate in the reading study because of lack of parental consent or because they were not in first or second grade at the second assessment time. Except for a slight age difference, there were no significant differences in the characteristics of these children based on the cohort intake measures (IQ, language comprehension, autism symptom severity, and adaptive functioning), which suggests that their sample is representative of the general population sample of children with ASD. This study explored reading profiles in individuals with ASD by examining predictors of reading skills within each profile. At around age 3, oral language ability (comprehension and production of words and sentences), cognitive/developmental level, and autism symptomatology, as well as adaptive, communicative, and social functioning were assessed as part of the ASD screening. At around age 8, assessments included oral language comprehension and production of words and sentences, phonological processing (nonword repetition), autism symptomatology, nonverbal cognitive ability, letter knowledge, and reading skills (Word Recognition/fluency and Reading Comprehension).

Exploration of reading profiles at the second assessment time revealed three different profiles. The first one was a profile of "Poor Readers," characterized by performance below the cutoff of – two Standard Deviations on Word Recognition and Reading Comprehension (25/53 children). Most children in this group were preliterate and had low performance even on the letter knowledge task. The second profile consisted of "Poor Comprehenders," who showed a discrepancy between Word Recognition and Reading Comprehension with scores above the cutoff for Word Recognition but below the cutoff for Reading Comprehension (10/53 children). The third profile encompassed a group of "Skilled Readers" who performed above the cutoff on both Word Recognition and Reading Comprehension (18/53 children). These results are in accordance with what is generally found in studies exploring the nature of reading profiles in individuals with ASD that have included samples with more restrictive inclusionary criteria, which reinforces this finding. They also replicated the findings of other studies showing wide heterogeneity in reading skills in individuals with ASD.

The authors then examined the performance of children in each of the three profiles on the other measures, obtained at the same assessment time (at around age 8) or earlier, at the first assessment time (around age 3). The results, summarized in Table 14.3, showed that the "Poor Readers" subgroup had general developmental limitations, with low nonverbal cognitive ability, low language skills, and more severe autism symptomatology. Children in the "Poor Comprehenders" subgroup showed more selective impairment in oral language skills and Reading Comprehension when compared to the skilled readers, which is in line with the Simple View of Reading. Taken together, the results of the "Poor Readers" and the "Poor Comprehenders" subgroups suggest that a variety of oral language skills measured around the age of 3 may predict (five years) later reading skills, notably Reading Comprehension, in children with ASD. Thus, supporting oral language skills in young children with ASD may help promote later reading skills.

Another interesting finding in this study concerns phonological processing skills. Phonological processing skills were shown to be low in the "Poor Readers"

Table 14.3 Comparison of the three reading profiles in Åsberg et al. 2019.

	Poor Readers 25/53 (47%)		Poor Comprehenders 10/53 (19%)		Skilled Readers 18/53 (34%)
Word Recognition (age 8)	Poor		Average		Average
Reading Comprehension (age 8)	Poor		Poor		Average
Nonverbal cognitive ability (age 8)	Poor Readers	<	Poor Comprehenders	=	Skilled Readers
Autism severity (age 8)	Poor Readers	>	Poor Comprehenders	=	Skilled Readers
Oral language skills (age 8)	Poor Readers	=	Poor Comprehenders	<	Skilled Readers
Phonological processing (age 8)	Poor Readers	<	Poor Comprehenders	=	Skilled Readers
Nonverbal cognitive ability (age 3)	Poor Readers	=	Poor Comprehenders	=	Skilled Readers
Autism severity (age 3)	Poor Readers	=	Poor Comprehenders	=	Skilled Readers
Oral language skills (age 3)	Poor Readers	=	Poor Comprehenders	<	Skilled Readers

Source: Åsberg et al. (2019). Reproduced with permission of Sage Publications.

but not in the "Poor Comprehenders." This suggests that phonology is intertwined with Word Recognition skills in individuals with ASD, similar to what is found in individuals without ASD.

Concerning autism symptom severity, although children in the "Poor Readers" subgroup had more severe symptoms before the age of 3, there was no difference in autism severity between the subgroups around the age of 8. The authors argue that this result suggests that it is hard to predict reading ability based on an early measure of autism severity. They interpret the higher autism severity measure in the "Poor Readers" subgroup at age 3 as a sign that this subgroup has more pervasive general developmental difficulties. Interestingly, there was no difference in autism symptom severity between the "Poor Readers" subgroup and the "Poor Comprehenders" subgroup. This finding does not support the hypothesis presented above according to which autism symptom severity is related to Reading Comprehension difficulties. This hypothesis suggests that autistic individuals' specific deficits in social and communication skills and in inference-making may impede Reading Comprehension, which was not the case in the Åsberg et al. study. Their result may be related, however, to the young age (8) of the children in the study, as the type of texts that are read in first and second grade may be less dependent on these skills.

In sum, this study, carried out with autistic children recruited through a general population sample screening, is consistent with the findings of other studies exploring reading profiles in individuals with ASD. It found three reading profiles in ASD, namely, "Poor Readers," "Poor Comprehenders," and "Skilled Readers." It also highlights the role of oral language (comprehension and production of words and sentences) and phonological processing in reading development in this population.

Conclusion

This chapter aimed to answer the following questions:

- How well do autistic individuals read?
- Is there a specific reading profile associated with autism?
- What are the factors that predict reading skills in individuals with autism?

Studies exploring reading skills in individuals with ASD have focused mainly on Reading Comprehension. Individuals with ASD have often been presented as having intact Word Recognition skills but impaired Reading Comprehension. However, studies examining reading profiles and individual abilities show high interindividual variability in this population. Reading Comprehension is often, but not universally, impaired in individuals with ASD, and Word Recognition skills can be impaired. The proportion of reading impairment affecting Reading Comprehension and/or Word Recognition is higher than what is observed in the general population.

In individuals with ASD, three different patterns of reading profiles are generally found. These correspond to a profile with intact Word Recognition and Reading Comprehension skills ("Skilled Readers"), a profile with intact Word Recognition but impaired Reading Comprehension ("Poor Comprehenders"), and a profile with impaired Word Recognition and Reading Comprehension ("Poor Readers"). Moreover, Word Recognition skills seem to predict Reading Comprehension skills, along with oral language skills, which is compatible with the Simple View of Reading. In addition to language skills, several other factors seem to predict reading performance, such as autism symptom severity, ToM (depending on the text that is being read), and known predictors of reading skills in the general population, such as phonological awareness and rapid automatized naming.

It is noteworthy, however, that despite the growth of the number of studies in the field, several methodological limitations of existing studies limit understanding of reading skills in individuals with ASD. These limitations concern mainly the sample size that is often insufficient, the inclusionary criteria of individuals with ASD that are often very restrictive, the characteristics of the control groups to which individuals with ASD are compared, and the tasks used. They result in inconsistent findings between studies, which add to the important interindividual differences inherent to ASD. In a nutshell, the results of studies on reading in individuals with ASD are in line with Towgood et al.'s (2009) claim that the most defining characteristic of individuals with ASD is variability.

> **What Do You Know Now?**
> Individuals with autism display a wide range of reading skills.
> - It is possible for individuals with ASD to access written language. Some individuals reach average to above-average performance in both Word Recognition and Reading Comprehension.
> - A significant proportion of individuals with ASD encounter reading difficulties. These difficulties may affect Word Recognition and/or Reading Comprehension. Reading Comprehension difficulties remain the most frequently reported difficulty. However, different reading profiles seem to exist in ASD.

Suggestion for Further Reading

If you are interested in learning more about reading in individuals with ASD, we recommend that you read Sorenson Duncan et al. 2021. It is a recent meta-analysis that reviews the state of knowledge on the different components of the Simple View of Reading in individuals with ASD. Like all meta-analyses, it combines the results of a number of studies. It also has the advantage of pointing out the methodological limitations in existing studies, and it is rather easy to read.

References

Åsberg, J. and Dahlgren Sandberg, A. (2012). Dyslexic, delayed, precocious or just normal? Word reading skills of children with autism spectrum disorders. *Journal of Research in Reading* 35 (1): 20–31.

Åsberg, J., Carlsson, E., Norbury, C. et al. (2019). Current profiles and early predictors of reading skills in school-age children with Autism Spectrum Disorders: a longitudinal, retrospective population study. *Autism* 23 (6): 1449–1459.

Åsberg, J., Fernell, E., Kjellmer, L. et al. (2022). Language/cognitive predictors of literacy skills in 12-year-old children on the autism spectrum. *Logopedics, Phoniatrics, Vocology* 47 (3): 166–170.

Brown, H.M., Oram-Cardy, J., and Johnson, A. (2013). A meta-analysis of the Reading Comprehension skills of individuals on the autism spectrum. *Journal of Autism and Developmental Disorders* 43: 932–955.

Catts, H.W., Hogan, T.P., and Fey, M.E. (2003). Subgrouping poor readers on the basis of individual differences in reading-related abilities. *Journal of Learning Disabilities* 36 (2): 151–164.

Coltheart, M. (2006). Dual route and connectionist models of reading: an overview. *London Review of Education* 4: 5–17.

Davidson, M.M. and Ellis Weismer, S. (2014). Characterization and prediction of early reading abilities in children on the autism spectrum. *Journal of Autism and Developmental Disorders* 24 (4): 828–845.

Frith, U. and Snowling, M. (1983). Reading for meaning and reading for sound in autistic and dyslexic children. *Journal of Developmental Psychology* 1: 329–342.

Gabig, C. (2010). Phonological awareness and Word Recognition in reading by children with autism. *Communication Disorders Quarterly* 31: 67–85.

Gough, P.B. and Tunmer, W.E. (1986). Decoding, reading, and reading disability. *Remedial and Special Education* 7 (1): 6–10.

Henderson, L.M., Clarke, P.J., and Snowling, M.J. (2014). Reading Comprehension impairments in Autism Spectrum Disorders. *L'Annee Psycholgique* 114: 779–797.

Jolliffe, T. and Baron-Cohen, S. (2000). Linguistic processing in high-functioning adults with autism or Asperger's syndrome: is global coherence impaired? *Psychological Medicine* 30: 1169–1187.

Lindgren, K.A., Folstein, S.E., Tomblin, J.B., et al. (2009). Language and reading abilities of children with Autism Spectrum Disorders and Specific Language Impairment and their first-degree relatives. *Autism Research* 2: 22–38.

Mayes, S.D. and Calhoun, S.L. (2006). Frequency of reading, math, and writing disabilities in children with clinical disorders. *Learning and Individual Differences* 16: 145–157.

McIntyre, N.S., Grimm, R.P., Solari, E.J. et al. (2020). Growth in narrative retelling and inference abilities and relations with Reading Comprehension in children and adolescents with Autism Spectrum Disorder. *Autism and Developmental Language Impairments* 5: 2396941520968028.

McIntyre, N.S., Oswald, T.M., Solari, E.J. et al. (2018). Social cognition and Reading Comprehension in children and adolescents with Autism Spectrum Disorders or typical development. *Research in Autism Spectrum Disorders* 54: 9–20.

McIntyre, N.S., Solari, E.J., Grimm, R.P. et al. (2017). A comprehensive examination of reading heterogeneity in students with high functioning autism: distinct reading profiles and their relation to autism symptom severity. *Journal of Autism and Developmental Disorders* 47 (4): 1086–1101.

Nally, A., Healy, O., Holloway, J. et al. (2018). An analysis of reading abilities in children with Autism Spectrum Disorders. *Research in Autism Spectrum Disorders* 47: 14–25.

Nation, K., Clarke, P., and Wright, B. (2006). Patterns of reading ability in children with Autism Spectrum Disorder. *Journal of Autism and Developmental Disorders* 36: 911–919.

Newman, T.M., Macomber, D., Naples, A.J. et al. (2007). Hyperlexia in children with Autism Spectrum Disorders. *Journal of Autism and Developmental Disorders* 37: 760–774.

O'Connor, I.M. and Klein, P.D. (2004). Exploration of strategies for facilitating the Reading Comprehension of high-functioning students with Autism Spectrum Disorders. *Journal of Autism and Developmental Disorders* 34: 115–127.

Ostrolenk, A., Forgeot d'Arc, B., Jelenic, P. et al. (2017). Hyperlexia: systematic review, neurocognitive modelling, and outcome. *Neuroscience & Biobehavioral Reviews* 79: 134–149.

Ricketts, J., Jones, C.R.G., Happé, F. et al. (2013). Reading Comprehension in Autism Spectrum Disorders: the role of oral language and social functioning. *Journal of Autism and Developmental Disorders* 43: 807–816.

Saldaña, D. and Frith, U. (2007). Do readers with autism make bridging inferences from world knowledge? *Journal of Experimental Child Psychology* 96: 310–319.

Smith, R., Snow, P., Serry, T. et al. (2021). The role of background knowledge in Reading Comprehension: a critical review. *Reading Psychology* 42 (3): 214–240.

Smith, N.V. and Tsimpli, I.M. (1995). *The Mind of a Savant: Language Learning and Modularity*. Hoboken, NJ: Blackwell.

Solari, E.J., Grimm, R.P., McIntyre, N.S. et al. (2019). Longitudinal stability of reading profiles in individuals with higher functioning autism. *Autism* 23 (8): 1911–1926.

Solari, E.J., Henry, A.R., Grimm, R.P. et al. (2022). Code-related literacy profiles of kindergarten students with autism. *Autism* 26 (1): 230–242.

Sorenson Duncan, T., Karkada, M., Deacon, S.H. et al. (2021). Building meaning: meta-analysis of component skills supporting Reading Comprehension in children with Autism Spectrum Disorder. *Autism Research* 14 (5): 840–858.

Towgood, K.J., Meuwese, J.D.I., Gilbert, S.J. et al. (2009). Advantages of the multiple case series approach to the study of cognitive deficits in Autism Spectrum Disorder. *Neuropsychologia* 47: 2981–2988.

Vale, A.P., Fernandes, C., and Cardoso, S. (2022). Word reading skills in Autism Spectrum Disorder: a systematic review. *Frontiers in Psychology* 13: 930275.

Welsh, C.M., Pennington, B.F., and Rogers, S. (1987). Word Recognition and comprehension skills in hyperlexic children. *Brain and Language* 32: 76–96.

Westerveld, M.F., Paynter, J., O'Leary, K. et al. (2018). Preschool predictors of reading ability in the first year of schooling in children with ASD. *Autism Research* 11: 1332–1344.

White, S., Frith, U., Milne, E. et al. (2006). A double dissociation between sensorimotor impairments and reading disability: a comparison of autistic and dyslexic children. *Cognitive Neuropsychology* 23: 748–761.

White, S., Hill, E., Happé, F. et al. (2009). Revisiting the strange stories: revealing mentalizing impairments in autism. *Child Development* 80: 1097–1117.

15

Brain, Language, and Autism

Caroline Larson and Inge-Marie Eigsti

> **What Do You Think?**
> You watch the movie *Rain Man* and the TV shows *The Good Doctor* and *Atypical*. Fictional depictions such as these portray unique abilities, such as rapid counting and exceptional drawing, and language differences, such as using only single words or very formal language to communicate, in autistic characters. They both reflect and shape societal views of neurodevelopmental conditions. You wonder, "Could the characters' differences be related to the way their brains work?"
>
> You attend a lecture on fMRI studies of language in ASD. Given that autism is diagnosed from behavior features alone, you wonder why we bother with such expensive and specialized methods.
>
> The key concept of this chapter is that differences in brain networks associated with language can reveal autistic differences in language comprehension and production. How do you think examining brain function can reveal information about the unique capabilities that individuals with autism have and about the core diagnostic features of autism? How might information derived from brain function differ from or clarify information derived from studies of behavior?

Introduction

Alongside the behavioral features of autism, this neurodevelopmental disorder is characterized by important differences in the neural circuitry underlying language processing. Regarding brain structure, most neurotypical individuals have larger left hemisphere volumes of brain regions that are important for language, compared to the same regions in the right hemisphere (the right

Language in Autism, First Edition. Edited by Jeannette Schaeffer et al.
© 2025 John Wiley & Sons Ltd. Published 2025 by John Wiley & Sons Ltd.

half of the brain). This asymmetry is due to the neural specialization of left hemisphere regions for the purpose of language functions. In contrast, the brains of autistic individuals seem to be more symmetrical, suggesting that language difficulties are associated with reduced left hemisphere specialization for language in the brain. The activity of brain regions involved in language also differs in autism. Examining brain activity reveals nuanced and important differences in the processes underlying language production and comprehension in neurotypical and autistic individuals, even when their language behavior appears similar.

This chapter addresses the following questions:

- How do language-related brain regions and networks differ between autistic and neurotypical individuals?
- How do language-related brain functions reflect behaviorally measured language skills and inform clinical practice?

Anchoring

As demonstrated in this book, the expression of thought in spoken language is complex. Brain imaging provides an exceptionally powerful tool for examining where and how language is processed in the brain. One widely used neuroimaging tool is **magnetic resonance imaging** (MRI), which uses the signal generated by blood flow in the brain to reveal the structure and function of the human brain. Anatomical, or structural, research has been carried out since the 1970s, but functional MRI (fMRI) research, first published by Kwong in the early 1990s, initiated a scientific revolution (Kwong et al. 1992). A review by Price (2010) described the brain regions consistently involved in language processing. This review was replicated and extended in a study of 1200 fMRI brain scans collected as part of the Human Connectome Project. This study described how those regions work together, forming **neural networks** that are critical for language function (Briggs et al. 2018).

> **Acronym and Terminology Reminder**
> **Default Mode Network:** The brain network that is activated when no particular task is being performed.
> **fMRI:** Functional Magnetic Resonance Imaging. An imaging technique whose purpose is to obtain images of cerebral activity by tracking the blood flow.
> **Global Connectivity (for Language):** Neural connectivity of brain regions that are classically associated with language function with regions that are not classically associated with language function.
> **Left/Right Hemisphere:** Left/right half of the brain.
> **Local Connectivity (for Language):** Neural connectivity among brain regions classically associated with language function.
> **MRI:** Magnetic Resonance Imaging. An imaging technique used to form pictures of the anatomy inside the body (organs, tissues, and bones).

Figure 15.1 depicts the left half (hemisphere) of the human brain. The highlighted regions associated with producing and understanding language form frontal (dark gray) and temporal (light gray) language networks. A large body of work has examined how these regions and networks become specialized for language function over the course of development. This work shows that the left and right hemispheres are both involved in language processing early in life, but the **left hemisphere** becomes increasingly dominant, or specialized, for language function. By early adulthood, 60% of individuals show no significant language-related

Neural Network: Functional connections between two or more brain regions that show a statistical association in activity, suggesting an enduring relationship.

Over-Connectivity: Greater connectivity between brain regions compared to neurotypical individuals.

RDoC: Research Domain Criteria. A research framework for studying mental health that de-emphasizes diagnostic categories and focuses instead on basic human functional domains (e.g. cognition, language, and social processes).

Resting-State Paradigm: An fMRI methodology where participants are asked to lie quietly and let their minds wander.

Task-Based Paradigm: An fMRI methodology where participants are asked to respond to a stimulus, typically by pressing a button on a hand-held response device.

Under-Connectivity: Less connectivity between brain regions compared to neurotypical individuals.

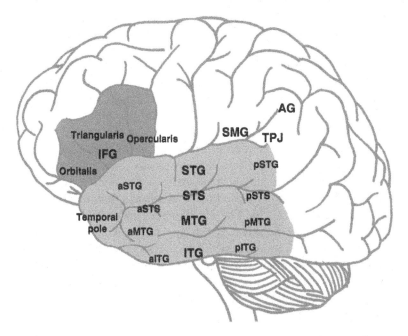

Figure 15.1 The language network includes brain regions involved in comprehending and producing language. *Source:* Larson et al. (2023). Reproduced with permission of Springer Nature.

activation in the right hemisphere (Olulade et al. 2020). Nearly all adults – about 95%, including most left-handed individuals – have highly dominant left hemisphere activation for language function, particularly in the regions depicted in Figure 15.1. For instance, inferior frontal gyrus functions (in dark gray) include articulatory phonology and linear morphosyntax, and temporal lobe functions (in light gray) include auditory phonology (posterior superior temporal gyrus), hierarchical lexical-syntactic (posterior middle temporal gyrus), and conceptual semantic processing (anterior temporal lobe; Matchin and Hickock 2020).

This knowledge of which brain regions and networks are associated with language function and how these regions and networks become specialized for language function contributes to our understanding of **language impairments** in autism (see below). Two fMRI methodologies are important for this research: resting-state and task-based paradigms. In **resting-state paradigms**, participants are asked to lie quietly and look at a still image such as a plus sign (a fixation cross) or at simple shapes that gently drift across the screen. Results show remarkable test-retest reliability (Chen et al. 2015). They are thought to reveal spontaneous brain activity during mind-wandering. Resting-state paradigms are thought to engage the **default mode network**, a task-negative network that is activated when we think about ourselves and when we process social information (Wang et al. 2021). A resting-state scan can provide a useful baseline for comparison with task-specific conditions. Many studies that have examined resting-state fMRI brain scans in autism used a large, multi-site database of thousands of autistic and non-autistic individuals aged 7–64 years, the Autism Brain Imaging Data Exchange (Di Martino et al. 2013).

In **task-based paradigms**, participants are asked to respond to a stimulus presented by eye, ear, or other sensory modality, typically by pressing a button on a hand-held response device (though many different responses are possible). Task-based paradigms compare **brain function** elicited by the task (the experimental condition) to brain function during a comparison task (the control condition) or to a resting-state baseline condition. Some studies use a subtractive design, where brain activity during the control condition is subtracted from brain activity during the experimental condition. The remaining activation is thought to reflect processing demands specific to the experimental task. Adaptive or stairstep paradigms are another design option. In such tasks, subsequent trials in a task become easier if the participant responds to a trial incorrectly or harder if the participant responds to a trial correctly. This approach reduces the impact of errors, fatigue, and comprehension challenges and is thought to probe the function of interest with greater sensitivity.

Task-based fMRI studies in the language domain typically home in on a specific linguistic domain or construct, such as phonology, semantics, or morphosyntax. Participants might judge whether a stimulus is a real word (lexical decision), categorize words (e.g. animate vs. nonanimate), categorize vowels (e.g. judge whether a speech sound was "sh" or "ss"), or listen to short stories. Some studies contrast neural responses to real speech with responses to acoustically comparable nonspeech (such as speech recordings that are acoustically "flipped," known as spectrally rotated speech). Recently, there have been advances in the validity and reliability of language tasks administered during fMRI. For instance, a study on adults with **aphasia** (a language disorder that results from brain injury) used an adaptive task-based paradigm to study language processing (Wilson, Yen, and Eriksson 2018). Participants judged the semantic similarity of related (e.g. *cash-money*) or unrelated (e.g. *age-night*) word pairs. In the nonlinguistic control condition, they judged the perceptual similarity of matching versus nonmatching (e.g. dᘔᔦNᔥ – ᔥᘔᔦNᔥ) symbol pairs. Use of this clever adaptive design meant that all participants performed at a similar level of accuracy, despite their heterogenous language abilities.

In addition to fMRI, brain function can be noninvasively studied using functional near-infrared spectroscopy (fNIRS), electroencephalography (EEG; see Vissers, Cohen, and Geurts 2012; Herringshaw et al. 2016), and magnetoencephalography (MEG). These methods identify regions of the brain that are active by measuring local changes in blood flow or changes in the strength of electrical currents generated by populations of neurons (see Lenartowicz and Poldrack's 2010 chapter for an excellent review).

Decades of functional neuroimaging research with neurotypical adults and individuals with aphasia highlight the regions that are central to language processing (Figure 15.1). In addition, studies of language development show that the left side of the brain (the left hemisphere) becomes specialized for language function by adolescence (Olulade et al. 2020). The brain regions that are most responsible for language function are in the left hemisphere and include the left inferior frontal gyrus (LIFG, also called Broca's area) and the left posterior superior temporal gyrus (LpSTG, also called Wernicke's area), and temporal lobe regions including superior temporal sulcus (STS), middle temporal gyrus (MTG), inferior temporal gyrus (ITG), middle and anterior STG, as well as parietal lobe regions next to the pSTG, including the temporoparietal junction (TPJ), angular gyrus (AG), and supramarginal gyrus (SMG); see Figure 15.1. This network of language regions is active during language processing tasks. Reflecting the Hebbian view that "cells that fire together, wire together," a neural network is defined in terms of functional connections, or two or more brain regions that consistently activate in synchrony (Vissers, Cohen, and Geurts 2012; Larson et al. 2023). This functional connectivity suggests enduring, systematic communication among brain regions. Reduced lateralization of language function to the left hemisphere, as we see in younger children with lower language ability relative to adults, is thought to be associated with poorer comprehension and production, likely because a language network that is more fragmented is less efficient. Complex behaviors, like language and social function, involve broad networks. To understand these behaviors, we must understand not only the individual regions involved but also how these regions interact (Vissers, Cohen, and Geurts 2012; Wang et al. 2021).

Language-Related Brain Function in Autism

Autism Spectrum Disorder (ASD) is a neurodevelopmental condition characterized by social interaction difficulties and the presence of restricted and repetitive interests and behaviors and sensory sensitivities (see Chapter 1 for details). One of the earliest signs of autism that parents report is a language delay. Autistic children often produce their first words at age 24–36 months, with first phrases even later (see Chapter 10). There is tremendous heterogeneity in language skills in autism. About a third of autistic individuals are minimally verbal, while others are verbally fluent with subtle difficulties in semantics, pragmatics, and discourse. Some have significant difficulties with structural language, including morphology (e.g. past-tense "-ed" use – see Chapter 11) and syntax (e.g. comprehension of center-embedded clauses, such as the portion in parentheses in the sentence *The store [that normally stocked batteries] ran out during the storm*). These difficulties are similar to those seen in the condition called **Developmental Language Disorder** (see Chapters 3 and 11). Co-occurring structural language impairment in ASD is referred to as "language disorder associated with autism" (Bishop et al. 2017). In part due to this linguistic heterogeneity, the most recent version of the DSM (American Psychological Association 2013) removed language impairment from autism diagnostic criteria, instead adding a specifier that notes whether the autism occurs with accompanying language impairment (see Chapters 1, 10, and 11 for further discussion, as well as Schaeffer 2018; Schaeffer et al. 2023).

In the next section, we start by addressing the first question raised in the introduction, namely how language-related brain regions and networks differ between autistic and neurotypical individuals, describing studies of language-related neural function in ASD. We describe a recent systematic review that shows a clear picture of the language network in autism (Larson et al. 2023) and talk about how this neural network connects to language abilities and autism features. We then discuss what this research means for clinical practice. In the next section, we highlight a recent study that adopts the framework of **Research Domain Criteria** (Insel et al. 2010) to study language ability and autistic features using fMRI (Larson et al. 2022). The Research Domain Criteria framework focuses on symptoms and characteristics (e.g. behavior and physiology) that cut across diagnostic categories by studying how a given characteristic, rather than a given diagnosis, maps onto genes, cells, and neural circuits.

How Do Language-Related Brain Regions and Networks Differ Between Autistic and Neurotypical Individuals?

Studies of brain functioning during language processing enhance our understanding of autism. For instance, a study comparing autistic and nonautistic adolescents reported striking differences in brain activation during sentence comprehension, even though their accuracy on the task was similar (Eigsti et al. 2016). Such differences in activation suggest that different neural processes are engaged in autism during this task that taps several language domains, including semantics and syntax. Though still in the early stages, this research should reveal how differences in neural specialization reflect the different language abilities and experiences of autistic individuals.

Recent research on autism has focused on neural networks: patterns of connection, or communication, among the regions identified in Figure 15.1 (Vissers, Cohen, and Geurts 2012; Di Martino et al. 2013). Neural networks become functionally connected over the course of development and are critical for complex behaviors like social and language functioning. Autism seems to be characterized by a unique neural network architecture. Resting-state studies show a more strongly connected network of regions important in sensory and motor functioning in autistic individuals of varied ages, with a more weakly connected network of other regions, including the default mode network, important in social functioning (Vissers, Cohen, and Geurts 2012; Wang et al. 2021).

In a recent systematic review of fMRI studies of language-related functional connectivity (Larson et al. 2023), the authors investigated the hypothesis that autism is characterized by differences in language-based functional connectivity. This hypothesis, based on seminal work by Casanova et al. (2002) and Just et al. (2004), states that **local over-connectivity** and **global under-connectivity** represent neurological markers of ASD. Over-connectivity is defined as greater connectivity between brain regions in autistic than neurotypical individuals, while under-connectivity is defined as less connectivity between brain regions in autistic than neurotypical individuals. Beyond the neural evidence, this hypothesis also reflects behavioral evidence that autistic individuals tend to focus on detailed, or local, information at the expense of more integrated, or global, information.

For instance, autistic individuals excel at picking out a picture that is embedded within a larger image but have difficulty identifying a complete image when only partial features are present (Booth and Happé 2018). The search terms used in the review by Larson et al. (2023) reflected this research question, including autism (the population), functional connectivity (the method/construct), and language (the more precise construct).

In this review, it was found that research studies have been inconsistent in how they define local and global connectivity (e.g. in terms of distance between regions and in terms of within vs. between network states). To address this inconsistency, the review developed consistent, network-based definitions for these constructs: local connectivity was defined as connectivity among regions within the language network (the gray areas in Figure 15.1); global connectivity was defined as connectivity between language regions (Figure 15.1) and out-of-network regions (i.e. regions not classically associated with language, including right hemisphere homologue regions). The systematic review included task-based and resting-state studies, measured functional connectivity, and examined language-relevant regions. The review distinguished between distinct language tasks (e.g. passive listening vs. sentence comprehension) to probe different aspects of brain activity that underlie language processing.

Results from task-based studies revealed that patterns of brain activity were not associated with a given task or language domain. Rather, there was strong evidence of local over-connectivity and global under-connectivity in ASD across studies employing different language tasks (e.g. lexical decision and narrative comprehension). Specifically, multiple task-based studies reported greater connectivity among language regions, such as LIFG (Broca's area) and LpSTG (Wernicke's area), in autistic individuals relative to neurotypical peers. In contrast, there was strong evidence of diminished global connectivity between language regions and out-of-network regions. For example, studies consistently reported under-connectivity of the LpSTG (in the language area) with visual regions and the right hemisphere MTG, and under-connectivity of LIFG (in the language area) with prefrontal regions and the right hemisphere pSTG. There was one exception to these patterns, in a finding of under-connectivity among language regions, namely between left MTG and LIFG, in response to more "social" language tasks (e.g. comprehending **nonliteral language**). This under-connectivity may reflect the social nature of these tasks, given that the MTG is a key region in the "social brain" and that social function is characterized by general patterns of under-connectivity in autism.

Across resting-state studies, where participants were engaged in mind-wandering, in contrast to language tasks, which necessitate a response, the systematic review provided more mixed evidence. Consistent with the task-based studies, multiple studies reported global under-connectivity in ASD between left hemisphere language and right hemisphere language homologue regions. However, some studies of autistic children and adolescents revealed a pattern of global over-connectivity of language regions with the default mode network and visual regions. This finding differs from the general pattern of global under-connectivity. Multiple studies in the review demonstrated mixed patterns of over- and under-connectivity in the default mode network in ASD relative to neurotypical peers. This pattern is broadly consistent with a spatial definition of local versus global connectivity (i.e. over-connectivity among proximal regions, under-connectivity among distal regions) rather than the network definition that was adopted in the review (i.e. local = within the language network, global = between language regions and regions outside the classic language network). These results were associated with ASD status but not with behavioral measures of language or social skills.

Three resting-state studies tested lateralization of language-related functional connectivity, which is of particular interest for this chapter. Two studies reported diminished left relative to right hemisphere connectivity in the language network in autistic relative to neurotypical peers (Cardinale et al. 2013; Nielsen et al. 2014), and the third study found no group differences (Gao et al. 2019). However, the regions tested in these studies differed. Cardinale et al. (2013) did not report specific regions within their language network, whereas Gao et al. (2019) and Nielson et al. (2014) included classic language regions (Figure 15.1) and out-of-network regions. Thus, while there is evidence of group differences in the neural specialization of the left hemisphere language network in autism, identifying precise differences requires evidence from future studies. Moreover, no studies to date have tested the lateralization of task-based functional connectivity of language networks.

Many of the studies in the systematic review examined associations between functional connectivity and behavior using resting-state designs. There was consistent evidence that both local over-connectivity and global under-connectivity were associated with more (or stronger) **autism features**, as measured by scores on diagnostic tests and measures of social communication and restricted and repetitive interests and behaviors. This finding supports the hypothesis that local over-connectivity and global under-connectivity during resting-state paradigms are important features of autism. Furthermore, there was consistent evidence that greater connectivity among language regions and between language and out-of-network regions was associated with relatively better language skills in ASD. Language skills were measured using normed clinical assessments such as the Clinical Evaluation of Language Fundamentals (CELF). The association between greater connectivity and better language abilities was evident across language task paradigms and resting-state paradigms. This finding differs from patterns of findings between connectivity and autism features, representing a dissociation between autism features and language skills (Table 15.1), similar to that observed in Larson et al. (2022), which is highlighted below.

Table 15.1 Model of language task-based connectivity in autism.

N.B. Positive association (+) indicates that greater connectivity is associated with more autism features and better language assessment scores; negative association (−) indicates that reduced connectivity is associated with relatively more autism features and poorer language assessment scores. The evidence does not support a clear model of language-related resting-state connectivity.

Language task-based connectivity	Autism vs. neurotypical connectivity	Associations with autism feature	Associations with language abilities
Within language network	−	+	+
Between language network and other regions	−	+	−

Caveat: Evidence of IFG and MTG under-connectivity within the language network in autism for tasks with social features

Source: Larson et al. (2023). Reproduced with permission of Springer Nature.

This systematic review revealed three conclusions and several methodological considerations that would not have been possible in an individual study. First, evidence clearly supports the hypothesis that ASD is characterized by local over-connectivity and global under-connectivity of the language network (Table 15.1). Second, modest evidence from the resting-state studies indicates global under-connectivity of the language network with language homologue regions. This under-connectivity suggests diminished integration processes that may negatively affect higher-level language skills (e.g. narrative comprehension) rather than lower-level language skills (e.g. single-word comprehension). There was also modest evidence from resting-state studies suggesting that global over-connectivity of language regions with default mode network and visual regions reflects autism features rather than language skills. Third, greater connectivity was consistently associated with better behavioral language skills. It is possible that the social context in which language is acquired and deployed affects the neural specialization for language function in autism, resulting in compensatory or supportive functions of language-specific connectivity during social interaction. Examining local over-connectivity and global under-connectivity remains a fruitful avenue for research on the neurobiological underpinnings of autism, though it is important to bear in mind the caveat that connectivity patterns depend on methodological details. The social demands within a given task, and the decision to analyze neural functions versus neuro-behavioral associations, are important methodological considerations in testing neural accounts of ASD.

Most studies examining language-related neural function in autism to date do not account for the possibility of significant impairment in morphosyntax (Eigsti et al. 2011) or other relevant co-occurring conditions (e.g. attention-deficit/hyperactivity disorder). They largely exclude individuals who are nonspeaking or have **intellectual disability**. Because most studies in the literature so far include only speaking individuals with age-appropriate cognitive abilities, the current literature ignores the tremendous linguistic heterogeneity in autism. This presents an exciting opportunity: identifying neural patterns specific to language impairment versus specific to autism may be highly informative. For instance, specialization for language may be quite different in autistic individuals with significant versus more subtle language differences (e.g. the use of more formal vocabulary or less varied prosody). Two studies have compared **brain structure** in autistic individuals with and without structural language impairment and included comparison groups with Developmental Language Disorder and neurotypical development. These studies found more left/right similarity of brain volumes in the language-impaired groups (De Fossé et al. 2004; Herbert et al. 2005), which suggests less neural specialization of the left hemisphere for individuals with language impairment. However, brain structure and brain function are not identical.

How Do Language-Related Brain Functions Reflect Behaviorally Measured Language Skills and Inform Clinical Practice?

Here, we describe how the evidence and the kind of basic scientific research described above can lead to a deeper understanding in the short term and, potentially, to clinical advances in the long term. First, examining neural function can reveal processes or mechanisms that underlie behavior, even when behavior looks similar in autistic and neurotypical individuals on the surface. In multiple studies (e.g. Eigsti et al. 2016; Larson et al. 2022), individuals with a history of autism who no longer have symptoms of autism (**Loss of Autism Diagnosis**; approximately 9–15% of individuals diagnosed with autism in childhood; e.g. Helt et al. 2008; Fein et al. 2013; Anderson, Liang, and Lord 2014) achieve language abilities similar to neurotypical peers but use alternate or compensatory neural circuitry while engaging in language comprehension. This result echoes findings from successfully remediated **dyslexia** (Eden et al. 2004), where formerly dyslexic readers with currently age-appropriate reading skills engage distinct neural systems during reading. Interventions that support the engagement and strengthening of alternative strategies (e.g. through targeted practice and alternative processing strategies) may lead to improved language comprehension and production, particularly in challenging contexts (e.g. in the classroom). For instance, if autistic students rely more heavily on nonlanguage brain regions during language processing, such as prefrontal regions associated with **Executive Function** (EF) processes (such as inhibition, memory, and decision-making), **interventions** that engage and strengthen those EF processes may have downstream effects on language processing. These findings highlight neural pathways that are less engaged in autistic individuals and thus represent potential treatment targets. Of course, this speculative proposal awaits empirical testing.

Functional neuroimaging research may also lead to the discovery of **neurobiological markers** of autism that help us identify and understand what it means to have this condition. For instance, the systematic review of language-related functional connectivity revealed that local over-connectivity and global under-connectivity are reliable characteristics of language-related neural function in autism (Larson et al. 2023). This finding was further validated by showing that these functional connectivity measures were associated with ASD features measured by tools used to diagnose autism in clinical settings (e.g. the Autism Diagnostic Observation Schedule [ADOS] and Autism Diagnostic Interview [ADI]). These findings link hot-off-the-press neuroimaging results to earlier behavioral theories of autism. Analyzing neural function allows researchers and clinicians to identify underlying processes and build and test hypotheses, which can then guide models of autism as a diagnostic entity and clinical practice (e.g. interventions that target improved global integration or higher-order processing such as figurative language and inferencing described in Chapter 6). Finally, the systematic review showed that connectivity associates differently with behavioral measures of language versus autism features. Greater connectivity of language-related regions with both language and nonlanguage-related brain regions (i.e. both local and global) was associated with better language skills, whereas greater local connectivity among language-related regions was associated with more pronounced autism features, and lesser connectivity between language and nonlanguage-related regions (e.g. less global connectivity) was associated with more pronounced autism features (recall Table 15.1). These findings suggest differences in the neurobiology of language impairment versus autism, as well as differences in treatment targets (e.g. local details and global language processing, but global and integrative social communication processing). Functional neuroimaging research contributes to our understanding of autism, generating hypotheses about clinical interventions that may be rigorously examined in translational studies.

In general, neuroimaging provides promising insights into the etiology and behavioral features of autism. No definitive biomarker (e.g. an objective, reliable, and accurate indication of a clinical condition) for autism has been established to date. There is no single test or symptom that can definitively establish the presence or absence of autism. However, most autistic individuals exhibit differences in brain structure and functioning, such as differences in cortical thickness and volume, brain surface area, gyrification (the formation of the folded structure of the cortex in the brain), and gray-white matter tissue contrast (Pretzsch and Ecker 2023), as well as clear and reliable differences in the trajectory of brain development, such as early brain overgrowth (Redcay and Courchesne 2005). Neuroimaging research is a promising means of connecting neuroanatomical profiles, or phenotypes, based on brain imaging, to behavioral, genetic, and developmental phenomena, and ultimately to our understanding of the causes and core features of autism. Given the importance of language delays and difficulties in autism, neuroimaging research that focuses on language processing, and the brain regions that are most important in language processing, is particularly promising in this regard.

Focus on a Specific Study

In this section, we highlight a recent study by Larson et al. (2022). This study was selected because it investigated language impairment in autism using the Research Domain Criteria (RDoC) classification system, which may lead to a better understanding of individual differences across behavioral, physiological, and other characteristics, and thus to precision-based clinical interventions. Unlike the DSM, whose goal is to define disorder categories around groups of core symptoms, the RDoC framework adopts a dimensional approach according to which characteristics pertaining to various domains (biology, cognition, etc.) combine with each other. This approach cuts across diagnostic categories and is a powerful way to study neurobiological and cognitive processes that fall along on a continuum. RDoC takes into account the heterogeneity inherent to neurodevelopmental disorders. An RDoC study, for example, could examine the neural networks underlying language by ignoring diagnostic groups (autistic vs. nonautistic) and focusing instead on individual differences in, e.g. morphosyntax. This approach allows scientists to make predictions that are specific to features (e.g. impairment in the use of past tense morphology) or symptoms (e.g. anxiety) rather than the presence versus absence of a diagnosis (e.g. autism or DLD). This approach has important clinical implications. For example, understanding the neural networks that could be modified by increasing exposure to a particular language construct could help us provide an individual with specific classroom supports or therapies. These supports may reduce mismatches between the individual and the environment (e.g. minimizing irrelevant sensory stimuli in the classroom and offering multimodal response formats), resulting in a more optimal functional context for the autistic individual. Support may also be critical in building skills.

Larson et al. (2022) measured structural language abilities in autistic and non-autistic neurotypical groups, and in a group of individuals who were diagnosed with autism in childhood using gold-standard diagnostic, but no longer met criteria in adolescence or young adulthood, referred to as Loss of Autism Diagnosis (Fein et al. 2013). Surprisingly, similar proportions of autistic and Loss of Autism Diagnosis participants met clinical criteria for structural language impairment (e.g. their scores on a standardized sentence recall task were in the clinically impaired range), suggesting that language impairment may be enduring even when ASD features are no longer present. The authors then compared lateralization of language function elicited by a sentence processing task in language impairment versus unimpaired groups, collapsing across autism status. Contrary to expectations, the structural language impairment group had more left hemisphere lateralization in frontal (e.g. IFG and inferior frontal sulcus) and temporal (e.g. pSTG and MTG) language regions. These findings held even after accounting for autism characteristics, suggesting that this result was specific to language impairment rather than autism. It was concluded that left hemisphere language-related brain regions may be "working harder" than their right hemisphere homologues during language processing in individuals with structural language difficulties and a history of autism, regardless of current ASD status or current ASD features. This study used an RDoC approach by focusing on features, including language, social skills, repetitive interests and behaviors, and attention, rather than ASD versus non-ASD status. There was no evidence that lateralization was associated with a coarse measure of attention difficulties. Thus, these findings were specific to language abilities in autism.

Naturally, language regions identified a priori based on research in neurotypical individuals (Figure 15.1) were examined. It is entirely possible that additional language regions that are not significantly active during language tasks in neurotypical individuals could play compensatory roles in language processing in individuals with language impairment. For instance, the medial prefrontal cortex is associated with Executive Functions and may play a supportive role in language function, particularly for individuals who struggle to understand and use language. Indeed, Eigsti et al. (2016) reported heightened activation of this region in a Loss of Autism Diagnosis group during language processing. The medial prefrontal cortex is not typically considered a language region, but it may be uniquely important in language impairment and could show unique patterns of lateralization. This question awaits further research.

Notably, findings from Larson et al. (2022) and Eigsti et al. (2016) converge on the interpretation that alternate, compensatory pathways develop as part of the neural specialization process for language in individuals with current or a history of autism. This clinically relevant finding suggests that autistic individuals without language impairment may produce language that, on the surface, appears similar to their nonautistic peers, but may have subtle differences in underlying processes that require ongoing support, particularly in challenging contexts (e.g. language use in social interaction). For autistic individuals with language impairment, alternate or compensatory processes may also be used to support language use. For example, individuals who rely on visual or associative brain regions during language processing may rely heavily on visual information. Though these clinical implications are preliminary, they are worth exploring in future studies. MRI methods are expensive and require a high degree of expertise. Furthermore, the narrow scanner bore, noisy environment, and requirements to remain motionless can all be difficult to tolerate, particularly for people with heightened sensory sensitivities. Despite these disadvantages, brain imaging is a critical tool for scientists to better understand how the brain works to support language development and language processing. Studies must carefully measure both autism severity and language impairments in study participants to capture the nature of neural specialization of language networks and the lateralization of functional connectivity in autism.

Conclusion

This chapter set out to address the following questions:
- How do language-related brain regions and networks differ between autistic and neurotypical individuals?
- How do language-related brain functions reflect behaviorally measured language skills and inform clinical practice?

Functional neuroimaging research aims to identify neurobiological markers of autism and to highlight mechanisms of change that are relevant for intervention. Studies of language-related functional connectivity in ASD suggest that the language network in autism is not left hemisphere dominant to the degree seen in neurotypical language. Studies of how language-related networks differ in autistic individuals show that greater global connectivity between language regions and regions outside the language network (e.g. right hemisphere homologue regions) is associated with relatively better language skills. The distributed language network in ASD is characterized by heightened connectivity among classically defined language regions (Figure 15.1) and diminished connectivity between language and regions outside the classic language network (see Table 15.1). In addition to a more distributed language network, ASD is generally characterized by diminished lateralization, with the exception of results from Larson et al. (2022), which found greater left hemisphere lateralization of language function in individuals with poorer language skills. This study analyzed only regions that are associated with language function based on neurotypical research, rather than examining lateralization of all brain activity. Future research is needed to replicate this result, which suggests different neural specialization rather than a lack of specialization. Furthermore, future research should examine the lateralization of functional connectivity in autism. For example, greater leftward lateralization of functional connectivity was associated with higher verbal IQ scores and fewer ASD features (Cardinale et al. 2013), consistent with the suggestion that functional connectivity lateralization is related to specialization. Moreover, we must test the impact of brain function in regions outside the language network in studies of language-related lateralization. Studies of the functional and structural connectivity of brain networks do not yet lead directly to specific clinical recommendations for autistic individuals. Future studies employing resting-state and adaptive functional paradigms may present a higher signal-to-noise ratio and allow researchers to sidestep task-related confounding factors such as effort, strategy use, or performance. Identifying group differences in MRI studies allows scientists to find functional differences associated with a disorder or condition and will eventually lead to treatments and targets for psychopharmacological and behavioral intervention (Fox and Greicius 2010), as well as environment-based interventions that foster a better functional match between individuals and environments and to sensitive measures of treatment effects.

What Do You Know Now?

The expression of thoughts in spoken language is highly complex. We still struggle to model spoken language. Examining the human brain with magnetic resonance imaging, MRI, is a powerful scientific tool. MRI studies can show how language is processed differently in autistic individuals. Identifying the typical and atypical brain structures and networks involved in language can reveal why many autistic individuals struggle with language. Here is what we have learned:

- Strengths and weaknesses in behavioral functioning are clearly tied to differences in brain organization. For example, neural lateralization is more strongly related to language skills than to ASD symptomology.
- Associations between language-related neural function and language-related behavior differ from associations between language-related neural function and ASD symptomology. It is critical to understand how behaviors (such as language abilities) are shaped by the underlying neural circuitry.
- Understanding the neural circuitry that contributes to language-related difficulties in autism is an important addition to our ability to diagnose

> and intervene in the behavioral challenges autistic individuals experience. Such research provides a window into how brain change is associated with improvements in functioning, how neural organization supports both strengths and weaknesses in functioning, and how neural structure and function in autism differ from neurotypical development.

Suggestions for Further Reading

If you are interested in learning more about language-related neural function in autistic individuals, we suggest several readings. Herringshaw et al. 2016 is a meta-analysis of language-related neural function in autism that focuses on lateralization. Eigsti et al. 2016 and Larson et al. 2022 are studies examining neural function elicited by a language task during fMRI in individuals with a current or past ASD diagnosis. If you are interested in learning more about functional connectivity and language networks in ASD, we suggest these readings: Just et al. 2004, Larson et al. 2023, and Vissers, Cohen, and Geurts 2012. Just et al. 2004 was the first study to describe language-related functional connectivity in autistic adults and broke new ground in suggesting that local over-connectivity and global under-connectivity were key features of language impairment in autism. Larson et al. (2023) tested and refined this theory in the form of a systematic review. Vissers, Cohen, and Geurts (2012) adopted a broader approach by conducting a systematic review of connectivity across constructs (e.g. language, visual attention, and Theory of Mind tasks) and neuroimaging techniques (e.g. fMRI, diffusion tensor imaging, and electroencephalography) and by focusing on methodological factors.

References

American Psychiatric Association. (2013). *Diagnostic and Statistical Manual of Mental Disorders-Fifth Edition*. American Psychiatric Association.

Anderson, D.K., Liang, J.W., and Lord, C. (2014). Predicting young adult outcome among more and less cognitively able individuals with Autism Spectrum Disorders. *Journal of Child Psychology and Psychiatry and Allied Disciplines* 55 (5): 485–494.

Bishop, D.V.M., Snowling, M.J., Thompson, P.A. et al. (2017). Phase 2 of CATALISE: a multinational and multidisciplinary Delphi consensus study of problems with language development: terminology. *Journal of Child Psychology and Psychiatry and Allied Disciplines* 58 (10): 1068–1080.

Booth, R.D.L. and Happé, F.G.E. (2018). Evidence of reduced global processing in Autism Spectrum Disorder. *Journal of Autism and Developmental Disorders* 48 (4): 1397–1408.

Briggs, R.G., Conner, A.K., Baker, C.M. et al. (2018). A connectomic atlas of the human cerebrum-Chapter 18: the connectional anatomy of human brain network. *Operative Neurosurgery (Hagerstown, Md.)* 15 (1): S470–S480.

Cardinale, R.C., Shih, P., Fishman, I. et al. (2013). Pervasive rightward asymmetry shifts of functional networks in Autism Spectrum Disorder. *JAMA Psychiatry* 70 (9): 975–982.

Casanova, M.F., Buxhoeveden, D.P., Switala, A.E. et al. (2002). Minicolumnar pathology in autism. *Neurology* 58: 428–432.

Chen, B., Xu, T., Zhou, C. et al. (2015). Individual variability and test-retest reliability revealed by ten repeated resting-state brain scans over one month. *PLoS One* 10 (12): e0144963.

De Fossé, L., Hodge, S.M., Makris, N. et al. (2004). Language-association cortex asymmetry in autism and Specific Language Impairment. *Annals of Neurology* 56 (6): 757–766.

Di Martino, A., Zuo, X.N., Kelly, C. et al. (2013). Shared and distinct intrinsic functional network centrality in autism and attention-deficit/hyperactivity disorder. *Biological Psychiatry* 74 (8): 623–632.

Eden, G.F., Jones, K.M., Cappell, K. et al. (2004). Neural changes following remediation in adult developmental dyslexia. *Neuron* 44 (3): 411–422.

Eigsti, I.M., de Marchena, A.B., Schuh, J.M. et al. (2011). Language acquisition in Autism Spectrum Disorders: a developmental review. *Research in Autism Spectrum Disorders* 5 (2): 681–691.

Eigsti, I.M., Stevens, M.C., Schultz, R.T. et al. (2016). Language comprehension and brain function in individuals with an optimal outcome from autism. *NeuroImage: Clinical* 10: 182–191.

Fein, D., Barton, M., Eigsti, I.M. et al. (2013). Optimal outcome in individuals with a history of autism. *Journal of Child Psychology and Psychiatry and Allied Disciplines* 54 (2): 195–205.

Fox, M. and Greicius, M. (2010). Clinical applications of resting state functional connectivity. *Frontiers in Systems Neuroscience* 4: 1443.

Gao, Y., Linke, A., Jao Keehn, R.J. et al. (2019). The language network in autism: atypical functional connectivity with default mode and visual regions. *Autism Research* 12 (9): 1344–1355.

Helt, M., Kelley, E., Kinsbourne, M. et al. (2008). Can children with autism recover? If so, how? *Neuropsychology Reviews* 18 (4): 339–366.

Herbert, M.R., Ziegler, D.A., Deutsch, C.K. et al. (2005). Brain asymmetries in autism and Developmental Language Disorder: a nested whole-brain analysis. *Brain* 128 (1): 213–226.

Herringshaw, A.J., Ammons, C.J., Deramus, T.P. et al. (2016). Hemispheric differences in language processing in Autism Spectrum Disorders: a meta-analysis of neuroimaging studies. *Autism Research* 9 (10): 1046–1057.

Insel, T., Cuthbert, B., Garvey, M. et al. (2010). Research domain criteria (RDoC): toward a new classification framework for research on mental disorders. *American Journal of Psychiatry* 167 (10): 748–751.

Just, M.A., Cherkassky, V.L., Keller, T.A. et al. (2004). Cortical activation and synchronization during sentence comprehension in high-functioning autism: evidence of underconnectivity. *Brain* 127: 1811–1821.

Kwong, K.K., Belliveau, J.W., Chesler, D.A. et al. (1992). Dynamic magnetic resonance imaging of human brain activity during primary sensory stimulation. *Proceedings of the National Academy of Sciences of the United States of America* 89 (12): 5675–5679.

Larson, C., Rivera-Figueroa, K., Thomas, H.R. et al. (2022). Structural language impairment in Autism Spectrum Disorder versus loss of autism diagnosis: behavioral and neural characteristics. *NeuroImage: Clinical* 34: 103043.

Larson, C., Thomas, H.R., Crutcher, J. et al. (2023). Language networks in Autism Spectrum Disorder: a systematic review of connectivity-based fMRI studies. *Review Journal of Autism and Developmental Disorders* 1–28.

Lenartowicz, A. and Poldrack, R.A. (2010). Brain imaging. In: *Encyclopedia of Behavioral Neuroscience* (eds. G.F. Koob, M.L. Moal, and R.F. Thompson), 187–193. Amsterdam, Netherlands: Elsevier Science.

Matchin, W. and Hickok, G. (2020). The cortical organization of syntax. *Cerebral Cortex* 30 (3): 1481–1498.

Nielsen, J.A., Zielinski, B.A., Fletcher, P.T. et al. (2014). Abnormal lateralization of functional connectivity between language and default mode regions in autism. *Molecular Autism* 5 (8): 1–11.

Olulade, O.A., Seydell-Greenwald, A., Chambers, C.E. et al. (2020). The neural basis of language development: changes in lateralization over age. *Proceedings of the National Academy of Sciences of the United States of America* 117 (38): 23477–23483.

Pretzsch, C.M. and Ecker, C. (2023). Structural neuroimaging phenotypes and associated molecular and genomic underpinnings in autism: a review. *Frontiers in Neuroscience* 17: 1172779.

Price, C.J. (2010). The anatomy of language: a review of 100 fMRI studies published in 2009. *Annals of the New York Academy of Sciences* 1191: 62–88.

Redcay, E. and Courchesne, E. (2005). When is the brain enlarged in autism? A meta-analysis of all brain size reports. *Biological Psychiatry* 58 (1): 1–9.

Schaeffer, J. (2018). Linguistic and cognitive abilities in children with Specific Language Impairment as compared to children with high-functioning autism. *Language Acquisition* 25 (1): 5–23.

Schaeffer, J., Abd El-Raziq, M., Castroviejo, E. et al. (2023). Language in autism: domains, profiles and co-occurring conditions. *Journal of Neural Transmission* 130 (3): 433–457.

Vissers, M.E., Cohen, M.X., and Geurts, H.M. (2012). Brain connectivity and high functioning autism: a promising path of research that needs refined models, methodological convergence, and stronger behavioral links. *Neuroscience and Biobehavioral Reviews* 36 (1): 604–625.

Wang, Q., Li, H.Y., Li, Y.D. et al. (2021). Resting-state abnormalities in functional connectivity of the default mode network in Autism Spectrum Disorder: a meta-analysis. *Brain Imaging and Behavior* 15: 2583–2592.

Wilson, S.M., Yen, M., and Eriksson, D.K. (2018). An adaptive semantic matching paradigm for reliable and valid language mapping in individuals with aphasia. *Human Brain Mapping* 39 (8): 3285–3307.

Conclusion

16

Building a Baseline Battery to Measure Language in Autism

Jeannette Schaeffer, Rama Novogrodsky, Alexandra Perovic, Philippe Prévost, and Laurice Tuller

The aim of this book was to compile current knowledge on how autistic people produce and comprehend language in terms accessible to a wide audience of interested parties – in other words, to "put language on the autism map." In so doing, we have taken care to unpack what we mean by "language," such that the different types of linguistic knowledge that together constitute language were examined domain by domain and across domains. Our hope is that, together, these chapters have provided a comprehensive (and comprehensible) overview of current understanding of language in autism. Attentive readers will have noticed that each of these chapters has pointed out issues in the study of language in autism that are methodological in nature. We propose to synthesize and discuss in this chapter, the most important methodological issues that have been raised: population sampling, scope and depth of language assessment, task-related biases, concomitant assessment of nonlinguistic cognitive skills, and study design. We then provide an example of the type of language assessment tools that we believe would allow for these issues to be taken into account. Finally, we summarize how we think that taking such methodological steps will allow the field to move forward in significant ways, not just with regard to our understanding of language in autism but also with the aim of showing that a linguistic perspective can advance our understanding of autism.

Methodological Issues Emerging from Studying Language in Autism

A major stumbling block in the study of language in autism is **participant selection**. Selection based solely on a diagnosis of autism results in very heterogeneous groups, which may nevertheless not be all-inclusive. The way in which people are diagnosed varies: sometimes diagnoses are made by multidisciplinary teams, other times by just a psychiatrist or a psychologist. In addition, there are people who have no clinical autism diagnosis but may display several characteristics that fit into a broader autism phenotype. Moreover, changes in the diagnostic criteria from older to more recent versions of the DSM, which have in some ways widened and in other respects narrowed the diagnosis of autism, have also increased the heterogeneity of population samples in studies across the years. Unless the population samples are very large, this makes it difficult to generalize, detect patterns, or draw conclusions with respect to autistic individuals' linguistic abilities. Heterogeneity in population sampling is often responsible for the conflicting results of studies on language in autism that have been frequently reported throughout this book.

At the same time, to get a picture of the different linguistic profiles that occur in autism, it is necessary to study autistic individuals across the spectrum, with and without co-occurring diagnoses (e.g. Disorder of Intellectual Development (DID), ADHD, epilepsy, sleep disorder), across ages, across intellectual and other nonlinguistic cognitive abilities (e.g. Theory of Mind [ToM], Executive Function [EF], Working Memory [WM], central coherence), across autism severity levels, and across language abilities. Recall that a substantial number of autistic people are minimally speaking (up to about 30%), but that it is not always clear what their receptive language abilities are or their extralinguistic cognitive skills. In addition, we have seen that autism severity does not predict language abilities; there are people with severe autism whose language skills are intact, and vice versa. Furthermore, many autistic people who do have fluent language have a structural (phonological, morphological, syntactic, and/or semantic) language impairment (ALI). As the chapters on pragmatics show (Chapters 6–8), the distinction between ALI and ALN (intact structural language abilities) is crucial for the assessment of pragmatic skills, since certain pragmatic difficulties may be related to impaired structural language. Furthermore, many autistic individuals are living with more than one language, as discussed in Chapter 13. One way to address the issue of heterogeneity is to identify subgroups according to, for example, autism severity, age, intellectual ability, nonlinguistic cognitive ability, general structural language abilities, and mono/multilingualism, or to somehow control for these characteristics. Although many recent studies discussed in this book have attempted to divide their population samples into subgroups along these lines, this can result in subgroups with very small numbers of participants. Small participant groups quite naturally make study replication difficult, as such small samples may not be representative of the larger population with similar characteristics. Yet, we believe that finding ways to take characteristics such as the ones mentioned above into account is crucial, as it is the only way to provide precise and comprehensive knowledge on the linguistic profiles of autistic people that is so urgently needed.

Some subgroups of autistic people are heavily underrepresented in existing research on language in autism (Lord et al. 2022). The reader may have noticed that the majority of studies discussed in this book are on children. Studies on the language of adolescents and adults, including older adults, on the autism spectrum are scarce (see Chapter 12). The same applies to autistic individuals who have DID, who are multilingual, or who are minimally verbal, who have a co-occurring condition (ADHD, epilepsy, etc.), or indeed any combination of these (see Chapters 10, 11, and 13). Few studies have included these important subgroups in their investigation of language. For minimally speaking autistic people, for example, it is far from clear what their linguistic skills are in the areas of language comprehension or reading. All these subgroups deserve much more attention in future research.

Assessment of different language domains constitutes another issue in linguistic research in autism. One frequently used method of obtaining language measures in studies on autism is through parental/caregiver questionnaires. Although these can be useful, their disadvantage lies not only in the indirect measurement of participants' skills, potentially providing inadequate insight into their current competence, but also in limiting which aspects of language abilities can be measured. Existing (usually standardized) language assessment tools that do test language abilities directly often do not adequately distinguish between the various language domains (e.g. yielding only a single omnibus score, or one score for expressive language and one for receptive language), and/or the testing method used relies strongly on nonlinguistic cognitive abilities (e.g. WM, ToM, EF). These tools, moreover, often entirely ignore one or more language domains, importantly, pragmatics, which is widely assumed to present difficulties in autism. Some standardized language tests that do assess only one language domain (for example, vocabulary) are used as proxies for language as a whole, which is problematic. Furthermore, vocabulary tests (such as PPVT) are sometimes used as measures for verbal mental age or verbal cognition. From a linguistic perspective, this is a bit surprising, as vocabulary skills are language skills, which can be dissociated from extralinguistic cognition, such as intellectual ability (see, for example, the case of Christopher, as described in Smith and Tsimpli 1985). Tools that measure vocabulary production through a picture-naming task or vocabulary comprehension via a picture-identification task, test vocabulary skills, but not structural language skills. These tools are moreover inadequate for probing the interface between the lexicon and syntax/semantics, or between semantics and pragmatics, areas that are often affected in autistic individuals. Moreover, specific words or pictorial stimuli used in standardized language tests for children may be inappropriate for adults, including older adults, for some cultures or languages, or for autistic people. Beyond standardized language tests, one way of assessing language abilities in autism that has yielded important results is analysis of **spontaneous language samples**. However, spontaneous language samples, despite their richness in certain respects (mostly in terms of information about the lexicon and structural language), often do not provide enough information about, for example, pragmatics, discourse or semantics, or the interface between different language domains. Yet, screening of abilities in each language domain is necessary, as one language domain may be impaired while another is intact, and difficulties in one domain (for example, structural language) can influence abilities in another domain (for example, pragmatics). Moreover, in spontaneous language, children and adults with various conditions/disorders (including autism) tend to (unconsciously) avoid aspects of language that are difficult for them (e.g. when complex syntax is impaired, they may communicate in simple sentences), or they may avoid communicating altogether, giving rise to scores not indicative of their true linguistic abilities. When this is the case, spontaneous speech samples cannot inform the researcher or the clinician about structural language competence, in particular, the more complex linguistic constructions.

A further aspect regarding how language in autism is studied concerns the **appropriateness of the way language tasks assess language**. Tasks must be appropriate for autistic participants across the spectrum, including people who are less verbal or have lower intellectual ability. For example, the length of tasks should be kept to a minimum, and pragmatic skills required by the task should be carefully controlled (e.g. a sentence repetition task requiring participants to repeat questions may see some autistic people answer these questions rather than repeat them). Cognitive demands should be minimal in order to avoid cognitive overload (e.g. deciphering a complex picture involving details and multiple colors while listening to the beginning of a sentence that needs to be completed in a way appropriate to part of the picture). Likewise, pointing can be problematic for at least some autistic participants. These different issues may lead to very low task completion rates (e.g. below 50% in Kjelgaard and Tager-Flusberg 2001), although completion rates are rarely reported. Taking into account all of these considerations would contribute to the design of language tasks that are autism-friendly across the spectrum. At the same time, we would like language tasks to provide a context that mimics natural language use as closely as possible since we know that language use in daily life is often more challenging for autistic people than in structured lab situations.

We have suggested that language task design needs to take into account potential bias from differences in extralinguistic cognition that are part of autism. Beyond this, there is an independent need for the **assessment of extralinguistic cognitive skills** in studies on language in autism. As seen in the preceding chapters, various extralinguistic cognitive functions are particularly important in the investigation of language (development) in autism, as they may (i) influence language (development), or vice versa and (ii) be different in autism. Autistic people may have their own ways of conceptualizing, thinking, and/or reasoning. This may be due to differences in cognitive functions such as ToM, EF, WM, central coherence, and intelligence. Nevertheless, sometimes these extralinguistic cognitive skills have not been tested independently of language in linguistic research on autism, even if a potential explanation of the linguistic results may appeal to differences in extralinguistic cognitive areas. It is crucial that extralinguistic cognitive skills such as ToM, EF, WM, and intelligence are tested independently of language and of each other. Preferably, this should be done nonverbally, as language impairment may bias scores on extralinguistic cognitive tests if they are administered through language. Similarly, potentially influencing co-occurring NDDs should be taken into account in the study of language in autism, as they may also influence the language (developmental) profile.

Beyond issues regarding participants and materials, research on language in autism would benefit from more attention to **study design**. As is the case for research on other aspects of autism, longitudinal studies of language are sorely needed. Language is part of the full profile of a baby or a toddler and is usually assessed after autism has been diagnosed. However, there is a need for language tests throughout the life of a person diagnosed with autism to better understand their development and (changing) need for support. While pan-lifespan tools are widely used to test, for example, intellectual abilities, analogous language tests are so far extremely limited.

The few **longitudinal language studies** in autism to date often do not use language tests that are comparable throughout life, precisely because such tools are so scarce. We thus cannot longitudinally track the development of language, specifically the various language domains: lexical, structural, and pragmatic abilities. Note that for some children with autism, a regression in language production is also reported (see Chapters 1 and 10), and there is not much evidence on the language of older autistic adults (Chapter 12), beyond the effects of aging. Age is another extralinguistic factor that affects language and might be an additional risk for older people with autism. Of note, to date there are very few appropriate language tests to assess the various language domains for adolescents, adults, including older adults, adding an additional challenge beyond the idea of language tools that are friendly for autism. These issues underscore the need for language tests that can be used across ages, which is elaborated in the following section "Addressing Methodological Challenges to the Study of Language in Autism: The LACA Baseline Battery."

Another type of study design that has so far been neglected is the study of **language in autism across languages and across countries**. Cross-language and cross-country studies will expand our understanding of language in autism from different angles. They will allow for the exploration of the effects of specific language properties on autism cross-linguistically, specifically those that differ across languages and those that are common in understudied languages (see Chapter 11). Similarities between languages within autism (whether showing typical patterns or atypical ones) will add to our understanding of how language is linked to autism. In addition, such studies will provide a baseline for exploring crosslinguistic influence in bilingual children with autism (Chapter 13), which may affect acquisition in different language domains, both positively and negatively. The study of language and language development in autistic people across languages and across countries can provide additional perspective to how we understand autism (Lord et al. 2022).

Addressing Methodological Challenges to the Study of Language in Autism: The LACA Baseline Battery

In order to address the methodological shortcomings raised in the previous section, the international LACA network[1] is in the course of developing a baseline battery consisting of tools it recommends for assessing different linguistic and extralinguistic domains in studies on (language in) autism: the LACA Baseline Battery (Prévost et al. 2023). The language components include the lexicon, structural aspects of language, pragmatics, and prosody. The extralinguistic domains comprise autism severity, EF, nonverbal IQ (NVIQ), central coherence, and ToM. As noted in Chapter 1 and in the section above on methodological issues, these extralinguistic abilities may interact with language (e.g. WM and/or ToM with morphosyntax (Chapter 3), ToM and/or central coherence with implicit meaning (Chapter 6), etc.), and are reported to be often different in autism compared to neurotypical development, as illustrated by many studies discussed in this book. The tools, which are either novel or existing (and often norm-referenced, standardized tests), are meant to be used as screening tools in order to identify individuals who have low linguistic and/or extralinguistic skills and the domain(s) where difficulties arise. They can be used in research studies, for example, to determine whether an autistic person has language impairment (ALI) or not (ALN). We believe that they could also be useful for clinical settings, although this requires further research.

In developing this battery, the LACA network surveyed a large number of assessment tools and established five inclusion criteria, as listed in (1):

(1) Criteria used for inclusion in the LACA Baseline Battery:
   a) Tools evaluating language skills should assess linguistic properties known to be potential sources of difficulties for autistic individuals, including those with language impairment.
   b) Tools assessing extralinguistic abilities should use a minimal amount of language, for example, in instructions, so as not to disadvantage

---

1 Language Abilities in Children with Autism. See the Preface of this book.

participants who struggle with language or who have DID and have trouble following verbal instructions.

c) Tools should be usable across the autism spectrum, including the lower intellectual ability end, and across ages, so that they can be administered to a wide range of autistic individuals and be used in studies comparing different age groups or following the same individuals over a period of time.

d) Tools should also be usable across languages and be appropriate for bilingual individuals. This is meant to (i) increase comparability across countries, (ii) enable pooling data to obtain larger datasets, and (iii) take into account the specificity of individuals living with more than one language, who represent the majority of individuals in the world.

e) Tools easily available to most researchers should be prioritized.

Following these criteria, several tools were selected for different linguistic and extralinguistic domains, which can be found in Tables 16.1 and 16.2, respectively. We would like to make it clear that the lists of tools appearing in these tables are not meant to be definitive. For some domains, there are ongoing efforts, particularly by members of the LACA network, to develop new tools that are even more appropriate than those identified so far. In particular, these concern pragmatics, prosody, and ToM (for a recently developed task assessing ToM, see Marinis et al. 2023). The lists are thus bound to change with time and integrate new tools as they become available.

Finally, although the tools that were selected were mainly identified for research studies on language in autism, some of them are also used in clinical settings, such as the PPVT-4, CELF-5, ADOS-2, WISC-V, and WAIS-IV. Other tools that are more experimental in nature, such as the LITMUS repetition tasks, need to be normed before they can be used clinically (and such efforts are already underway in some countries). In general, further developments of the LACA Baseline Battery should include tools that could be easily integrated into clinical practice.

We would like to illustrate the approach adopted by the LACA network in developing the Baseline Battery by focusing on the LITMUS tools of sentence repetition (SR) and nonword repetition (quasi-universal) (NWR-QU). These tools assess **structural language abilities** such as morphosyntax and phonology, respectively, and are available, for free, in many languages.[2] They are short in duration (five minutes), and their instructions are simple and easily understandable ("Repeat exactly what you hear"). They include morphosyntactic and phonological structures known to be sensitive to language difficulties and language impairment. The potential effects of other abilities on performance are

---

[2] Information on available versions and how to access them can be found at https://www.litmus-srep.info (for SR) and at https://www.bi-sli.org/qu-nonword-repetition (for NWR-QU).

Table 16.1 LACA Baseline Battery – tools recommended for assessing language in autism.

Domain	Tools
Lexicon	Peabody Picture Vocabulary Test (PPVT) (Dunn and Dunn 2007)
Structural language (morphosyntax and phonology)	• LITMUS Sentence Repetition (Marinis and Armon-Lotem 2015) • LITMUS-Quasi Universal-Nonword Repetition (dos Santos and Ferré 2018)
Pragmatics	• Autism Diagnostic Observation Schedule-2 (ADOS-2; Lord et al. 2012) • Clinical Evaluation of Language Fundamentals-5 (CELF-5) Pragmatic profile (Wiig et al. 2013) • Children's Communication Checklist-2 (CCC-2; Bishop 2006)
Prosody	• ADOS-2 • Profiling Elements of Prosody in Speech-Communication (PEPS-C; Peppé and McCann 2003)

Table 16.2 LACA Baseline Battery – tools recommended for assessing extralinguistic cognition related to language in autism.

Area	Recommended tests
Autism severity	• ADOS Calibrated Severity Score (Gotham, Pickles, and Lord 2009) • Social Responsiveness Scales (SRS) (Constantino and Gruber 2007)
Executive Function	• Cambridge Neuropsychological Test Automated Battery (CANTAB 2023), notably Intra-Extra Dimensional Set Shift (IED) and Spatial Working Memory (SPW) • Digit Span, notably from WISC-V (Wechsler 2014) and WAIS-IV (Wechsler 2008)
Nonverbal IQ	• Raven's Progressive Matrices, Second Edition (Raven's 2) (Raven et al. 2018) • Block Design, Matrix Reasoning (WAIS-IV, Wechsler 2008; WISC-V, Wechsler 2014)
Central coherence	Navon – Global-Local Visual Processing Task (Navon 1977)
Theory of Mind	Belief Attribution Task (Forgeot d'Arc and Ramus 2011)

limited. For example, pragmatic influence on SR is minimized by having participants repeat decontextualized sentences, and the effect of lexical knowledge and WM on NWR is minimized by making sure that the items, the nonwords, do not resemble existing words in the language and by restricting the length of each nonword. The LITMUS SR and NWR tasks have been used with a wide range of autistic individuals, including those with DID. High completion rates (over 80%) have been reported, meaning that when participants start repeating sentences or nonwords, they are very likely to continue to the end of the task. This suggests that LITMUS tools are particularly appropriate for the autistic population (Silleresi et al. 2020; Manenti et al. 2023). We would like to point out that echolalia, the unsolicited repetition of a language form produced by another person (e.g. a word or a phrase), which is frequently found in ASD, does not seem to boost performance on repetition tasks in autistic children (Silleresi 2023). In Silleresi's study, for example, children with the lowest repetition scores on LITMUS-SR in fact displayed the highest scores for echolalic language. The LITMUS repetition tasks are also appropriate for multilingual individuals, as they were specifically developed to test language skills in this population. The items they contain, while targeting structures known to be sources of difficulties for children with language impairment, were selected so as to limit how language experience (such as length of exposure and use), which can vary greatly across bilingual individuals, may affect performance.[3] Finally, while originally created for assessing language skills of children aged 5–12 (for SR) and 4–12 (for NWR-QU), they are easily adaptable to other ages, as the length and complexity of the items may be manipulated according to the targeted population. The complexity or length of the task can be reduced for assessing the language skills of toddlers or increased in order to be used with adolescents and adults (Manenti et al. 2023). This makes LITMUS tools good candidates for longitudinal studies of language development in autism.

Concerning measures of **intellectual abilities**, the LACA network recommends using tasks that are not language-based, since many autistic individuals have difficulties with language. Intellectual development can be measured by different types of tasks that vary in how much language is involved. Some tasks are clearly language-based, such as the tests that make up the Verbal Comprehension Index of the WISC-V (Vocabulary and Similarities). Using such tasks may

---

3 This notwithstanding, it is strongly recommended that language assessment in multilingual individuals be crossed with measures of language experience, age of acquisition, and other variables (for a more elaborate discussion, see Chapter 13). These measures can be obtained through questionnaires that can be administered to the parents of the participants or to the participants themselves, such as the LITMUS Parental Bilingual Questionnaire (PABIQ, https://www.bi-sli.org/pabiq) or the Quantifying Bilingual Experience questionnaire (Q-Bex, https://www.q-bex.org).

therefore underestimate the intellectual capacities of individuals with language impairment. In contrast, some IQ tasks are nonverbal, in that participants may be asked to complete a pattern by identifying a missing element (e.g. Raven's Progressive Matrices) or by reproducing a pattern using cubes (e.g. Block Design of the WISC-V). These tasks, which measure abstract reasoning, employ succinct instructions, making them particularly appropriate for individuals who struggle with language. In some cases, a task may be conceptually nonverbal but requires a verbal answer. This is the case of the Picture Concepts subtest of the WISC-IV for which participants are asked to single out pictures from rows of pictures and explain, verbally, what they have in common. Such tasks may not be most suitable for measuring the intellectual capacities of many autistic individuals.

A few final notes on language assessment in autism are in order here. As hinted at above, evaluations taking place under standardized conditions (e.g. in a lab situation) often render results that differ from evaluations taking place under more ecological conditions. This suggests that we will need to search for possibilities to turn our targeted language tasks into "living lab" situations (Archibald et al. 2021), so as to mimic natural language use as closely as possible. We believe that only this way will we arrive at a more complete picture of autistic people's language abilities. Furthermore, it is important to find ways to embed detailed and nuanced language assessment in autism into a participatory research framework. This involves the incorporation of all autistic people's (including, e.g. minimally speaking and intellectually disabled people) perspectives and needs about what sort of research should be conducted, how it is carried out, and how it is implemented (Cornwall and Jewkes 1995). One final challenge concerns investigation into if and how technological innovations can facilitate the implementation of large-scale language assessments in both clinical and research settings.

Advancing the Linguistic Perspective on Autism

Although referring to **heterogeneity** as the hallmark of autism has become ubiquitous, consensus in the field has failed to emerge regarding the nature/cause of this heterogeneity and the best way to grapple with it (Mottron 2021a and 2021b). Is autism best regarded as a broad, all-inclusive category, ASD, consisting of a dimension along which various profiles can be observed, or as a collection of distinct clinical entities, some/one of which is central and others peripheral? Very much part of these questions is whether the categorical vision of NDDs inherent in current diagnostic classification (APA 2022; WHO 2022), which distinguishes, for example, ASD from Developmental Speech and Language Disorders, is the most useful way to study and understand these conditions. Or, rather, is the optimal strategy one that follows a **dimensional approach** in which behavioral dimensions are studied along their full range of functioning levels so that specific processes such as language ability are studied across traditional diagnostic categories? Another paradigm shift in the study of autism has stemmed from the **neurodiversity** movement, which emerged in the 1990s and which has promoted inclusion and acceptance of all individuals. This concept embodies the view that the observed array of how people develop, behave, and experience the world corresponds to ways in which the brain works that are simply different, and that do not consist of some ways labeled as "normal" or "typical" and others as "deficient."

Each of these issues is closely tied to how we study language in autism. We believe that appropriate language study methodology, explicitly outlined and argued for in the preceding sections of this chapter, will galvanize progress toward our understanding of language in autism by allowing researchers to seriously take into consideration the issues raised by autism heterogeneity, NDD dimensionality, and neurodiversity. In so doing, we can hope to move forward in our understanding of the nature and cause(s) behind the variety of language abilities observed in autism, notably language impairment, as well as offer a needed linguistic perspective on our understanding of autism.

Autism Heterogeneity and NDD Dimensionality

We begin with the issues of **autism heterogeneity and NDD dimensionality** from a linguistic perspective. As seen throughout the different chapters of this book, language ability constitutes a major ingredient in the high heterogeneity observed across the autism spectrum. Language ranges from entirely absent or extremely minimal to structurally rich; its development may conform to ordinary language milestones, but very often does not. In individuals who do develop language, difficulties are not always restricted to aspects of pragmatics, at least some of which can be linked to core autism features in rather obvious ways (e.g. difficulty with social interaction and communication). Structural language abilities may be impaired (ALI) or not (ALN), and linking these to core autism features is much less obvious. On the other hand, pragmatic difficulties and/or structural difficulties are observed in many other NDDs and in some medical conditions (e.g. epilepsy).

Tackling the issue of language in **autism heterogeneity** entails careful delineation of subgroups and language profiles. The "with accompanying functional language impairment '/'without accompanying functional language impairment" specifier in the DSM and the ICD is clearly insufficient from a linguistic perspective, as language profiles most probably differ in quite subtle ways, and only when these are studied in and of themselves can we come to grips with heterogeneity. For example, there may be possible links between selective phonological impairment and specific aspects of Restricted and Repetitive Behaviors (RRB), i.e. sensitivity to sensory stimuli is part of RRB and phonology relies on auditory stimuli. Such links may be obscured if this profile is not studied separately, in terms of both participants and language assessment tools. This profile, like others, would most likely be lost in the sea of very heterogeneous language profiles. The LACA Baseline Battery presented above includes language assessment tools designed for their capacity to narrowly test language components separately and across the autism spectrum. Tools of this type are what is needed to identify meaningful language profiles for further investigation.

Tackling the larger question of **NDD dimensionality**, and indeed dimensionality in "mental disorders" more generally, is the overall aim of the RDoC (Research Domain Criteria) project, instigated in 2009 by the U.S. Institute of Mental Health (see Cuthbert and Insel 2013). This project has proposed that, for research purposes, a more fertile alternative to traditional categories based on collections of symptoms, as in the DSM and the ICD, is one in which study is concentrated on behavioral dimensions that cut across traditional nosographic categories such as ASD and DLD. In other words, the idea behind the RDoC approach is that studying dimensions will serve to increase understanding of each currently proposed diagnostic manual category and ultimately to determine if it is appropriate to even talk about comorbidity between, say, autism and DLD (see Schaeffer et al. 2023).

In the RDoC research classification system, language is one of the identified dimensions: it is a fundamental behavioral component that may be affected in multiple disorder categories and that furthermore is associated with an identified neural underpinning. Clearly, this type of investigation also requires assessment tools capable of targeting specific abilities as narrowly as possible and tools that are useable across disorder categories, such that they do not bias language scores (introduce measurement artifacts) due to disorder-related nonlinguistic difficulties (attention deficits, social pragmatic difficulties, focus on visual details, etc.). This is precisely what the LACA Baseline Battery proposes: a battery of autism-friendly tools, where autism-friendly in fact also means NDD-friendly. As explained above, the LITMUS repetition tasks were developed to screen for DLD in bilingual children, and have been shown to be useable for language in autism, yielding high completion rates and reliable results. These specific types of language assessment tools, SR and NWR, selected for this battery receive support from the study of other NDDs, beyond DLD. For example, researchers working on language abilities in ADHD have also pleaded for the use of language assessment tools that both target specific core linguistic domains and do not "penalize" these children's language performance due to properties of ADHD. Redmond (2016) argues in particular for the use of short (16-item) repetition tasks (NWR and SR) as well as tasks focusing on specific linguistic structures (tense-marking in English). The LACA Baseline Battery has come to these same conclusions for the identification of language impairment across the autism spectrum, suggesting that the choice of these tools is a promising one. The basic need for tools useable across diagnostic categories requirement corresponds to RDoC Aim #3 – "Develop reliable and valid measures of fundamental components of mental disorders" (Cuthbert and Insel 2013). The precision inherent in such tools provides the necessary base for the exploration of dimensional neural correlates (RDoC Aim #4) and for the study of the full range of behavioral variation within a given dimension. Studying the full range in this way will furthermore lay the groundwork for identification and understanding of the point at which language differences are so great that there is reason to conclude that there is language impairment and that appropriate, individualized support could be put in place.

Neurodiversity and Language Abilities in Autism

Consider how looking at autism through a **neurodiversity** lens (see Chapter 1) may have consequences for how we investigate language, study design, and materials. The neurodiversity approach suggests that language in autism be viewed as the result of alternative developmental paths, whether the focus is on language outcomes that resemble neurotypical language patterns or on those that are the most neurodivergent. The most obvious cases of alternative paths to language so far appear to be rare (see Kissine, Saint-Denis, and Mottron 2023). A coherent first step in the elucidation of these alternative paths has consisted of carefully documenting case studies, such as the language savant Christopher, and the more recently reported cases of unusual bilingual language development (Kissine 2020 and Chapter 15). The next step requires efforts to pool these cases together, from across labs/cultures/countries, to identify commonalities, and to explore seriously what different ways of developing language look like and are based on (Mottron, Ostrolenk, and Gagnon 2021). Kissine, Saint-Denis, and Mottron (2023) emphasize that the concept of neurodiversity in fact "requires the scientific community to keep an open mind as to the existence of language learning mechanisms specific to autism – however, unusual they may appear from what we know about nonautistic minds."

Exciting work in neurolinguistics suggests that the view of autism entailing different paths leading to superficially similar skills may receive support from the neural underpinnings for language (see Chapter 15). Bringing forth evidence that neural specialization for language in autism could be different rather than simply lacking, Larson et al. (2022) have argued that superficially ordinary language production may in fact differ in subtle ways in underlying processes, meaning that, contrary to appearances, even these autistic individuals may benefit from ongoing support. Although this particular result requires confirmation, it is clear that this type of work is needed and that it can only proceed when grounded in language measures coming from robust and carefully focused linguistic assessment tools.

Investigating language in autism from the angle of neurodiversity leads quite naturally to the wider angle of diversity in all of its meaning. Despite autism being a global public health challenge, there exists a significant gap in research focusing on language (and other aspects of development) in autistic individuals outside of high-income countries (Franz et al. 2017; Lord et al. 2022). To understand differences in the course of language development in autism, it is crucial to consider diverse cultural and linguistic contexts. For instance, the widely studied concept of joint attention and its purported relation to language development may be of different value in cultures in which caregivers interact in different ways with children. Structural aspects of language can differ markedly in speakers of different languages, as we know from decades of sophisticated linguistic research literature detailing language development in individuals with DLD. The dearth of research in low and middle-income countries can be attributed to limited resources, alongside the pervasive stigma surrounding autism diagnosis (Gillespie-Lynch et al. 2019; Han et al. 2022; Lord et al. 2022). It is thus crucial to support the neurodiversity attitude, which entails fostering inclusion of individuals in diverse cultures who may escape diagnosis because of stigma or the lack of public and professional awareness that may contribute to negative attitudes, more common in some countries than in others. Taking into account cultural influence entails including large numbers of participants so that the full array of profiles is represented and the variables that distinguish them can be studied. As mentioned above, inter-country/culture comparisons mean pooling data from different labs, which therefore must use the same tools. These kinds of comparisons are particularly vital for the study of language in autism because different countries/cultures involve different languages, whose structural aspects can differ markedly. Once again, this enterprise is feasible only when we consider the nature of language assessment tools: not only do such tools need to be autism-friendly and test all language domains, including pragmatics, they also need to be sensitive to subtle aspects of the linguistic structures found in diverse languages that may be indicative of language impairment.

The Nature and Cause(s) of Language Features Found in Autism

Turning, finally, to the nature and cause of language impairment and, more generally, language features found in autism, consider how this endeavor intimately stems from how we choose to study language. Understanding language in autism entails thorough and reliable characterization of the range of language abilities found in autism as well as bringing forth evidence for their underlying causes. What is language impairment in autism? What does it look like, linguistically? Are its properties specific to autism or shared with other disorders/conditions in which language impairment occurs? Is the underlying cause autism-specific or not? In other terms, is language impairment in autism (ALI) a dimensional property found in various disorders for various reasons but having similar linguistic manifestations, or is ALI in fact the manifestation of multiple diagnoses ("comorbidity" of two separate diagnostic categories "autism" and "DLD")?

As the reader was forewarned in Chapter 1, the goal of this book was not to grapple with these questions but, rather, to present what we know about language in autism, how it is studied, and why the linguistic perspective is important to understanding autism. This having been said, it is fitting that the final chapter of this book revisit these fundamental questions. Achieving these aims and answering questions like these is predicated on the appropriate study of language. Describing the full range of language abilities found in autism requires appropriate population sampling of autistic individuals and comparison groups; this entails the use of autism-friendly and pan-spectrum-friendly linguistic tools that narrowly target specific aspects of linguistic abilities. Moreover, drawing conclusions about the autism specificity of particular language features, an important contribution to general understanding of autism, entails testing population samples across language acquisition contexts (without autism), including detailed study of language impairment across NDDs and medical conditions (epilepsy, deafness, etc.) – again, with tools appropriate to individuals with very different disabilities/conditions.

In sum, we can hope to reach explanatory adequacy in our understanding of language in autism, notably, language impairment (explaining the data and accounting for how autistic people's differing states of knowledge of language are obtained) if, first of all, we succeed in achieving descriptive adequacy more closely. Achieving descriptive adequacy means using appropriate, targeted ways of testing language and testing not only across the autism spectrum but across neurodevelopmental disorder categories. In other words, more adequate methods for the study of language in autism are the foundation for advancing our understanding of language in autism and providing a linguistic perspective on our understanding of autism.

References

American Psychiatric Association (APA) (2022). *Diagnostic and Statistical Manual of Mental Disorders*, 5e, Text Rev. American Psychiatric Association.

Archibald, M.M., Wittmeier, K., Gale, M. et al (2021). Living labs for patient engagement and knowledge exchange: an exploratory sequential mixed methods study to develop a living lab in paediatric rehabilitation. *BMJ Open* 11: e041530.

Cambridge Cognition (2023). *CANTAB® [Cognitive assessment software]*. Available at: www.cambridgecognition.com (accessed 2 June 2024).

Constantino, J.N. and Gruber, C.P. (2007). *Social Responsiveness Scale (SRS)*. Los Angeles, CA: Western Psychological Services.

Cornwall, A. and Jewkes, R. (1995). What is participatory research? *Social Science & Medicine* 41: 1667–1676.

Cuthbert, B.N. and Insel, T.R. (2013). Toward the future of psychiatric diagnosis: the seven pillars of RDoC. *BMC Medicine* 11: 1–8.

dos Santos, C. and Ferré, S. (2018). A nonword repetition task to assess bilingual children's phonology. *Language Acquisition* 25 (1): 58–71.

Dunn, L.M. and Dunn, D.M. (2007). *Peabody Picture Vocabulary Test (Fourth Edition)*. San Antonio, TX: Pearson.

Forgeot d'Arc, B. and Ramus, F. (2011). Belief attribution despite verbal interference. *The Quarterly Journal of Experimental Psychology* 64 (5): 975–990.

Franz, L., Chambers, N., von Isenburgh, M. et al. (2017). Autism Spectrum Disorder in Sub-Saharan Africa: a comprehensive scoping review. *Autism Research* 10: 723–749.

Gillespie-Lynch, K., Daou, N., Sanchez-Ruiz, M.J. et al. (2019). Factors underlying cross-cultural differences in stigma toward autism among college students in Lebanon and the United States. *Autism: The International Journal of Research and Practice* 23 (8): 1993–2006.

Gotham, K., Pickles, A., and Lord, C. (2009). Standardizing ADOS scores for a measure of severity in Autism Spectrum Disorders. *Journal of Autism and Developmental Disorders* 39 (5): 693–705.

Han, E., Scior, K., Avramides, K. et al. (2022). A systematic review on autistic people's experiences of stigma and coping strategies. *Autism Research* 15 (1): 12–26.

Kissine, M. (2020). Autism, constructionism, and nativism. *Language* 97 (3): e139–e160.

Kissine, M., Saint-Denis, A., and Mottron, L. (2023). Language acquisition can be truly atypical in autism: beyond joint attention. *Neuroscience and Biobehavioral Reviews* 153: 105384.

Kjelgaard, M.M. and Tager-Flusberg, H. (2001). An investigation of language impairment in autism: implications for genetic subgroups. *Language and Cognitive Processes* 16 (2–3): 287–308.

Larson, C., Rivera-Figueroa, K., Thomas, H.R. et al. (2022). Structural language impairment in Autism Spectrum Disorder versus loss of autism diagnosis: behavioral and neural characteristics. *NeuroImage Clinical* 34: 103043.

Lord, C., Charman, T., Havdahl, A. et al. (2022). The Lancet Commission on the future of care and clinical research in autism. *The Lancet* 399 (10321): 271–334.

Lord, C., Rutter, M., DiLavore, P.C. et al. (2012). *Autism Diagnostic Observation Schedule, Second Edition (ADOS-2)*. Los Angeles, CA: Western Psychological Services.

Manenti, M., Tuller, L., Houy-Durand, E. et al. (2023). Assessing structural language skills of autistic adults: focus on sentence repetition. *Lingua* 294: 103598.

Marinis, T. and Armon-Lotem, S. (2015). Sentence repetition. In: *Methods for Assessing Multilingual Children: Disentangling Bilingualism from Language Impairment* (eds. S. Armon-Lotem, J. de Jong, and N. Meir), 95–124. Bristol, UK: Multilingual Matters.

Marinis, T., Andreou, M., Bagioka, D.V. et al. (2023). Development and validation of a task battery for verbal and non-verbal first- and second-order Theory of Mind. *Frontiers in Language Sciences* 1: 1052095.

Mottron, L. (2021a). A radical change in our autism research strategy is needed: back to prototypes. *Autism Research* 14 (10): 2213–2220.

Mottron, L. (2021b). Progress in autism research requires several recognition-definition-investigation cycles. *Autism Research* 14 (10): 2230–2234.

Mottron, L., Ostrolenk, A., and Gagnon, D. (2021). In prototypical autism, the genetic ability to learn language is triggered by structured information, not only by exposure to oral language. *Genes* 12 (8): 1112.

Navon, D. (1977). Forest before the trees: the precedence of global features in visual perception. *Cognitive Psychology* 9: 353–383.

Peppé, S. and McCann, J. (2003). Assessing intonation and prosody in children with atypical language development: the PEPS-C test and the revised version. *Clinical Linguistics and Phonetics* 17: 345–354.

Prévost, P., Tuller, L., Schaeffer, J. et al. (2023). The LACA Baseline Battery for the evaluation of language and nonlinguistic cognition in individuals with ASD. Poster presented at the Meeting on Language in Autism (MoLA), Durham, USA.

Raven, J., Rust, J., Chan, F. et al. (2018). *Raven's 2 Progressive Matrices, Clinical Edition (Raven's 2)*. San Antonio, TX: Pearson.

Redmond, S.M. (2016). Language impairment in the attention-deficit/hyperactivity disorder context. *Journal of Speech, Language, and Hearing Research* 59 (1): 133–142.

Schaeffer, J., Abd El-Raziq, M., Castroviejo, E. et al. (2023). Language in autism: domains, profiles and co-occurring conditions. *Journal of Neural Transmission* 130: 433–457.

Silleresi, S. (2023). *Developing Profiles in Autism Spectrum Disorder*. Amsterdam: John Benjamins.

Silleresi, S., Prévost, P., Zebib, R. et al. (2020). Identifying language and cognitive profiles in children with ASD via a cluster analysis exploration: implications for the new ICD-11. *Autism Research* 13 (7): 1155–1167.

Wechsler, D. (2008) *Wechsler Adult Intelligence Scale – Fourth Edition (WAIS-IV)*. APA PsycTests.

Wechsler, D. (2014). *Wechsler Intelligence Test for Children – Fifth Edition (WISC-V)*. Bloomington, MN: Pearson.

World Health Organization (WHO) (2022). ICD-11: International Classification of Diseases (11th revision). https://icd.who.int/ (accessed 11 April 2024).

Author Index

a

Abatzoglou, G. 259
Abbot-Smith, K. 170, 178
Abdelaziz, A. 40, 44, 45
Abd El-Raziq, M. 4, 278, 281, 318, 346
Adams, C.V. 215, 233
Adams, L. 84, 85
Adani, F. 159, 171, 172, 173
Adani, S. 216
Aiad, F. 14, 280
Aishworiya, R. 229
Allen, D.A. 18, 55, 87
Almazan, M. 238
Alpers-Leon, N. 217
Ammons, C.J. 317, 329
Anderson, D.K. 14, 252, 253, 254, 323
Andreou, M. 146, 150, 151, 152, 153, 154, 277, 284, 341
Andrés-Roqueta, C. 125, 127, 128, 129, 130, 133, 137
Andrianopoulos, M.V. 192, 193
Angelov A. 229
An, I. 280
An, S. 109, 110
Annaz, D. 127
Archibald, M.M. 344
Arciuli, J. 186
Ariel, M. 281, 284

Armon-Lotem, S. 274, 279, 342
Arnold, J.E. 150, 173–177
Arosio, F. 61
Arunachalam, S. 116
Asaro-Saddler, K. 178
Åsberg, J. 302, 303, 304, 306, 307
Asghari, S.Z. 192
Assumpção, F.B.J. 193
Augustyn, A. 182, 187, 189, 194, 199
Avramides, K. 348
Avram, L. 61
Axbey, H. 133, 134, 137

b

Backes, B. 213
Baghdadli, A. 253, 259
Bagioka, D.V. 341
Baird, C. 37, 38
Baird, G. 88
Baixauli, I. 149, 151, 156
Baker, C.M. 314
Bal, V.H. 209, 210, 214, 260
Baldimtsi, E. 150, 151, 277, 284
Ballaban-Gil, K. 260
Ballard, K.J. 186
Bambini, V. 107, 108, 127, 132
Bang, J.Y. 38
Baraka, N. 218

Barbarroja, N.   104, 107
Barbieri, L.   61
Barger, B.D.   212, 213
Barnes, L.L.   252
Barnhart, M.   31
Baron-Cohen, S.   8, 62, 124, 147, 148, 211, 250, 299
Barron, K.L.   41
Barry, J.G.   90
Barthélémy, C.   3
Barthez, M.A.   59
Bartolucci, G.   109, 110, 190, 191, 256
Barton, M.   323, 326
Bashirian, S.   192
Bavin, E.L.   105, 106, 107, 148
Baxter, L.C.   256, 261
Baxter, R.   238
Beaumont, R.   150
Becker, K.   147
Bedford, R.   212, 213, 222
Begeer, S.   19
Beitchman, J.   3
Bellavance-Courtemanche, M.   165
Belletti, A.   61
Belliveau, J.W.   314
Bemis, R.H.   193
Benders, T.   185
Bennetto, L.   146, 147, 150, 173–177, 194
Bentea, A.   60, 63
Berger, F.   164
Berg, I.J.   261
Berman, R.   164, 171, 173
Bernard, C.   164
Bernard, F.A.   188
Bertrand, J.   229
Betz, S.K.   230, 244
Bilenberg, N.   192
Bishop, D.V.M.   16, 83, 90, 126, 148, 230, 233, 238, 318, 342
Bishop, S.L.   9, 209, 210, 214

Bjørnstad, P.G.   229
Black, L.M.   193
Bleses, D.   43
Bolton, P.   215
Bonneh, Y.S.   181
Boo, C.   217
Boorse, J.   150
Booth, R.D.L.   320
Bosa, C.A.   213
Boterberg, S.   213
Bottema-Beutel, K.   19, 40
Botting, N.   149, 218
Boucher, J.   87, 89
Boucher, M.   192, 193
Bowler, D.M.   60, 260, 262
Branchini, C.   61
Brants Yosefy, D.   276
Bredin-Oja, S.L.   230
Breheny, R.   122
Bremner, R.   256
Brennan, C.   94
Briggs, R.G.   314
Brignell, A.   14, 84, 216, 266
Brock, J.   105, 107
Brown, H.M.   15, 38, 213, 254, 295, 297, 298, 302
Brownlie, E.   3
Bryan, K.M.   209
Bryson, S.   255, 259
Buckwalter, P.   230
Buijsman, R.   19
Buitelaar, J.   107, 108, 255, 258
Bush, H.H.   3
Buxhoeveden, D.P.   319

C

Çalhoun, S.L.   297
Campbell, J.M.   212, 213
Candan, A.   101
Cano-Chervel, J.   126

Cao, A. 39
Cappell, K. 323
Caramazza, A. 34, 40, 43
Cardinale, R.C. 321, 328
Cardoso, S. 296, 304
Carlier, S. 126
Carlsson, E. 302, 304, 306, 307
Carruthers, S. 217
Casanova, M.F. 319
Casillas, M. 185
Castro, S.L. 165, 178
Castroviejo, E. 4, 104, 107, 278, 318, 346
Catts, H.W. 300
Cepanec, M. 216
Cerquiglini, A. 213, 218
Chahboun, S. 127, 132
Chakrabarti, B. 207
Chambers, C.E. 316, 317
Chambers, N. 348
Chan, F. 342
Charman, T. 3, 37, 38, 84, 211, 213, 214, 336, 340, 348
Chatzidimitriou, C. 259
Chen, A. 164, 178
Chenausky, K.V. 84, 85, 213
Chen, B. 316
Chen, L. 109, 110
Chen, Y. 187, 199
Cherkassky, V.L. 319, 329
Chesler, D.A. 314
Chevallier, C. 108, 183, 189, 190, 194
Chien, Y.C. 235, 240, 242, 244
Chierchia, G. 102, 116
Chilton, H. 3
Chin, I. 37, 38
Choi, B. 287
Chomsky, N. 233
Chondrogianni, V. 63, 279
Christophe, A. 185
Christou, N. 104, 107

Churchill, D.W. 18
Cicchetti, D. 8
Clahsen, H. 238
Clarke, P.J. 297
Cleave, P.L. 237
Cleland, J. 84, 187
Coene, M. 61
Cohen, D.J. 126–127
Cohen, M.X. 329
Cola, M. 150
Colle, L. 147, 148
Colomer, C. 149, 151, 156
Coltheart, M. 293, 294
Condouris, K. 55
Conner, A.K. 314
Constantino, J.N. 8, 342
Cooper, J. 178, 212
Cornwall, A. 344
Cortesi, F. 213, 218
Costa, J. 61
Courchesne, E. 325
Cox, C.R. 212
Crago, M. 61
Crain, S. 102
Creemers, A. 167–168
Crompton, C.J. 133, 134, 137
Crutcher, J. 315, 318, 319, 320, 322, 324, 329
Crystal, D. 230
Cuthbert, B.N. 319, 346, 347

d

Dahlgren Sandberg, A. 304
Dai, H. 109, 110
D'Ambrose Slaboch, K. 190
Daniels, A. 261
Daou, N. 348
Dautriche, I. 185
Davidson, M.M. 302
Davids, R.C. 261

Davis, E.   153
Davis, M.H.   188
DaWalt, L.S.   254, 260
Dawson, G.   209, 210
Dawson, M.   191
Deacon, S.H.   297, 298, 308
Dean-Pardo, O.   181
DeBrabander, K.M.   133, 134, 137
de Carvalho, A.   185
De Cat, C.   164
De Fossé, L.   323
De Houwer, A.   271
Delafield-Butt, J.   84
Delage, H.   56, 60, 61, 62, 65, 66, 67, 68
Deliens, G.   127, 128, 147
de Marchena, A.B.   38, 323
Dennis, M.   148
Dent, C.H.   123
de Pape A.-M.R.   178
Deramus, T.P.   317, 329
Deserno, M.K.   260, 262
Deutsch, C.K.   15, 323
de Villiers, J.   126
de Villiers, J.G.   60
Devoti, M.   43
Devouche, E.   184
Diehl, J.J.   146, 147, 150, 173–177, 193, 194–196, 198
DiLavore, P.C.   8, 342
Di Martino, A.   316, 319
Djaja, D.   186
dos Santos, C.   342
Douard, E.   212
Drew, A.   37, 38, 211, 214
Dubé, R.V.   16, 144, 145
Dubé, S.   61
Duku, E.   255, 259
Dunn, D.M.   16, 342
Dunn, L.M.   17, 342
Dunn, M.A.   18, 42, 55, 87

Durrleman, S.   49, 56, 57, 58, 59, 60, 62, 63, 65, 66, 67, 70, 151, 255
Dworzynski, K.   215

e

Ecker, C.   325
Edelson, L.R.   148, 150, 169, 281–282
Eden, G.F.   323
Edmunds, S.R.   212, 213
Edwards, M.L.   87, 94
Edwards, S.   63
Efron, D.   217
Egger, E.   275
Ehlen, F.   42
Eigsti, I.M.   38, 313, 319, 323, 326, 329
Einav, S.   105, 107
Eisenhower, A.   3
El Akiki, C.   291
Ellawadi, A.   40, 41, 43, 44
Ellis Weismer, S.   89, 94, 212, 213, 302
Eriksson, D.K.   317
Evans-Williams, C.V.   133, 134, 137
Ewen, J.B.   217–218

f

Falkum, I.L.   123, 132
Faloppa, F.   14
Farashi, S.   192
Fein, D.   39, 40, 41, 43, 44, 45, 106, 107, 109, 110, 323, 326
Fenson, L.   15
Ferguson, H.J.   122
Fernandes, C.   295, 296, 304
Fernell, E.   211, 222, 303, 304
Ferré, S.   56, 60, 75, 87, 88, 89, 181, 342
Fey, M.E.   300
Fielding-Gebhardt, H.   230
Filipe, M.G.   165, 178
Filippova, E.   123
Fine, J.   190, 191

Finegan, E.   21
Finnegan, E.G.   178
Fishman, I.   321, 328
Fletcher, P.T.   321
Fletcher-Watson, S.   279
Floris, D.L.   15
Fok, M.   260
Foldager, M.   41, 42, 43, 44
Foley, M.   186
Folstein, S.E.   302
Fombonne, E.   3, 9, 261
Foppolo, F.   97
Forgeot d'Arc, B.   299, 342
Fox, M.   328
Foy, K.   3
Francis, K.   56, 63, 65, 165, 166
Franck, J.   14, 57, 58, 59, 60
Franz, L.   348
Freed, J.   215
Friedberg, C.   194–196, 198
Friedman, L.   254, 260
Friedmann, N.   54
Frith, U.   62, 105, 124, 132, 298, 299, 304
Frota, S.   165, 178
Fuentes, J.   3
Fuerst, Y.   87, 88, 94
Fusaroli, R.   192
Fyndanis, V.   151

g

Gabig, C.   303
Gagarina, N.V.   143, 144
Gagnon, D.   9, 212, 347
Gale, M.   344
Galley, K.   277
Gao, Y.   321
Garufi, M.   185
Garvey, M.   319
Gastgeb, H.Z.   40, 41
Gavarró, A.   56, 70

Geelhand, P.   141, 147
Gelman, S.A.   34, 39
Gemmell, T.   137, 149
Genesee, F.   61
Georgiadès, S.   214, 218
Georgieff, N.   110, 111, 112
Gernsbacher, M.A.   127, 136
Geurts, H.M.   261, 329
Giannotti, F.   213, 218
Gibbon, F.E.   186, 187
Giesen, J.   90, 92, 93
Gilbert, S.J.   308
Gilhuber, C.S.   277
Gillberg, C.   222
Gillespie-Lynch, K.   348
Ginsberg, G.   190, 191
Girolamo, T.   254, 255
Giustolisi, B.   127
Gladfelter, A.   41
Gleitman, L.   31, 39, 102
Glenn, C.   143
Goldberg, B.   256
Gomes, H.   42
Gomot, M.   188
Gonzalez-Barrero, A.M.   151, 279, 287
Gorman, K.   90
Gotham, K.   211, 342
Gough, P.B.   292
Grandgeorge, M.   212
Gratier, M.   184
Green, D.   84
Green Snyder, L.   261
Greicius, M.   328
Grice, H.P.   120
Grimm, R.P.   296, 297, 298, 300, 301, 302, 303
Groen, Y.   261
Groenman, A.P.   262
Grohmann, K.K.   104, 107
Grosjean, F.   271, 273

Grossman, R.B.   192, 193
Gruber, C.P.   8, 342
Gualmini, A.   102, 113
Guasti, M.T.   70, 102, 230, 232, 244
Guelminger, R.   110, 111, 112
Guo, L.Y.   99

h

Haebig, E.   37, 212
Hagoort, P.   107, 108, 255, 258
Hall, G.B.C.   178
Hamann, C.   61
Hamner, T.   230, 240
Hampton, S.   272, 287
Han, E.   348
Hanley, M.   195
Hantman, R.M.   287
Happé, F.G.E.   108, 124, 125, 127, 132, 135, 147, 183, 189, 190, 194, 303, 320
Hartman, C.A.   168, 169, 170, 172, 173, 176
Hartwick, K.   287
Hattersley, C.   19
Hausberger, M.   212
Havdahl, A.   3, 336, 340, 348
Hawi, Z.   14, 216
Hayward, D.   16, 144, 145
Healy, O.   299, 301
Heaton, P.F.   190, 199, 262
Hedvall, Å.   211, 222
Helt, M.   323
Henderson, L.M.   297
Hendriks, P.   159, 168, 169, 170, 172, 173, 176
Henry, A.R.   296, 303
Henry, C.   61
Hepburn, S.   230
Herbert, M.R.   15, 323
Herringshaw, A.J.   317, 329
Heshmati, Y.   56
Hickman, L.   19

Hickmann, M.   85
Hickok, G.   316
Hill, A.P.   90
Hill, E.   303
Hills, T.T.   37
Hilvert, E.   230, 244
Hindi, I.   280
Hinerman, C.M.   185
Hippolyte, L.   255
Hodge, S.M.   323
Hodson, B.W.   91
Hoff, E.   32
Hoff-Ginsberg, E.   32
Hogan, T.P.   300
Holbrook, S.   199
Holloway, J.   299, 301
Hornby, P.A.   164
Horvath, S.   39
Houy-Durand, E.   255, 259, 343
Howlin, P.   3, 252, 256, 259, 260, 262–264, 266
Hübscher, I.   185
Hudry, K.   272, 278
Huettig, F.   100, 105
Hulk, A.   275
Hull, L.   215, 222
Hunter J.   229
Hupp, J.M.   185
Hurewitz, F.   102

i

Igarashi, M.   188
Insel, T.R.   319, 346, 347
Israelsen, M.   199
Iverson, J.M.   191

j

Jakubowicz, C.   54
Jakubowski, K.   190, 199
Jao Keehn, R.J.   321
Jarvinen-Pasley, A.   190

Jelenic, P. 299
Jewkes, R. 344
Jiménez, E. 37, 212
Johnson, A. 15, 295, 297, 298, 302
Johnson, C. 3
Jolliffe, T. 299
Jones, C.R.G. 303
Jones, D.R. 133, 134, 137
Jones, K.M. 323
Jorba, M. 132
Joseph, R.M. 210, 214
Jungers, M.K. 185
Just, M.A. 319, 329
Jylkkä, J. 151

k

Kalandadze, T. 127, 132, 136
Kalb, L. 214
Kambanaros, M. 104, 107
Kamp-Becker, I. 147, 210, 216
Kanner, L. 132
Kapp, S.K. 19
Karkada, M. 297, 298, 308
Karsten, A.M. 178
Kasari, C. 3, 210
Kasirer, A. 127, 132
Katsos, N. 119, 122, 125, 127, 128, 129, 130, 133, 137, 272, 278
Katz, T. 209, 210, 214
Kaufman, N.R. 84
Kauschke, C. 216
Keating, C.T. 19
Keller, T.A. 319, 329
Kelley, E. 106, 107, 323
Kelly, C. 316, 319
Kenny, L. 19
Kent, R. 259
Key, A.P. 190
Kidd, E. 105, 106, 107
Kinsbourne, M. 323
Kirchner, R.M. 230

Kissine, M. 14, 67, 126, 128, 129, 280, 347
Kjelgaard, M.M. 41, 55, 338
Kjellmer, L. 211, 222, 303, 304
Klein, P.D. 299
Klein-Tasman, B.P. 230, 240
Klin, A. 182, 187, 189, 194, 199
Klop, D. 143, 144
Klostermann, F. 42
Köder, F. 123
Koegel, L.K. 209
Kohnert, K. 272, 273
Korkman, M. 16, 89
Korrel, H. 217
Kotsopoulou, A. 168, 239, 281
Kovarski, K. 188
Kover, S.T. 40, 44, 45, 212, 213
Kuijper, S.J. 168, 169, 170, 172, 173, 176
Kunnari, S. 144
Kuntay, A.C. 101
Kuriki, S. 188
Kwok, E.Y. 38, 213, 254
Kwong, K.K. 314

l

Lai, M.C. 207, 250
Lammertink, I. 185
Landa, R.J. 85, 86, 154
Landau, B. 153
Larson, C. 313, 315, 318, 319, 320, 321, 322, 323, 324, 325, 326, 327, 329, 347
Lassen, J. 41, 42, 43, 44
Latinus, M. 188
Law, K. 217–218
Laws, G. 238
Lazenby, A.L. 148
LeBarton, E.S. 85, 86
Le Couteur, A. 8
Lécuyer, R. 85
Ledbetter, P.J. 123
Lee, N.R. 240

LeGrand, K.J.   255, 260
Lehtonen, M.   151
Lenartowicz, A.   317
Leslie, A.M.   62, 124
Lester, J.N.   19
Leung, J.   19
Levanon, Y.   181
Levinson, S.   3
Lewis, M.   39
Li, H.Y.   316, 318, 319
Li, Y.D.   316, 318, 319
Liang, J.W.   323
Lidz, J.   102, 112
Lindgren, K.A.   302
Lind, S.   60
Line, E.A.   255
Linke, A.   321
Lockwood Estrin, G.   215
Lockyer, L.   148
Lombardo, M.V.   207
Loomes, R.   215
Lord, C.   3, 8, 9, 14, 210, 211, 214, 252, 253, 254, 255, 260, 323, 336, 340, 342, 348
Loucas, T.   88
Luffin, X.   14, 280
Lyons, M.   189

m

Ma, H.   105, 107
Macomber, D.   299
Magiati, I.   252, 266
Mak, E.   274
Makris, N.   323
Malkin, L.   170, 178
Mandy, W.P.L.   215, 222
Manenti, M.   89, 249, 255, 259, 343
Mani, N.   100, 105
Mann, C.C.   178
Manolitsi, M.   149
Manwaring, S.S.   214

Mar, R.A.   153
Marchman, V.A.   15
Marinis, T.   14, 49, 56, 57, 58, 59, 63, 65, 165, 166, 168, 170, 239, 281, 341, 342
Marschik, P.B.   88, 192, 213
Martin, G.E.   193
Marvin, A.R.   217-218
Mashal, N.   127, 132
Matchin, W.   316
Mathy, P.   214
Mawhood, L.   256, 260
May, T.   14, 216
Mayer, J.L.   262
Mayer, M.   16, 144, 169
Mayes, S.D.   297
Mazzaggio, G.   127
Mccann, J.   186, 342
McConnell-Ginet, S.   116
McCormack, T.   195
McDermott, E.   39
McDonough, J.D.   212, 213
McGovern, C.W.   253, 260
McGregor, K.K.   99
McIntyre, N.S.   217, 296, 297, 298, 300, 301, 302, 303
McKeever, L.   84
McNicholas, P.D.   214, 218
Mcsweeny, J.L.   189, 191
Meir, N.   172, 271, 274, 276, 277-279, 280, 281, 282, 283, 284
Mervis, C.B.   229, 230, 240
Mesite, L.   109, 110
Meuwese, J.D.I.   308
Meyer, E.   55
Michel, C.   132
Michelon, C.   253, 259
Milne, E.   304
Milner, V.   215
Milton, D.E.   133
Minshew, N.J.   40, 41
Misquiatti, A.R.   193

Modyanova, N. 56, 109, 110, 168, 237, 239, 240, 241
Mofid, Y. 188
Molins, B. 19
Monjauze, C. 61, 68
Montgomery, L. 279
Morgan, A.T. 84, 266
Morgan, J.L. 185
Morra, L. 133
Morris, J. 229
Morrison, K.E. 133, 134, 137
Moss, P. 3, 259, 262–264
Mottron, L. 9, 191, 344, 347
Mueller, K.L. 217
Mullen, E.M. 16
Mundy, P.C. 37
Munson, J. 209, 210
Musolino, J. 102, 112
Myers, B. 126

n

Nadig, A.S. 38, 151, 279, 287
Nærland, T. 127, 136
Næss, K.A.B. 127, 132
Naigles, L.R. 29, 32, 37, 38, 39, 40, 41, 43, 44, 45, 103, 106, 107, 109, 110, 115
Nally, A. 299, 301
Naples, A.J. 299
Nation, K. 297
Navon, D. 342
Nayar, K. 193
Nespodzany, A. 256, 261
Newcombe, P. 150
Newman, T.M. 299
Nichelli, F. 43
Nichiporuk Vanni, N. 274
Nicoladis, E. 275
Nielsen, J.A. 321
Norbury, C.F. 105, 107, 127, 132, 134–136, 137, 148, 149, 233, 136, 302, 304, 306, 307

Norton, A. 213
Noveck, I.A. 110, 111, 112, 183, 189, 190, 194
Novogrodsky, R. 3, 148, 150, 169, 172, 271, 274, 276, 277–279, 281, 281–282, 283, 284, 335
Nuske, H.J. 148

o

Oatley, K. 153
O'Connor, I.M. 299
Ohayon, S. 61
O'Leary, K. 302, 304
Olivati, A.G. 193
Olulade, O.A. 316, 317
Oram-Cardy, J. 15, 295, 297, 298, 302
Orvig, A.S. 164
Ostashchenko, E. 130
Ostrolenk, A. 299, 347
Oswald, T.M. 303
Overweg, J. 168

p

Pan, B.A. 45
Panzeri, F. 97, 127
Papafragou, A. 102
Papastamou, F. 127, 128, 147
Paradis, J. 61, 274, 287
Patel, S.P. 193
Paul, R. 87, 88, 94, 126–127, 137, 149, 181, 182, 187, 189, 191, 193, 194–196, 198, 199
Paynter, J. 302, 304
Pearl, L.S. 103
Pennington, B.F. 296
Peppé, S. 186, 187, 342
Peristeri, E. 141, 146, 150, 151, 152, 153, 154, 277, 278, 284, 287
Pernon, E. 253, 259
Perovic, A. 3, 56, 109, 110, 168, 227, 234, 237, 238, 239, 240, 241, 242, 335

Pescosolido, M.F. 218
Peterson, M. 15
Petrides, K.V. 215, 222
Petrolini, V. 132
Phillips, L. 124
Pickles, A. 14, 84, 211, 212, 213, 222, 252, 253, 254, 342
Pierce, S.J. 109, 110
Pijnacker, J. 107, 108, 255, 258
Piotroski, J. 45
Plate, S. 150
Pokorny, F.B. 88, 192
Poldrack, R.A. 317
Pomper, R. 89, 94
Pond, R.E. 16
Portner, P.H. 116
Potrzeba, E.R. 39, 40
Pouscoulous, N. 123
Prendergast, L.A. 105, 106, 107
Pretzsch, C.M. 325
Prévost, P. 3, 14, 56, 59, 60, 65–68, 87, 88, 89, 210, 222, 249, 259, 276, 278, 287, 335, 340, 343
Price, C.J. 314
Prieto, P. 185
Prigge, M.B.D. 15
Pripas-Kapit, S.R. 127, 136
Prisecaru, A. 60, 63
Prizant, B.M. 84
Pronina, M. 185
Protic, D.D. 229
Protopapas, A. 152
Prud'hommeaux, E.T. 193

r

Rabagliati, H. 272, 287
Rabins, P.V. 261
Radhoe, T.A. 262
Ramsay, G. 87, 88, 94
Ramstad, K. 229
Ramus, F. 190, 342
Rapin, I. 18, 55, 87, 260
Rapin, L. 165
Raulston, T.J. 277
Raven, J. 342
Records, N.L. 230
Redcay, E. 325
Redmond, S.M. 346
Rees, R. 238
Reilly, K. 39
Rekun, O. 276
Renfrew, C.E. 16, 144
Rescorla, L. 37
Reznick, J. 54
Riby, D.M. 195
Rice, M.L. 16, 55, 109, 110, 230, 236, 237, 244, 254, 255
Riches, N.G. 88
Ricketts, J. 303
Rinaldi, M.L. 191
Riva, D. 43
Rivera-Figueroa, K. 319, 321, 323, 325, 326, 327, 329, 347
Rivero-Arias, O. 229
Rivière, J. 85
Rizzi, L. 52, 54
Robb, M.P. 186
Roberts, J.A. 55, 109, 110, 237
Roberts, J.M.A. 148, 149
Robinson, B.F. 229
Rodríguez, A. 212, 222
Roepke, S. 42
Roestorf, A. 260, 262
Rogers, S. 178, 212, 296
Ronald, A. 215
Ropar, D. 133, 134, 137
Roselló, B. 149, 151, 156
Rost, G.C. 99
Rumpf, A.-L. 147
Rundblad, G. 127

Rust, J. 342
Rutter, M. 8, 18, 256, 260, 342
Ruytenbeek, N. 127, 128

S

Sadiq, S. 217
Saffran, J. 89, 94
Safyer, P. 37
Saiegh-Haddad, E. 272, 281
Saint-Denis, A. 347
Salcedo-Arellano, M.J. 229
Saldaña, D. 127, 132, 298
Salvadó, B. 212, 222
Sanchez-Ruiz, M.J. 348
Sanoudaki, E. 242
Santos, C. 75
Saulnier, C.A. 8
Savage, S. 3, 262–264
Schaeffer, J. 3, 4, 167–168, 278, 318, 335, 340, 346
Schaeken, W. 107, 108
Scheeren, A.M. 19
Schiller, J. 3
Schneider, J.A. 252
Schneider, P. 16, 144, 145
Schoen Simmons, E. 189
Schopler, E. 8
Schuh, J.M. 323
Schuller, B. 88, 192
Schultz, R.T. 319, 323, 326, 329
Sciberras, E. 217
Scior, K. 348
Scontras, G. 103
Scorah, J. 3
Sebastian, M.J. 42
Secord, W.A. 16
Semel, E. 16
Serry, T. 295
Sevaslidou, I. 259
Seydell-Greenwald, A. 316, 317

Sharp, M. 133, 134, 137
Sheinkopf, S.J. 191
Shih, P. 321, 328
Shriberg, L.D. 85, 189, 191
Sideridis, G. 152
Sigman, M. 253, 260
Silk, T. 217
Silleresi, S. 14, 89, 151, 205, 207, 208, 210, 222, 259, 343
Simonoff, E. 259
Sizaret, E. 61
Skinner, R. 8
Skwerer, D.P. 193
Slušná, D. 212, 222
Smith, A.B. 186
Smith, L.B. 31, 39, 40
Smith, M.D. 261
Smith, N.V. 205, 209, 211, 291
Smith, R. 295
Smyth, H. 186
Smyth, R.E. 38, 213, 254
Snedeker, J. 195, 196
Snowling, M.J. 83, 297, 299, 318
Snow, P. 295
Solari, E.J. 296, 297, 298, 300, 301, 302, 303
Sorace, A. 272, 287
Sorenson Duncan, T. 297, 298, 308
Soulières, I. 191
Spain, D. 215
Sparrow, S.S. 8
Stainton, R.J. 126
Stegenwallner-Schütz, M. 171, 172, 173
Stein, N. 143
Steiner, V.G. 16
Sterling, A. 230, 238, 244, 254, 260
Sterling, L. 209, 210
Stevens, M.C. 319, 323, 326, 329
Strand, E. 85
Strauss, M.S. 40, 41

Streiner, D. 109, 110
Stringer, D. 259
Strømme, P. 229
Stroth, S. 210
Sturrock, A. 3, 215
Su, L.Y. 108
Su, P.L. 209
Su, Y.E. 106, 107, 108, 109, 110
Suanda, S.H. 31
Sukenik, N. 29, 44, 45
Swensen, L.D. 103, 106, 107, 109
Swineford, L. 214
Switala, A.E. 319
Syrett, K. 116
Szatmari, P. 255, 256, 259
Szendrői, K. 164

t

Tager-Flusberg, H. 3, 18, 41, 55, 85, 109, 110, 178, 210, 212, 213, 214, 237, 338
Tait, P.A. 214, 218
Talantseva, O.I. 280
Talcott, J.B. 280
Tamura, Y. 188
Tay, X.W. 252, 266
Taylor, E. 211, 214
Taylor, L. 217
Tecoulesco, L. 41, 45
Tek, S. 37, 38, 39, 44, 109, 110
Terzi, A. 56, 63, 65, 159, 165, 166, 168, 170, 239, 281
Thal, D.J. 15
Thomas, H.R. 315, 318, 319, 320, 321, 322, 323, 324, 325, 326, 327, 329, 347
Thompson, P.A. 83, 318
Thorson, J.C. 185
Thurm, A. 214
Tomasello, M. 32, 123
Tomblin, J.B. 230, 302

Tordjman, S. 212
Torenvliet, C. 262
Tovar, A.T. 109, 110, 115
Towgood, K.J. 308
Triche, E.W. 218
Trudeau-Fisette, P. 165
Tsang, W.F. 190, 199
Tsimpli, I.M. 141, 143, 146, 151, 152, 153, 154, 205, 209, 211, 275, 278, 287, 291
Tuchman, R. 260
Tuller, L. 3, 14, 44, 45, 56, 59, 60, 61, 65–68, 87, 88, 89, 205, 208, 255, 259, 273, 274, 276, 278, 287, 335, 340, 343
Tunmer, W.E. 292

u

Uljarević, M. 272, 278

v

Vach, W. 43
Vale, A.P. 295, 296, 304
Van Bourgondien, M.E. 8
van der Beek, B. 216
van der Fluit, F. 230, 240
Van Haeren, M. 107, 108
Van Santen, J.P. 90, 193
van Witteloostuijn, M. 167–168
Varlokosta, S. 61, 242
Velleman, S.L. 192, 193
Vestergaard, M. 41, 42, 43, 44
Vicente, A. 104, 107, 119, 132
Vilà-Giménez, I. 185
Viscidi, E.W. 218
Vissers, M.E. 261, 329
Vivanti, G. 19, 240
Vogelzang, M. 151, 278, 287
Vogindroukas, I. 152
Volden, J. 124
von Isenburgh, M. 348

Vulchanov, V. 127, 132, 280
Vulchanova, M. 280

W

Wagner, L. 103, 109
Wagner, M. 40, 44, 45
Wallace, G.L. 190
Walsh, M.J.M. 256, 261
Walton, K.M. 230
Wang, Q. 316, 318, 319
Warren, S.F. 230, 244
Watson, D. 194
Watt, H.J. 255
Wechsler, D. 342
Wehberg, S. 43
Weil, L.W. 255, 260
Wellman, G.J. 8
Welsh, C.M. 296
Westby, C. 143
Westerveld, M.F. 148, 149, 302, 304
West, K.L. 85
Wexler, K. 16, 56, 109, 110, 168, 227, 231, 232, 233, 235, 236, 237, 239, 240, 241, 242, 244
Wheelwright, S. 8, 147, 148
Whitehouse, A.J. 90, 255
White, S. 303, 304
Wiesner, D. 144
Wiig, E.H. 16, 342
Williams, D. 170, 178
Wilson, A.C. 126
Wilson, D. 108
Wilson, R.S. 252
Wilson, S.M. 317
Wise, E.A. 261
Wittmeier, K. 344
Wodka, E.L. 214
Wojcik, E.H. 34
Wolf, L. 256

Wolff, N. 210
Wolk, L. 87, 90, 92, 93, 94
Woolfenden, S. 266
Worek, A. 38
Wright, B. 297
Wright, N. 212, 213, 222
Wu, J. 229

X

Xu, S. 187, 199
Xu, T. 316

Y

Yang, X. 274
Yeh, Y.C. 101
Yen, M. 317
Young, E.C. 146, 147
Yu, B. 272, 276
Yuan, S. 195, 196

Z

Zafeiri, A. 170
Zajic, M.C. 178
Zanon, R.B. 213
Zebib, R. 14, 65–68, 89, 210, 222, 291, 343
Zeidan, J. 3
Zeribi, A. 212
Zhan, L. 105, 107
Zhang, F. 230
Zhang, M. 187, 199
Zhou, C. 316
Zhou, P. 105, 107
Zhukova, M.A. 280
Ziegler, D.A. 15, 323
Zielinski, B.A. 321
Zimmerman, I.L. 16
Zufferey, S. 255
Zuo, X.N. 316, 319

Subject Index

a

accent   164, 182–186, 189, 193, 198, 275
accusative clitic. *see* clitic
acoustic   76, 79, 85, 182, 183, 186–187, 190–192, 197, 317
  cues   197
  features   187, 192
affective prosody. *see* prosody
agent (grammar)   32, 51, 99, 101, 303
aging   211, 249–251, 257, 260–262, 265, 266, 339
ALI. *see* Autism with Language Impairment
allocentric pragmatics. *see* pragmatics
ALN. *see* Autism without language impairment
aphasia   317
Arabic
  Modern Standard   280–281
  Palestinian   281
  Tunisian   280
article   167
  definite   130, 144, 151, 161, 167–168
  indefinite   130, 143, 161, 167–168
articulation, articulatory   76–81, 83–87, 90, 91, 93, 182, 192, 316
  disorder   83, 86
  skills   83–84

aspect, aspectual   98, 103, 108–110, 113–114, 115
  imperfective   109
  perfective   103, 109–110
  progressive   103, 109–110
assimilation (phonological)   80, 81, 89
autism, autistic
  features   135, 206, 208–211, 214, 220, 318–319, 321–322, 324, 345
  girls   206, 215–216, 220
  severity, severity of, symptom severity   5–6, 20, 42, 87–89, 93, 94, 107, 188–189, 192, 206–207, 210–211, 214, 218–222, 238, 249–250, 259, 266, 281, 286, 301–302, 304–308, 327, 336, 340, 342
  with language impairment, ALI   18, 51, 55, 60, 62–66, 68, 69–70, 77, 88, 90, 98, 104, 113, 114–115, 121, 127, 135, 167, 207, 209, 229, 235–244, 336, 340, 345, 349
  without language impairment, ALN   18, 51, 55, 60, 62, 64–66, 69–70, 77, 88, 90, 98, 104, 114, 121, 135, 207, 209–210, 214, 229, 235–243, 336, 340, 345

Subject Index

autism diagnosis   4–10, 15, 18–19, 84, 104, 105, 107, 181, 192, 205, 210, 215, 216, 218–221, 227, 230, 238, 250–251, 255, 262, 286, 297, 329, 335, 336, 348
  autism diagnostic criteria   5, 261, 318
  diagnosis process   3, 4–10
  first dimension   5, 206, 207, 208, 210–211, 214, 220
  loss of autism diagnosis   323, 326
  restricted and repetitive behavior, RRB   5, 8, 206, 207, 210–211, 345–346
  second dimension   5, 206, 207, 208, 210–211, 220, 303
  social communication, social interaction, SI   3, 5–8, 13, 31, 37, 115, 165, 184, 187, 198, 205–207, 210, 216, 256, 259, 318, 321, 322, 324, 327, 345

b

babbling   87, 184
bilingual, bilingualism   151, 155, 156, 271, 273–285, 287, 340, 341, 343, 346–347. *see also* multilingual, multilingualism
  unexpected bilingual acquisition   280–281
binding   231, 233, 235, 239–240, 244
  Binding Theory   229, 240
biomarker   191
brain   5, 14, 15, 188, 190–191, 199, 313–329, 345
  function   313, 316, 317, 318–325, 327–328
  imaging   188, 199, 314, 316, 325, 327
  structure   15, 313–314, 323, 325, 328

Broca's area   317, 320
Bulgarian   280

c

canonical word order. *see* word order
Case
  accusative   101
  nominative   67
causal information   152
c-command   229, 233–234
central coherence   14, 105, 150, 336, 338, 340, 342
  weak central coherence   298–299
  weak central coherence processing   132
  Weak Central Coherence Hypothesis   105, 114
Childhood Apraxia of Speech   77, 84–85
clause   50, 51–54, 144, 174–176, 212, 234
  complement   50, 51, 53–54, 59–60, 69, 70, 152–154
  embedded   51, 53–54, 59–60, 152, 154, 318
  main   51, 53
clinical marker   61, 236
clitic   50, 51, 54, 60–70, 232
  accusative   51, 61–63, 65–68
  object   54, 60–63, 65
coda   77, 79, 82, 86, 87, 88
code-mixing. *see* code-switching
code-switching   273–276
cognitive
  decline   249, 250, 251, 257, 262, 265
  flexibility. *see* executive function
  load   173, 176, 293, 294, 295
cohesive ties   142–145, 153, 155, 156

communication, communicative abilities, skills   8, 85, 146, 256, 258, 259, 277, 307
  competence   184, 186
  function   122–123, 141, 182
  impairment   3, 56, 205
  verb   51, 53, 59–60
comorbid, comorbidity   4, 7, 20, 188, 207, 215–218, 230, 243, 346, 349. see also co-occurring condition
complement clause. see clause
complexity   51–54, 58–59, 61, 90, 114, 205, 218, 255, 281, 293, 294, 343
  conceptual   124
  derivational   110
  linguistic   295
  morphosyntactic   51–54, 57, 61, 63, 66, 69, 70, 277
  phonological   79, 88, 90
  segmental   82
  story grammar   153, 154
  structural   142, 143, 146, 150
  syllabic   82, 87, 89
  syntactic   57
  task   172–173, 177, 178, 338, 343
compositionality (semantics)   98
compound (word)   98–99, 104, 107, 189
conceptual complexity. see complexity
connective, connectives. see relational ties
connectivity (brain)   314, 318–324, 327–329
  functional   318–321, 324, 327–329
  over-connectivity   315, 319–322, 324, 329
  under-connectivity   315, 319–322
consonant cluster   82, 85, 88
content word   97–98, 113–114, 115

co-occurring. see also comorbid, comorbidity
  condition   4, 9, 14, 20, 206–208, 211, 213, 216, 217, 219–222, 260, 323
  diagnoses   216, 336
  factors   205, 213, 214
  intellectual disability   165
  language impairment   172–173, 318
  NDDs   339
crosslinguistic influence   273–276, 284, 286, 340

d

Danish   42, 43
definite article. see article
definiteness   151, 282, 284
  marker, marking   273, 282, 284
demonstrative   164, 282
derivational complexity. see complexity
developmental change   207, 208, 211
Developmental Language Disorder, DLD   7, 54, 55, 57, 59, 61–63, 65–66, 68, 70, 77, 86, 88–90, 93, 94, 99, 104, 107, 109, 114, 128, 135–136, 148, 217, 227–232, 235–239, 243, 257, 278–279, 318, 323, 325, 346, 348, 349
diagnostic criteria. see autism diagnosis
diagnostic process. see autism diagnosis
DID. see Disorder of Intellectual Development
digit span   176, 279, 342
diglossia, diglossic   272, 273, 280
dimensionality, dimensional
  approach   4, 325, 344–345
  diagnostic. see autism diagnosis
  NDD   345–347
discourse   12, 16, 61–62, 65, 98, 106, 144, 148, 152, 159–178, 184, 253, 273, 282, 292, 318, 338
  discourse prominence   163

Disorder of Intellectual Development, DID. *see* intellectual disability
diversity   20, 134, 348
  children across the spectrum, in all their diversity   221
  language abilities   280
  language skills   66
  lexical diversity   34–35
  methodologies used   187, 197
  neurodiversity   19, 134, 136, 345, 347–348
  results   188
  syllable types   87
  terminological   18, 20
  types of sentences   32
  verb   260
DLD. *see* Developmental Language Disorder
double delay   272, 273, 277–279, 284, 285
double dissociation   209
double empathy problem   133
Down Syndrome, DS   227, 228–230, 235, 238, 239, 242, 243
DS. *see* Down Syndrome
Dutch   19, 55, 107–108, 164, 167, 169, 185, 236, 275
dyslexia   323
dyspraxia   84, 85

e
echolalia, echolalic   17, 84, 261, 343
EEG. *see* electroencephalography
EF. *see* executive function
egocentric pragmatics. *see* pragmatics
elderly   14
electroencephalography, EEG   217, 317, 329
embedded clause. *see* clause
emergence. *see* language
emotional prosody. *see* prosody

English   11, 15, 19, 22, 30–31, 43, 51–53, 61, 76–82, 89, 90, 98, 101, 103, 106–109, 111–112, 122–123, 161, 162, 164, 167, 169, 174, 183, 185, 231–233, 236, 239, 242, 271, 273–276, 280, 282, 293, 346
epilepsy   14, 205, 206, 208, 213, 216–218, 220, 221, 336, 337, 345, 349
executive dysfunction. *see* executive function
executive function, EF   14, 87, 113, 134, 136, 142, 150–152, 155, 195–198, 251, 261, 278, 285, 324, 326, 336–340, 342
  attention switching, switching   14, 36, 113, 251, 278–279
  cognitive flexibility, flexibility   84, 142, 150–151, 155, 266, 278
  executive dysfunction   132
  inhibition   14, 87, 113, 142, 150, 251, 261, 278, 324
  set-shifting   278
  shifting   62, 65–68, 132, 151, 183, 195–196, 198, 278
existential quantifier. *see* quantifier
explicit meaning. *see* meaning
eye-tracking   35, 39, 177, 194, 196

f
F_0. *see* fundamental frequency
figurative language. *see* meaning
figurative speech. *see* meaning
finiteness. *see* tense
first dimension. *see* autism diagnosis
fMRI   313–317, 319, 329. *see also* MRI
focus   160–162, 164–167
  focalized   166
Fragile X Syndrome, FXS   216, 228–230, 235, 238–239
French   43, 51, 53–54, 56–57, 59, 60–61, 65–66, 68, 80–82, 86, 88, 110–112, 164, 185, 231–233, 236, 271, 275, 282

full noun phrase. *see* noun phrase
functional connectivity. *see* connectivity
functional neuroimaging. *see* neuroimaging
function word   98–99, 101–102, 107–108, 110–111, 113–115
fundamental frequency   182, 183, 190–193
FXS. *see* Fragile X Syndrome

g

gender (biological)   5, 7, 108, 174, 182, 192, 206, 208, 215, 220, 222, 240, 301, 304
gender (grammatical)   51, 61–62, 65, 163, 275
German   79, 80, 164, 169, 171–172, 277, 280
global processing. *see* processing
goal-attempt-outcome   143
grammar   8, 10, 62, 105, 123, 126, 149, 163, 167, 227–232, 235–244, 255, 280
grammatical prosody. *see* prosody
grapheme   292–294
Greek   51, 63, 65, 104, 151, 152, 162, 165–166, 169–170, 232, 239, 242, 275, 277

h

Hebrew   43, 169, 172, 271, 276–278, 280, 282–284
heritage language   272, 273, 275, 280
heterogeneity   4, 18, 41, 44, 69, 88, 187, 189, 192, 193, 197, 205, 214–215, 219, 220, 227, 235, 238–240, 243, 251, 253, 256–257, 264, 280, 296, 305, 318, 323, 325, 336, 344–346
home language   272, 274, 281
hyperlexia. *see* reading

i

ID. *see* Intellectual Disability
imageability   31, 33–34
implicature   121–122, 124, 126, 130, 132
   quantity   121–122, 128, 130
   relevance   121, 122, 126
   scalar   121–122, 125–126, 129–130
implicit meaning. *see* meaning
indefinite article. *see* article
indirect speech act. *see* speech act
inference. *see also* pragmatic, pragmatics
inference skills, inferencing skills   146, 293–295, 298, 304
information structure   160, 161, 163–168, 177–178
inhibition. *see* executive function
input   30, 32, 37, 43, 105, 191, 211, 233, 235, 272, 274–275, 279–281, 285, 286
   noninteractional   38, 280
intellectual abilities, ability   14, 17, 206, 208–211, 214, 215, 217, 220, 221, 222, 250, 255, 261, 302, 304, 336–339, 341, 343–344
intellectual disabilities, disability, ID   3, 9, 18, 104, 107, 114, 152, 165, 194, 196, 206, 207, 227–229, 235, 242, 244, 257, 285, 303, 323
   Disorder of Intellectual Development, DID   5, 6, 10, 14, 172, 206, 207, 209, 210, 213–218, 220, 221, 250, 254–257, 261, 264, 304, 336, 337, 341, 343
intelligence   105, 151, 174, 205, 211, 213–214, 219, 240, 264, 266, 338–339
   Intelligence Quotient, IQ   42, 56–57, 59, 63, 91, 104, 105, 130, 151, 152, 155, 174, 205, 214, 218, 250, 253–260, 263, 264, 281, 296, 302, 305, 328, 344
   Nonverbal Intelligence Quotient, NVIQ   57, 59, 63, 104, 108, 130, 174, 207, 214, 229, 235, 238, 281, 302, 340, 342

Intermodal Preferential Looking, IPL 31, 35, 38–40, 99, 100–101, 103, 106, 109–110, 115
internal state language, internal state terms 142, 143, 145, 147, 149–150, 152–155
intonation 12, 130, 161–164, 181–186, 190–191, 256
IPL. *see* Intermodal Preferential Looking
IQ. *see* Intelligence Quotient
irony 5, 120–121, 123–125, 127–130, 133, 182, 183, 186
Italian 43, 162, 232, 238, 271, 276

j

jargon 91, 184
joint attention 31, 32, 37–40, 115, 260, 348

l

language
  comprehension 13, 15–16, 135, 213, 220, 305, 313, 323–324, 337
  dominance 274, 285, 286
  expressive 6–8, 15–17, 85–86, 91, 149, 207, 212–214, 230, 238, 240, 250, 251, 252, 254, 256, 263–264, 304, 337
  impairment, LI 3–4, 6–10, 13, 18, 37, 92, 99, 105, 109, 110, 172–173, 205–207, 209, 211, 216–218, 220, 221, 236, 249, 251, 254–256, 261, 265, 277–278, 281, 303, 316, 318, 323, 324, 325–327, 329, 339, 341, 345, 347–349
  language-specific 232, 274, 282, 284, 286, 322
  language-universal 282, 284, 286
  late emergence 9, 54, 61, 114, 211–212, 213, 229
  network 315, 318, 320, 321–322, 327–328
  preference 19
  processing. *see* processing
  receptive 7–8, 15–16, 38, 89, 91, 109, 207, 213, 214, 230, 240, 250–252, 254, 256, 263–264, 292–294, 336, 337
  regression 6, 126, 135, 207, 211–213, 339
  structural 8, 10, 13, 49, 55, 70, 75–76, 83, 86, 88, 93–94, 115, 121, 123, 125–130, 132, 135–137, 142, 149, 154–155, 165, 173, 182, 207, 209–211, 219, 273, 278, 281, 300, 318, 323, 326, 336–342, 345, 348
  trajectory, trajectories 206, 207, 211–215, 220, 222, 252
language-mixing. *see* code-switching
late language emergence. *see* language
lateralization 318, 321, 326–329
letter knowledge. *see* reading
lexical
  access 292, 293, 296–297
  restriction 99–100, 105
  stress. *see* stress
lexicon 10–13, 29–45, 82, 154, 250, 251, 255, 275, 337–338, 340, 342
  mental 29–31, 34–35, 44, 251
LI. *see* language impairment
linguistic complexity. *see* complexity
linguistic pragmatics. *see* pragmatic, pragmatics
linguistic prosody. *see* prosody
listening comprehension. *see* reading
literal meaning. *see* meaning
literalist bias 127, 132
local processing. *see* processing

longitudinal 214, 252
  change 206, 207, 262
  studies 218, 252, 255, 257–259, 264–265, 300, 303, 304, 339, 343
long-term memory 293
loss of autism diagnosis. *see* autism diagnosis

m

macrostructure. *see* narration, narrative
Mandarin, Mandarin Chinese 101, 105–110
mapping 31, 38, 106
meaning
  explicit 120
  figurative 120, 121
  implicit 11, 119–137, 340
  literal 120, 121, 123, 132
  nonliteral 132
  pragmatic 119, 123, 127, 129, 130, 132, 135–137
metaphor 49, 120, 121, 123–125, 127, 130, 132, 133, 135–137
minimally speaking 3, 55, 206, 209–215, 220–222, 336, 337, 344
minimally verbal 20, 55, 84, 85, 91, 104, 107, 110, 114, 212, 227, 229, 257, 318, 337
monolingual 151, 273, 275–284, 286
morpheme 55, 99, 102, 103, 109, 110, 115, 236
morphology 33, 50, 76, 82, 98, 108, 114, 115, 121, 123, 142, 207, 255, 273, 318, 325, 336
morphosyntax 10–13, 16, 49–70, 75, 76, 93, 107, 108, 125, 135, 149, 154, 155, 160, 164, 212, 228, 230, 231, 236, 250, 255, 265, 275, 283, 284, 316, 317, 323, 325, 340–342

morphosyntactic complexity. *see* complexity
motor
  dysfunction 85, 216
  skills 85, 86, 90, 91, 260, 302
  speech disorder 76, 77, 84–86
MRI 314, 327, 328. *see also* fMRI
multilingual, multilingualism 14, 144, 150–152, 155, 271–287, 336, 337, 343
  acquisition 272, 343
  sequential 272
  simultaneous 272
  unbalanced 273, 278
mutual exclusivity 31, 32, 38

n

narration, narrative 11, 16, 124, 137, 141–156, 168–170, 172, 174–175, 216–217, 266, 277, 282, 320, 322
  coherence 144
  macrostructure 141–143, 146–155
NDD. *see* Neurodevelopmental Disorder
negative quantifier. *see* quantifier
neural
  function 318, 322–324, 328, 329
  network 15, 314, 315, 317–319, 325
  pathway 324
neurobiological markers. *see* biomarkers
Neurodevelopmental Disorder, NDD 3–5, 14, 17, 20, 216, 227–244, 250, 313, 325, 339, 344–346, 349
neurodiversity. *see* diversity
neuroimaging 314, 317, 324, 325, 327, 329
noncanonical word order. *see* word order
nonliteral meaning. *see* meaning
nonnormative 126
Nonverbal Intelligence Quotient. *see* intelligence

nonword 16, 132, 133, 258, 293, 296, 297, 303, 305, 341–343. *see also* pseudoword
noun phrase 51, 59, 99, 101, 106, 143–144, 148, 150, 152, 161, 162, 164, 166–170, 172–176, 178, 229, 231, 233–235, 241, 242, 273
null subject. *see* subject
number (grammatical) 36, 51, 163, 275
numerical quantifier. *see* quantifier
NVIQ. *see* intelligence

o

object (grammar) 11, 39, 50–54, 57–63, 65, 67, 69, 70, 99–101, 105–107, 161, 162, 165–167, 170, 172, 174, 175, 194, 232, 255
   direct object 39, 51, 61, 101, 161, 167, 174
object clitic. *see* clitic
object relative clause. *see* relative clause
object wh-question. *see* wh-question
OI. *see* Optional Infinitive
Optional Infinitive, OI 55, 229, 231, 232, 236, 237, 244
outcome predictors 256, 259–260
over-connectivity. *see* connectivity

p

passive 50, 51, 56–57, 69, 70, 255
patient (grammar) 32, 51, 99, 101
person (grammatical) 51, 52, 59, 61–63, 65–68
personal pronouns. *see* pronouns
phoneme, phonemic 30, 76–82, 84–87, 89, 91–94, 182, 251, 261, 292–294
   phonemic inventory 87, 91, 92
phonetic, phonetics 76–78, 82–84, 86, 91, 93–94, 230, 251, 258
   disorder 76, 82, 93

phonological awareness 294, 301, 303, 308
phonological decoding. *see* reading
phonology, phonological 10–13, 16, 31, 49, 50, 55, 70, 75–94, 121, 123, 142, 207, 212, 230, 258, 273, 275, 292, 300, 307, 316, 317, 341, 342, 346
   complexity. *see* complexity
   disorder 76, 82, 86–87, 93
   feature 77
   process 77, 80–82, 88, 90–92, 94, 305–307
   representation 31, 33, 82
pitch 165, 181–183, 185, 187, 189–192, 198
Portuguese 81, 165
pragmatic, pragmatics 6, 7, 10–13, 59, 67, 98, 107, 110, 113, 119–125, 127–137, 142, 146, 159, 160, 182–184, 187, 197, 206, 212, 215–217, 227, 235, 239, 240, 242, 244, 250, 255, 256, 258, 265, 277, 281–283, 285, 286, 318, 336–343, 345, 346, 348
   allocentric pragmatics 128, 129
   egocentric pragmatics 128, 129
   linguistic pragmatics 121, 129–131, 160, 161, 165, 166, 173, 178
   social pragmatics 129–133, 159, 160, 165, 277, 281, 282, 285, 346
pragmatic
   inferencing skills 146
   meaning. *see* meaning
   prosody. *see* prosody
processing 14, 40, 41, 43, 44, 89, 105, 106, 113, 115, 132, 133, 175, 177, 185, 187, 188, 190, 191, 194, 195, 197, 198, 216, 251, 261, 298, 303, 305–307, 313–317, 319, 320, 324–327
   global processing 41

local processing 132
weak central coherence processing. *see* central coherence
pronoun, pronouns 54, 59, 51, 61, 63, 64, 67, 68, 142–144, 148, 150, 161–164, 166, 168–170, 172–176, 231–236, 239–243, 276, 277
  ambiguous 148, 150, 161, 169, 170, 276
  personal 163, 164, 229, 234, 236, 239, 240
  reflexive 63–64, 229, 231, 233–234, 239–240
  relative 51, 52, 191
prosody 12, 13, 55, 84, 85, 130, 161, 162, 164–166, 168, 177, 178, 181–199, 256, 261, 323, 340–342
  affective/emotional prosody 182, 183, 188, 190
  grammatical prosody 183, 184
  linguistic prosody 183, 184, 191, 193
  pragmatic prosody 184
  prosodic deficit 182, 186, 193, 197, 198
pseudoword. *see* nonword

q

quantifier 98, 99, 101, 102, 107–108, 111–114, 120, 121, 125, 130
  negative 102
  numerical 101–102
  quantifier domain restriction 120
  universal 99, 102, 107, 108, 111, 112
quantity implicature. *see* implicature

r

RAN. *see* Rapid Automized Naming
Rapid Automized Naming, RAN 293, 294, 301, 304, 308
RDoC. *see* research domain criteria

reading 5, 14, 15, 18, 291–309, 323, 337
  hyperlexia 299
  letter knowledge 293, 294, 301, 303–305
  listening comprehension 292–294, 299, 300
  phonological decoding 292, 293, 296, 297
  reading comprehension 15, 292–295, 297–308
  reading profiles 299–308
  sight word recognition 293
  word recognition 15, 292–294, 296–305
reference, referential 32, 114, 123, 143–145, 148–152, 154, 160, 161, 163–165, 167–174, 176–178, 228–231, 233, 234, 239, 243, 282–284
  chain 143
  expression 156, 273, 281–284
  referent 31–36, 61, 62, 65, 163, 148, 161, 167–177, 185, 273, 276, 282, 284, 298
  ties 142–145, 147, 148
reflexive pronouns. *see* pronouns
regression 6, 207, 211–213, 339. *see also* language
relational ties. *see* connectives
relative clause 50–53, 57–59, 69, 70, 152–154, 171, 251, 255
  object relative clause 52, 53, 58, 69, 70, 255
  subject relative clause 52, 53, 58
relative pronoun. *see* pronoun
relevance implicature. *see* implicature
Research Domain Criteria, RDoC 315, 319, 325, 326, 346–347
restricted and repetitive behavior. *see* autism diagnosis
rhythm 12, 161, 182–184, 190, 193, 198

rigidity   42, 132
risk marker   192
root infinitive. *see* optional infinitive
Russian   151, 271, 276, 277, 280, 282, 284

S

scalar implicature. *see* implicature
scope   99, 102
  ambiguity   102
  inverse   99, 102, 112
  surface   99, 102, 112, 113
scrambled   167
second dimension. *see* autism diagnosis
segmental complexity. *see* complexity
semantic, semantics   10–13, 30, 33, 34, 40–42, 50, 97–115, 215, 231, 261, 317–319, 337, 338
  categories   31, 40, 44, 252
  fluency   42, 261
  network   31, 33, 36, 133
  representation   31, 33, 136, 293
  sentence-level   12, 55, 104, 114, 155
sentence repetition   90, 255, 258, 277, 338, 341, 342
sentence structure   16, 49, 51, 57, 76, 160, 165, 178, 250, 258
Serbo-Croatian   242
SES. *see* Socioeconomic Status
set-shifting. *see* executive function
severity of autism. *see* autism
shape bias   31, 32, 39, 40, 45
shifting. *see* executive function
short-term memory   87, 89, 90, 279
  deficit in   90
sight word recognition. *see* reading
social cognition   14, 150, 197, 198, 278, 298
social communication. *see* autism diagnosis
social integration   182
social interaction. *see* autism diagnosis

social pragmatics. *see* pragmatics
Socioeconomic Status, SES   142, 150–152, 155, 156, 233
Spanish   104, 162, 232, 274–276
Specific Language Impairment, SLI   228, 232, 237. *see also* Developmental Language Disorder
specifier, specifiers   4, 6, 8, 10, 206, 219, 318, 345
  clinical   219
  descriptive   206
  language impairment   8, 10, 318, 345
  trajectory   219
speech   6, 11–13, 76, 77, 83–86, 89, 93, 94, 181, 182, 183, 184–186, 190–193, 197, 198, 205, 207, 212, 213, 256, 259, 262, 293, 294, 317
  caregiver speech measures   34
  disorder. *see* phonetic disorder
  figurative   124
  parent   32, 34
  samples   34, 54
  sound   11, 13, 77–78, 83–84, 86, 93, 183, 258, 294
  spontaneous   34, 54, 55, 56, 60, 69, 92, 164, 165, 230, 235, 236, 338
speech act   121, 122, 185
  indirect speech act   123, 128
story grammar   143, 145, 146, 149, 152–155
stress   12, 13, 161, 162, 166, 183–186, 189, 190, 193, 198, 256
structural complexity. *see* complexity
structural language. *see* language
subject (grammar)   11, 32, 39, 49, 50, 52–53, 57–59, 67, 101, 106, 161–162, 164, 169, 170, 172, 174–176, 232–234, 237, 255, 276
  clitic. *see* clitic
  null   170, 232

subject relative clause. *see* relative clause
subject wh-question. *see* wh-question
Subject-Verb-Object, SVO. *see* word order
syllabic, syllable   11–13, 76–80, 82, 85–90, 93–94, 183–184, 186, 192, 232, 294
  complexity. *see* complexity
  structure   79, 82, 86, 88, 89
syntactic, syntactically, syntax   11, 31–34, 39, 50, 54, 57, 61, 68, 76, 82, 83, 86, 90, 98, 100, 114, 115, 121, 123, 142, 162, 163, 165, 166, 168, 177, 178, 183–185, 189, 193–195, 197, 207, 216, 219, 233, 251, 255, 260, 273, 295, 316, 318, 319, 336–338
  syntactic complexity. *see* complexity
syntactic bootstrapping   31, 32, 39

t

task complexity. *see* complexity
temporal marker   98, 99, 103
tense   11, 16, 17, 55, 99, 103, 228, 229, 232, 236–238, 243, 346
  finiteness   229, 231–233, 236–238
  future   11, 99, 103
  past   11, 50, 99, 103, 232, 237, 238, 318, 325
  present   11, 99, 103, 232, 237, 238
thematic role   99, 101, 106
  agent   32, 51, 99, 101, 303
  patient   32, 51, 99, 101
Theory of Mind, ToM   14, 15, 51, 54, 55, 60, 62, 63, 65, 66, 69, 121, 122, 124–137, 142, 147, 149–155, 160, 161, 163, 165, 167, 168, 170, 172, 173, 176–178, 185, 278, 279, 285, 293, 301, 303, 304, 308, 336–341
ToM. *see* Theory of Mind
topic   123, 124, 143, 159–162, 164–167, 170, 176, 178, 184, 275, 295
  topicalized   165, 166

trajectory, trajectories   206, 211–215, 218–220, 222, 252, 260, 274, 325
  developmental   5, 14, 106, 207, 208, 211, 213, 219, 257, 259, 263, 265, 266
  of language acquisition. *see* language
Turkish   101

u

under-connectivity. *see* connectivity
universal quantifier. *see* quantifier

v

verbal communication
  skills   5–8
verbal fluency   31, 36, 41, 42, 250–252, 261–262. *see also* semantic fluency
verbal praxis   84
vocabulary
  expressive vocabulary   152, 215, 264, 302
  receptive vocabulary   31, 37–38, 100, 104–105, 108, 174, 215, 218, 256, 260, 264, 300, 302
voice   85, 181–182, 187, 188, 191–193
  quality   182

w

weak central coherence. *see* central coherence
Weak Central Coherence Hypothesis. *see* central coherence
weak central coherence processing. *see* processing
Wernicke's area   317, 320
wh-question   50, 53, 57–59, 69
  object wh-question   53, 58, 69, 70
  subject wh-question   53, 58
Williams Syndrome, WS   228, 229, 238, 240–244
WM. *see* Working Memory

word order 11, 51–54, 61, 101, 106–107, 114, 115, 162, 167, 237, 282
   canonical 51–53, 59, 61
   noncanonical 51–52, 54, 69, 70
   Subject-Verb-Object, SVO 51, 52, 54, 99, 61, 101, 106–107, 162, 277–278

word recognition. *see* reading

Working Memory, WM 14, 51, 53–55, 57, 61–63, 65, 69, 134, 142, 150, 161, 163, 170, 172, 173, 176, 177, 251, 278, 279, 293–295, 336–340, 342, 343

WS. *see* Williams Syndrome